PEARLS
of WISDOM

I0027514

Otolaryngology and Facial Plastic Surgery
BOARD REVIEW

Second Edition

Mary Talley Bowden, M.D.

McGraw-Hill
Medical Publishing Division

New York Chicago San Francisco Lisbon London
Madrid Mexico City Milan New Delhi
San Juan Seoul Singapore
Sydney Toronto

Otolaryngology and Facial Plastic Surgery Board Review, Second Edition

Copyright © 2006 by The McGraw-Hill Companies, Inc. All rights reserved. Printed in the United States of America. Except as permitted under the United States Copyright Act of 1976, no part of this publication may be reproduced or distributed in any form or by any means, or stored in a data base or retrieval system, without the prior written permission of the publisher.

4 5 6 7 8 9 0   IBT/IBT   1 9 8 7 6 5 4 3 2 1 0

ISBN 0-07-146440-9

The editors were Catherine A. Johnson and Marsha Loeb.
The production supervisor was Phil Galea.
The cover designer was Handel Low.
IBT Global was printer and binder.

This book is printed on acid-free paper.

Cataloging-in-Publication data for this title is on file at the Library of Congress.

INTERNATIONAL EDITION ISBN: 0-07-110879-3

DEDICATION

To Peter for his love and support.

Mary Talley Bowden

EDITOR:

Mary Talley Bowden, M.D.
Memorial Northwest Otolaryngology –
Head and Neck Surgery Associates
Houston, TX
www.mnwent.com

FIRST EDITION CONTRIBUTORS:

William T. Adamson, M.D.
Pediatric Surgery Fellow
The Children's Hospital of Philadelphia
Philadelphia, PA

Gwenda Lyn Breckler, D.O.
Department of Surgery
Chicago Medical School
Mt. Sinai Hospital
Chicago, IL

Edward Buckingham, M.D.
Department of Otolaryngology
University of Texas Medical Branch
Galveston, TX

Dennis D. Diaz, M.D.
Assistant Professor of Surgery
Department of Otolaryngology
Head and Neck Surgery
Penn State Geisinger Health systems
Penn State University
Hershey, PA

Gerard M. Doherty, M.D.
Assistant Professor of Surgery
Washington University School of Medicine
St. Louis, MO

Robert J. Gewirtz, M.D.
Assistant Professor of Neurosurgery
Department of Surgery
University of Kentucky
Chandler Medical Center
Lexington, KY

Jeffrey S. Jacobs, M.D.
Assistant Professor of Anesthesiology
Miami VA Medical Center
Jackson memorial Hospital
University of Miami
Miami, FL

Roger J. Levin, M.D.
Assistant Professor of Surgery
Section of Otolaryngology
Head and Neck Surgery
Penn State Geisinger Health System
Penn State University
Hershey, PA

Kimball I. Maull, M.D.
Director
The Trauma Center at Carraway
Carraway Methodist Medical Center
Birmingham, AL

Ravi Moonka, M.D.
Staff Surgeon
Puget Sound Veterans Affairs Medical Center
Clinical Instructor
Department of Surgery
University of Washington Medical Center
Seattle, WA

Michael L. Nance, M.D.
Schnaufer Senior Surgical Fellow
The Children's Hospital of Philadelphia
Philadelphia, PA

Juan B. Ochoa, M.D.
Assistant Professor of General Surgery
Section of Trauma and Critical Care
University of Kentucky
Lexington, KY

Carlos A. Pellegrini, M.D.
Professor and Chairman
Department of Surgery
University of Washington Medical Center
Seattle, WA

Laurie Reeder, M.D.
Section of General Thoracic surgery
University of Washington School of Medicine
Seattle, WA

Elizabeth Rosen, M.D.
Department of Otolaryngology
University of Texas Medical Branch
Galveston, TX

Andrew Shapiro, M.D.
Department of surgery
Penn State Geisinger Health System
Penn State University
Hershey, PA

Karen L. Stierman, M.D.
Department of Otolaryngology
University of Texas Medical Branch
Galveston, TX

Eric Vallieres, M.D.
Section of General Thoracic surgery
University of Washington School of Medicine
Seattle, WA

Boris Vinogradsky, M.D.
Section of Trauma and Critical Care
University of Kentucky
Lexington, KY

Douglas E. Wood, M.D.
Director
Section of General Thoracic surgery
University of Washington School of Medicine
Seattle, WA

John H. Yim, M.D.
Resident in General Surgery
Washington University School of Medicine
St. Louis, MO

INTRODUCTION

Congratulations! *Otolaryngology and Facial Plastic Surgery Board Review: Pearls of Wisdom* is designed to help you prepare you for the Board Examination in Otolaryngology. This book is one in a series of *Pearls of Wisdom* texts which include all areas of medicine. Before you get started, a few words are appropriate discussing the intent, format, limitations and proper use of this book.

Since *Otolaryngology and Facial Plastic Surgery Board Review* is primarily intended as a study aid, the text is structured in a question and answer format. Most of the questions are short with short answers. This is to facilitate moving through a large body of information. Such a format, while quite unlike the format used in the actual Board Examination, is useful to enable you to assess your strengths and weaknesses in a particular area. This allows you to concentrate further studies on areas of interest or weakness. Emphasis has been placed on distilling trivia and key facts that are easily overlooked, that are quickly forgotten, and that somehow seem to occur frequently on board examinations.

It must be emphasized that any question and answer book is most useful as a learning tool when used in conjunction with a subject-specific textbook. Truly assimilating these facts into a framework of knowledge absolutely requires further reading on the surrounding concepts. The more active the learning process, the better the understanding. Use this book with your preferred source texts handy and open. When you encounter a question that you cannot recall the answer or that you find of particular interest, you are strongly encouraged to review the pertinent area in the textbook at hand.

The chapters are organized to include all aspects of otolaryngology. Some areas are covered more thoroughly than others. The questions within each chapter are randomly arranged to simulate board examinations and the way questions arise in real life. There are several areas of redundancy. This is intentional – redundancy is a good thing when preparing for board examinations.

This book does have limitations. While great effort has been made to verify that the questions and answers are accurate, discrepancies and inaccuracies sometimes occur. Most often this is attributable to variance between original sources. We have tried to verify in several references the most accurate information. Keep in mind that some answers may not be the answers you would prefer. In addition, this book risks accuracy by aggressively pruning complex concepts down to the simplest level; the dynamic knowledge base and clinical practice of medicine is not like that. Furthermore, new research and practice occasionally deviates from that which likely represents the correct answer for test purposes. Remember, this book is designed to maximize your score on a test. Refer to your most current sources of information and mentors for direction in practice.

Each question is preceded by a hollow bullet. This permits you to check off areas of interest, weakness or simply note that it has been read. This also allows for re-reading without having uncertainty about what was reviewed earlier.

We welcome your comments, suggestions and criticism. Please make us aware of any errors you find. We hope to make continuous improvements and would greatly appreciate any input with regard to format, organization, content, presentation, or about specific questions. We are also interested in recruiting new contributing authors and publishing new textbooks. We look forward to hearing from you!

Study hard and good luck on the Boards!

M.T.B.

TABLE OF CONTENTS

BULLET REVIEW

○ **Where are most esophageal foreign bodies found?**

Just below the cricopharyngeus muscle.

○ **A 3-year-old sustains bilateral subcondylar fractures of the mandible. Occlusion is normal and radiological studies demonstrate minimal displacement. What is the recommended management?**

A soft diet and physical therapy aimed at maintaining range of motion.

○ **What is the most common cause of massive hemoptysis (greater than 600 ml of blood in 24 hours)?**

Tuberculosis.

○ **An 8-year-old boy has a draining ear filled with friable tissue. CT demonstrates a punched out lytic lesion of the temporal bone. Biopsies show only lipid laden histiocytes. What is the most likely diagnosis?**

Histiocytosis X.

○ **A patient presents with gingival pain and a foul mouth odor. Physical examination reveals fever, lymphadenopathy, bright red gingiva and ulcerated papillae with a gray membrane. What is the most likely diagnosis?**

Acute necrotizing ulcerative gingivitis; also known as trench mouth or Vincent's disease.

○ **What fungus produces a granulomatous tissue reaction and can cause the triad of pneumonitis, erythema nodosum and arthralgias known as valley fever?**

Coccidioidomycosis.

○ **What is the most common cause of vertigo in a child?**

Otitis media.

○ **A patient with a frontal sinusitis presents with a large forehead abscess. What is the most likely diagnosis?**

Pott's puffy tumor.

○ **What physical features constitute the Pierre-Robin sequence?**

Glossoptosis, micrognathia and cleft palate.

○ **An ill-appearing patient presents with a fever of 103 °F, bilateral chemosis, 3rd nerve palsy and sinusitis. What is the most likely diagnosis?**

Cavernous sinus thrombosis.

○   **Retropharyngeal abscess is most common in what age group?**

6 months to 3 years (retropharyngeal lymph nodes regress in size after the age of three).

○   **What is a ranula?**

A mucous retention cyst involving the sublingual gland in the floor of the mouth characterized by a bluish surface.

○   **A 48-year-old male presents with a high fever, trismus, dysphagia and swelling inferior to the mandible in the lateral neck. What is the most likely diagnosis?**

Parapharyngeal space abscess.

○   **T/F: A patient can lose more of the upper lip than the lower lip without cosmetic problems.**

False. Up to one-third of the lower lip can be avulsed or debrided and the patient may still have an acceptable cosmetic appearance. The upper lip is less forgiving due to the relationship with the columella, alar bases and philtrum.

○   **What are the components of the CHARGE sequence?**

Coloboma, heart defects, choanal atresia, retarded growth, genital hypoplasia and ear anomalies.

○   **What is scrofula?**

Tuberculous or nontuberculous cervical adenopathy.

○   **What % of parotid and submandibular gland calculi are radiopaque on CT scan?**

10% and 90%, respectively.

○   **In which Le Fort fracture is CSF rhinorrhea most common?**

III.

○   **What is the treatment of choice for bullous myringitis?**

Erythromycin.

○   **In which salivary gland are stones most likely to occur?**

The submandibular gland.

○   **What organism causes Lemierre's syndrome?**

Fusobacterium necrophorum.

○   **A toddler sustains an electrical injury to the commissure of his mouth after biting through an electrical cord from a floor lamp. What post-injury warning should be given to the parents?**

The labial artery may hemorrhage if the overlying soft tissue of the commissure breaks down. The parents should be instructed to hold digital pressure on the lip with their thumb and index finger to control the bleeding and seek help immediately.

O   **Fourth and sixth arch derivatives are innervated by which nerves?**

Superior laryngeal nerve and recurrent laryngeal nerve, respectively.

O   **Nystagmus is defined by which component?**

Fast component.

O   **What syndromes are associated with hearing loss and renal abnormalities?**

Alport, Branchiootorenal, Fanconi Anemia, Turner, and Weil.

O   **A 6-year-old boy is referred because of hearing loss. Audiometric studies reveal a 40 dB conductive hearing loss in the left ear. He is also noted to have downward sloping palpebral fissures, depressed cheek bones, deformed pinnas, receding chin and a large *fishmouth*. What is the most likely diagnosis?**

Treacher Collins syndrome.

O   **A 32-year-old sailor presents with a 6 month history of vertigo. On evaluation he has rotary nystagmus, scanning speech, an intention tremor and bilateral intranuclear ophthalmoplegia. What is the most likely diagnosis?**

Multiple sclerosis.

O   **An 88-year-old white male presents with a painless mass just below his ear that has been slowly enlarging over 2 to 3 years. Pathology shows round, plump, granular eosinophilic cells with small indented nuclei. What is the most likely diagnosis?**

Warthin's tumor.

O   **Where would you expect to find the parathyroid glands in a 10-year-old patient with a lingual thyroid gland?**

In the tracheoesophageal groove.

O   **A 3-year-old boy presents with a midline anterior neck mass just below the hyoid bone that moves with deglutition and tongue protrusion. What is believed to be the cause of this congenital mass?**

Failure of complete obliteration of the thyroglossal duct.

O   **An infant presents with coughing, choking and cyanosis during feeding. This clinical triad suggests what process?**

A tracheoesophageal fistula.

O   **What is the minimum systolic arterial pressure required to maintain cerebral perfusion?**

50 mm Hg.

O   **What diagnosis must be investigated in a patient presenting with pulsating exophthalmos?**

Carotid-cavernous fistula.

O   **What are the disadvantages of using technetium scans to monitor therapy for necrotizing otitis externa?**

It reflects osteoblastic activity and bone remodeling but is not specific for osteomyelitis. It also has poor spatial resolution and may remain positive long after clinical resolution.

O   **Why is facial electroneurography (ENoG) an unreliable prognostic indicator more than 3 weeks after the onset of facial paralysis?**

Asynchronous discharge from regenerating nerve fibers can give a false-positive or false-negative report of nerve status.

O   **Bilateral facial paralysis associated with progressive ascending motor neuropathy of the lower extremities and elevated CSF protein is characteristic of what clinical entity?**

Guillain-Barré syndrome.

O   **How would you grade facial nerve function in a patient with facial asymmetry at rest, incomplete eye closure and minimal motion of the mouth with maximal effort?**

House Grade V.

O   **In the tonotopic organization of the cochlea, where are the low frequencies located?**

At the cochlear apex.

O   **Recurrent facial paralysis, facial edema, furrowed tongue and cheilitis are consistent with what diagnosis?**

Melkersson-Rosenthal syndrome.

O   **T/F: A narrow internal auditory canal is a contraindication for cochlear implantation.**

True.

O   **In a child with bilateral congenital aural atresia, how is normal sensorineural hearing confirmed in the ear to be operated on first?**

Detection of an ipsilateral wave I on bone conduction ABR.

O   **T/F: Most acoustic neuromas are inherited on chromosome 22.**

False.

O   **What is the most common tumor of the middle ear?**

Glomus tumor.

O   **What is the most common site of origin of glomus tympanicum tumors?**

Jacobson's nerve.

O   **What is the primary treatment for erysipelas involving the ear?**

Oral or intravenous antistreptococcal antibiotics.

O   **What do neurofibromatosis, tuberous sclerosis and von Hippel-Lindau disease have in common?**

These are phakomatoses, a group of hereditary syndromes with neural, ocular and cutaneous manifestations.

O   **What is the most common type of tracheo-esophageal fistula?**

A blind-ending proximal esophageal pouch with a fistula from the lower esophagus to the trachea (85%).

O   **A 3-year-old male presents with a firm neck mass. Examination reveals Horner's syndrome. What is the most likely diagnosis?**

Neuroblastoma.

O   **A 4-month-old female has had a progressive barking cough and inspiratory stridor for 2 months. Examination reveals a raised, bright red lesion on her back that has been gradually enlarging. High kilovoltage x-rays of her neck demonstrate asymmetric narrowing of the subglottic region. What is the most likely diagnosis?**

Subglottic hemangioma.

O   **A 9-year-old male presents with headaches and a rock hard left posterior triangle mass. Examination is significant for mouth breathing and bilateral serous otitis media. Fine needle aspiration of the neck mass reveals poorly differentiated malignant cells. What is the most likely source of the tumor?**

The nasopharynx.

O   **A 7-year-old female presents for evaluation of florid warty lesions growing from both tonsils. Biopsy demonstrates well differentiated, nonkeratinizing squamous epithelium growing over a fibrovascular stalk. What is the most likely diagnosis?**

Papillomatosis.

O   **What etiology must be considered in the above patient?**

Sexual abuse.

O   **An 11-year-old underwent excisional biopsy of a midline cyst adjacent to the hyoid bone. He continues to experience drainage and breakdown of his surgical wound. What is the treatment of choice?**

A Sistrunk procedure, the definitive procedure for thyroglossal duct cysts.

O   **Which autoimmune disease causes both SNHL and interstitial keratitis?**

Cogan's syndrome.

O   **What organism is most commonly involved in bacterial tracheitis?**

Staphylococcus aureus.

O   **What is the most common cause of primary hypercalcemia?**

Parathyroid adenoma.

O   **Six days after parotidectomy, your patient develops a fluid collection at the angle of the mandible. What test would be most helpful in determining the etiology of the fluid?**

Amylase (to differentiate between sialocele and seroma).

O   **From which pharyngeal pouch is the tympanic membrane derived from?**

1st.

O   **T/F: Vancomycin does not cross the blood-brain barrier.**

True.

O   **T/F: Cephalosporins are contraindicated in patients with a history of anaphylaxis to penicillin.**

True.

O   **What is the drug of choice for *pseudomonas enterocolitis*?**

Metronidazole (less expensive than oral vancomycin).

O   **What is the most common complication of acute mastoiditis?**

Subperiosteal abscess.

O   **What is the most common presenting symptom in patients with Zenker's diverticulum?**

Dysphagia.

O   **What benign skin lesion capable of undergoing malignant transformation is characterized by irregular scattering of epidermal melanocytes with deepened rete ridges?**

Lentigo maligna.

O   **Two months after autograft hair transplantation, all of the hair falls out. What do you tell your patient?**

New hair should start to grow about 10 – 16 weeks after surgery.

O   **Which organ in the head and neck is most sensitive to radiation?**

The lens.

O   **What is the most common complication of recurrent cholesteatoma?**

Labyrinthine fistula.

O   **What is the primary blood supply to the trapezius muscle?**

Transverse cervical artery.

O   **What is the treatment of choice for granular cell tumor of the larynx?**

Endoscopic excision.

O   **What is the initial treatment for a patient with suspected air embolism?**

Placement of the patient in the left lateral decubitus position and Trendelenburg.

O   **What is the most common cause of a widened dorsum after rhinoplasty?**

Greenstick fractures from osteotomies.

O   **What is the most common reason for rhinoplasty revision?**

"Polly Beak" deformity or supratip swelling.

O   **What is the most common complication of blepharoplasty?**

Ectropion.

O   **What is the most common complication of rhytidectomy?**

Hematoma.

O   **What is the most common complication of the phenol peel?**

Cardiotoxicity.

O   **What precautions should be taken to prevent cardiotoxicity during phenol peel?**

IV fluid hydration and treatment of the face in separate units, 30 minutes apart.

O   **What are the most common complications of dermabrasion?**

Milia and hypopigmentation.

O   **What is the most common complication of tissue expanders?**

Implant exposure.

O   **What is the most common cause of flap failure?**

Venous thrombosis.

O   **When is arterial thrombosis most likely to occur?**

1st 72 hours.

O   **What is the initial treatment for any free flap that appears to be failing?**

Immediate reexploration.

O   **What is the significance of time to reexploration and flap survival?**

If flaps are reperfused in 1 – 4 hours, 100% survival is likely. If reperfusion is established by 8 hours, 80% survival is likely. If reperfusion is not reestablished by 12 hours, flap survival is unlikely.

O   **Where is the defect through which a nasal dermoid protrudes?**

Foramen cecum.

O   **What is the diagnosis and treatment for a patient presenting with nasal obstruction and progressive destruction of the septal wall who is negative for c-ANCA?**

Lethal midline granuloma; radiation.

O   **What is the basic structure of IgA?**

Dimer.

O   **What disorder is characterized by deficiency of C1q esterase inhibitor?**

Angioneurotic edema.

O   **What happens if Jacobson's nerve is divided?**

Loss of parasympathetic stimulation to the parotid gland.

O   **What cell bodies are contained within the geniculate ganglion?**

Cell bodies of somatic and visceral afferents of the mucous membranes of the nose, palate, and pharynx through the greater superficial petrosal nerve.

O   **Which part of the facial nerve would be divided if lacrimation and the stapedial reflex are preserved, but movement of the muscles of facial expression and taste to the anterior 2/3 of the tongue are absent?**

Tympanic.

O   **What part of the nerve unit is affected by Wallerian degeneration?**

Distal axon to the motor end plate and proximal axon to the 1st node of Ranvier.

O   **What is the function of vitamin C?**

Hydroxylation of proline and lysine.

O   **What two congenital malformations of the cochlea are contraindications to a cochlear implant?**

Michel aplasia and small internal auditory canal syndrome.

O   **What is the treatment for alar retraction of >2 mm?**

Auricular microcomposite graft.

O   **What is the most common cause of voice failures after TEP?**

Pharyngoesophageal spasm.

O   **What is class I occlusion?**

Mesiobuccal cusp of the maxillary 1st molar is in occlusion with the buccal groove of the mandibular 1st molar.

O   **After a knife wound to the cheek just inferior to the medial canthus, the patient has buccal branch paralysis. How is this managed?**

Observation; exploration is not warranted if the injury occurs medial to the lateral canthus.

O   **What complication is seen more often with cricothyroidotomy than tracheotomy?**

Subglottic stenosis.

O   **What is the mechanism of action of botulinum A toxin?**

Inhibition of the release of acetylcholine at the presynaptic nerve terminal.

O   **What is the most feared complication of septal hematoma?**

Saddle nose deformity.

O   **What muscles create vertical glabellar rhytids?**

Corrugator supercilii muscles.

O   **What is the anterior limit of the hiatus semilunaris?**

Uncinate process.

O   **What is rollover?**

A decrease in speech discrimination at high intensities suggestive of a retrocochlear lesion.

O   **What % of tympanocentesis specimens are sterile despite apparently active disease?**

20 – 30%.

O   **What is Griesinger's sign?**

Edema and tenderness over the mastoid cortex associated with thrombosis of the mastoid emissary vein secondary to lateral sinus thrombosis.

O   **What is the most common cause of chronic cervical adenopathy in children and adolescents?**

Cat-scratch disease.

O   **What is the etiology of a nasal dermal sinus?**

Defective obliteration of the dural projection through the foramen cecum and entrapment of epithelium as the dural tract resorbs.

O   **What is the blood supply to the sternocleidomastoid flap?**

Occipital artery, superior thyroid artery, transverse cervical artery, inferior thyroid artery.

O   **Where is verrucous carcinoma most likely to arise?**

Buccal mucosa.

O   **What is another name for papillary cystadenoma lymphomatosum?**

Warthin's tumor.

O   **What do biopsy specimens of rhinoscleroma show?**

Mikulicz' cells, histiocytes, and Russell bodies.

O   **What bacterium is associated with rhinophyma?**

Demodex follicularis.

O   **Where is tuberculosis of the larynx most commonly found?**

Interarytenoid area and laryngeal surface of the epiglottis.

O   **What tumors are psyaliferous cells seen in?**

Chordomas.

O   **What is the most common benign tumor of the esophagus?**

Leiomyoma.

O   **How long does it take for the dermis to normalize after chemical face peeling?**

10 months.

O   **T/F: Children are more likely than adults to form hypertrophic scars.**

True.

O   **Which nevi have the propensity for malignant degeneration?**

Junctional nevi.

O   **What finding on biopsy specimen distinguishes Sjögren's syndrome from lymphoma?**

Myoepithelial cells are only seen in Sjögren's syndrome.

O   **Acute, branching, septate hyphae are characteristic of which fungus?**

Aspergillus fumigatus.

O   **Which mandibular cyst forms around impacted molars?**

Dentigerous cysts.

O   **For which penetrating cervical injuries is angiography indicated in almost all cases?**

Injuries involving zone 1 or 3.

O   **What is a hamartoma?**

Circumscribed overgrowth of tissues, normally present in that part of the body.

O   **What laboratory values are abnormal in patients with von Willebrand's disease?**

Bleeding time and PTT.

O   **Where are the cell bodies of special visceral afferent nerves from taste buds in the anterior 2/3 of the tongue?**

Geniculate ganglion.

O   **Between what structures does a Killian-Jamieson dehiscence occur?**

Cricopharyngeus and circular fibers of the esophagus.

ANATOMY AND EMBRYOLOGY

SINUS ANATOMY

O **Where does the nasolacrimal duct lie in relation to the ostium of the maxillary sinus?**

3 – 6 mm anteriorly.

O **The majority of posterior ethmoid cells empty into which meatus?**

Superior meatus.

O **What % of the population has a supreme nasal concha?**

60%.

O **What are the 5 basal or ground lamella of the paranasal sinuses?**

Uncinate process, bulla ethmoidalis, basal lamella of the middle turbinate, lamella of the superior turbinate, lamella of the supreme turbinate (if present).

O **What structure separates the anterior and posterior ethmoid complexes?**

Basal lamella of the middle turbinate.

O **What is the name of the space between the bulla ethmoidalis and the middle turbinate?**

Hiatus semilunaris superioris.

O **Where does the natural ostium of the maxillary sinus empty?**

Ethmoid infundibulum.

O **What is the most posterior part of the middle turbinate attached to?**

Crista ethmoidalis of the perpendicular process of the palatine bone.

O **In what ways is the middle turbinate an important surgical landmark?**

Separates the cribriform plate from the fovea ethmoidalis; anterior tip marks the limit of the anterior dissection of maxillary antrostomy; basal lamella identifies entrance into the posterior ethmoids; lower half and insertion into the choanae help identify entrance into the sphenoid sinus.

O **Where does the anterior portion of the middle turbinate most often attach superiorly?**

Laterally onto the lamina papyracea (may also attach to the skull base).

O **What is an agger nasi cell?**

Pneumatized area of the lateral nasal wall immediately anterior and superior to the insertion of the middle turbinate.

O   **What problem can an enlarged agger nasi cell cause?**

Narrowing of the frontal recess.

O   **What is the term for a persistent, non-pneumatized second basal lamella?**

Torus ethmoidalis/lateralis.

O   **What is the term for a pneumatized second basal lamella?**

Bulla ethmoidalis.

O   **When may the suprabullar recess extend into the retrobullar recess?**

If the posterior wall of the bulla lamella is not in contact with the basal lamella of the middle turbinate.

O   **What is the bulla lamella?**

Lamella of bone that when pneumatized forms the ethmoid bulla.

O   **What is another name for retrobullar recess?**

Sinus lateralis.

O   **What is the most posterior aspect of the anterior ethmoids?**

Retrobullar recess.

O   **What does the retrobullar recess drain into?**

Hiatus semilunaris superior.

O   **What are the borders of the suprabullar recess?**

Superiorly, the ethmoid roof; laterally, the lamina papyracea; inferiorly, the roof of the ethmoid bulla; posteriorly, the basal lamella of the middle turbinate.

O   **What recess does the suprabullar recess open into?**

Frontal recess; anteriorly it is separated from the recess by the bulla lamella.

O   **Through which area can the suprabullar and retrobullar recesses be accessed medially and inferiorly?**

Hiatus semilunaris superior.

O   **What are the borders of the ethmoid infundibulum?**

Medially, the uncinate process; laterally, lamina papyracea and frontal process of the maxilla; posteriorly, ethmoid bulla.

○ **Into what does the ethmoid infundibulum drain posteriorly?**

Hiatus semilunaris inferior.

○ **Where does the maxillary sinus ostium lie in relation to the ethmoid infundibulum?**

At the floor and lateral aspect of the infundibulum between its middle and posterior 1/3.

○ **T/F: The frontal recess is synonymous with the nasofrontal duct.**

False, the nasofrontal duct bridges the frontal recess with the frontal sinus.

○ **What is the frontal recess?**

The most anterior and superior part of the anterior ethmoid complex.

○ **Which structures can narrow the frontal recess?**

Posteriorly, ethmoid bulla/bulla lamella; anteriorly, a pneumatized agger nasi cell.

○ **What defines the configuration of the ethmoid roof?**

The length of the lateral lamella of the cribriform plate, which determines the depth of the olfactory fossa.

○ **What are the 4 possible configurations of the ethmoid roof described by Keros?**

Type I: olfactory fossa 1 – 3 mm deep.
Type II: olfactory fossa 4 – 7 mm deep.
Type III: olfactory fossa 8 – 16 mm deep.
Asymmetric skull base

○ **What are the nasal fontanelles?**

Bony dehiscences of the lateral nasal wall usually above the insertion of inferior turbinate where the nasal mucosa approximates the mucoperiosteum of the maxillary sinus.

○ **What is the thinnest bone of the anterior skull base?**

Lateral lamella of the cribriform plate, where the anterior ethmoid artery crosses from the medial orbital wall to the cribriform.

○ **What is a concha bullosa?**

Pneumatized middle or superior turbinate.

○ **What is a Haller cell?**

Infraorbital ethmoid cell at the roof of maxillary sinus.

○ **What structures can a Haller cell potentially narrow?**

Maxillary sinus ostium or ethmoid infundibulum.

○ **What is the osteomeatal complex?**

Final common pathway for drainage and ventilation of the frontal, maxillary, and anterior ethmoid cells.

○   **What is the sphenoethmoid recess?**

Space between the superior (and supreme, if present) turbinate laterally, the cribriform plate superiorly, septum medially, anterior face of the sphenoid posteriorly, inferior margin of the superior turbinate inferolaterally.

○   **What are sphenoethmoid or Onodi cells?**

Pneumatized posterior ethmoid cells, superolateral to the sphenoid sinus.

○   **What % of people have a sphenoethmoid cell?**

12%.

○   **What important structures may run through an Onodi cell?**

Optic nerve and carotid artery.

○   **Where does the sphenoid sinus lie in relation to the most posterior ethmoid cell?**

Inferior and medial.

○   **Where is the natural ostium of the sphenoid sinus in relation to the superior turbinate?**

Medial, and within millimeters of its inferior border.

○   **What % of patients have a bony dehiscence of the cavernous portion of the carotid canal?**

22%.

○   **When does aeration of the frontal sinus begin?**

Age 4 – 5 and continues into the late teens.

○   **What are the normal dimensions of the frontal sinus?**

28 mm (length) x 24 mm (width) x 20 mm (depth) (Van Alyea).

○   **What is the incidence of frontal sinus agenesis?**

Unilateral agenesis 4%; bilateral agenesis 5%.

○   **Where is the anterior ethmoid artery found intranasally?**

Anterior to the vertical portion of basal lamella, immediately below the skull base, and posterior to the frontal recess.

○   **What % of patients have a bony dehiscence of the canal covering the anterior ethmoid artery?**

20 – 40%.

○   **What is the distance from the posterior ethmoid artery to the optic foramen?**

5 – 10 mm.

○   **What is the optic nerve tubercle?**

Bony protuberance on the medial surface of the optic foramen.

○   **What are the 3 types of sphenoid sinuses as described by Hamberger?**

Sellar (67 – 76%): sella turcia bulges into a well-developed sinus.
Presellar (23 – 28%): cancellous bone extends from under the sella to the anterior aspect of the floor.
Conchal (0 – 5%): sphenoid sinus is entirely filled with cancellous bone.

○   **T/F: Presence of a conchal sphenoid is an absolute contraindication to transsphenoidal hypophysectomy.**

False (the bone can be drilled out to permit access).

○   **What bony structure is found posterior to the sphenoid?**

Clivus.

○   **What structures are found within the cavernous sinus?**

Internal carotid artery, venous channels, III, IV, VI, V1, V2.

○   **Which of these nerves is closely associated with the lateral wall of the ICA?**

VI.

○   **Where is the optic canal in relation to the sphenoid?**

Anterolateral aspect of the sphenoid roof.

○   **What % of patients have a very thin or absent bone of the optic canal?**

4%.

○   **T/F: Tumors isolated to the sphenoid sinus and sella are best approached transpalatally.**

False, best approach is transseptal or transethmoid unless the tumor extends into the nasopharynx.

○   **From anterior to posterior, what structures comprise the medial orbital wall?**

Frontal process of the maxilla, lacrimal bone, lamina papyracea, sphenoid bone to optic nerve foramen.

○   **What is the blood supply to the retina?**

Choroid chorio capillaries (outer half) and central retinal artery and branches.

○   **Where does the sphenoid ostium lie in relation to the chonal bridge?**

1.5 cm above or 1/3 distance from chonae to the skull base.

○   **Where are the natural ostia of the sphenoid sinus?**

2/3 of the way from the vaginal process to the top of the anterior sphenoid wall.

○   **What is the normal angle of a line drawn from the nasal spine to the sphenoid ostium?**

30 degrees.

NEURO-OTOLOGIC ANATOMY

○   **What is the foramen of Huschke?**

An embryologic remnant that normally obliterates in the anteroinferior portion of the medial bony external auditory canal (EAC).

○   **What is the clinical significance of the foramen of Huschke?**

Serves as a potential route for spread of tumor from the parotid gland to the temporal bone.

○   **What is the foramen of Morgagni?**

Gap between superior constrictor muscle and skull base.

○   **What is the clinical significance of the foramen of Morgagni?**

Serves a potential route for spread of nasopharyngeal tumors to the skull base and brain.

○   **Where is the tympanic notch of Rivinus?**

Superior portion of the tympanic ring (squamous portion of temporal bone).

○   **What are the four parts of the temporal bone?**

Squamous, tympanic, petrous, mastoid.

○   **Which wall of the EAC is shorter-the anteroinferior or posterosuperior?**

Posterosuperior (approximately 25 mm whereas anteroinferior wall is 31 mm).

○   **How much of the EAC is cartilaginous?**

1/3.

○   **How much of the eustachian tube (ET) is cartilaginous?**

2/3.

○   **At what month gestation does the ear canal open?**

7.

○   **What are the dimensions of the tympanic membrane (TM)?**

9 – 10 mm vertically; 8 – 9 mm horizontally.

O **What is the pars tensa?**

Portion of the TM inferior to the mallear fold and prominence.

O **What are the layers of the TM?**

Squamous epithelium, radiating fibrous layer, circumferential fibrous layer, mucosa.

O **What is the sensory innervation of the auricle?**

Greater auricular nerve (C3), auriculotemporal nerve (V3), lesser occipital nerve (C2,3), auricular branch of the vagus, and sensory branches of VII and IX.

O **What is Hitzelberger's sign?**

Hypoesthesia of the postauricular area associated with VIIth nerve compression secondary to an acoustic neuroma.

O **Which has greater sensory innervation-pars tensa or pars flaccida?**

Pars flaccida.

O **What are the three nerves of the tympanic plexus?**

V3, IX (Jacobson's nerve), X.

O **Which ossicles can be found in the epitympanic recess?**

Head of the malleus, body and short process of the incus.

O **Which ossicle has the most tenuous blood supply and is most prone to necrosis?**

Long process of the incus.

O **What structure is found in Meckel's cave?**

Gasserian ganglion of V.

O **Where is Dorello's canal and what nerve does it contain?**

Between the petrous tip and the sphenoid bone; contains VI and inferior petrosal sinus.

O **What is Gradenigo's syndrome?**

Petrositis involving VI in Dorello's canal causing retro-orbital pain, diplopia and otorrhea.

O **What is the scutum?**

Lateral wall of the epitympanum.

O **What structures are superior to the falciform crest in the internal auditory canal (IAC)?**

Facial nerve and superior branch of the vestibular nerve.

O   **What structures are inferior to the falciform crest in the IAC?**

Cochlear nerve and inferior branch of the vestibular nerve.

O   **What are the four openings into the temporal bone?**

IAC, vestibular and cochlear aqueducts, and subarcuate fossa.

O   **Where is the primary auditory cortex?**

Brodmann's area 41 in the superficial portion of the temporal lobe.

O   **What are the boundaries of the epitympanum?**

Superiorly, the tegmen; inferiorly, the fossa incudis; anteriorly, the zygomatic arch; posteriorly, the aditus; medially, the lateral semicircular canal and VII; laterally, the scutum.

O   **What are the boundaries of the tympanic cavity?**

Superiorly, the tegmen; inferiorly, the jugular wall and styloid prominence; anteriorly, the carotid wall, eustachian tube, and tensor tympani; posteriorly, the mastoid, stapedius, pyramidal prominence; medially, the labyrinthine wall; laterally, the TM and scutum.

O   **What structure separates the epitympanic recess from the cranial cavity?**

Tegmen tympani.

O   **What is the inferior boundary of the tympanic cavity?**

Jugular bulb.

O   **What structures are anterior to the tympanic cavity?**

The carotid artery, ET, and the canal for the tensor tympani muscle.

O   **What structures are posterior to the tympanic cavity?**

Aditus, posterior sinus, chorda tympani, fossa incudis, pyramidal prominence, stapedial tendon.

O   **What is the promontory?**

Elevation of the medial wall of the tympanic cavity formed by the basal turn of the cochlea.

O   **What structures create three small depressions in the posterior portion of the medial wall of the tympanic cavity?**

Subiculum, ponticulus.

O   **What structure is located inferior to the subiculum and posteroinferior to the promontory?**

Round window.

O   **What structure lies between the subiculum and ponticulus?**

Sinus tympani.

○   **What structure lies superior to the ponticulus?**

Oval window.

○   **What structure lies between the prominence of the lateral semicircular canal (SCC) and the promontory/oval window?**

Prominence of the facial canal.

○   **What proportion of the population has a pneumatized petrous pyramid?**

1/3.

○   **What is the upper limit of normal diameter of the IAC?**

8 mm.

○   **What are the two most important landmarks in the middle fossa approach to the IAC?**

Arcuate eminence and hiatus for the greater superficial petrosal nerve.

○   **What is the most anterior structure of the medial wall of the tympanic cavity?**

Cochleariform process.

○   **Cochleariform process: tensor tympani...... pyramidal process:_____?**

Stapedius.

○   **Which ossicles develop from the first branchial arch (Meckel's cartilage)?**

Head and neck of the malleus, body and short process of the incus.

○   **Which ossicles develop from the second branchial arch (Reichert's cartilage)?**

Manubrium of the malleus, long process of the incus, stapes (except footplate).

○   **What does the stapes footplate develop from?**

Otic mesenchyme.

○   **Which ossicular component develops from membranous bone?**

Anterior process of the malleus.

○   **Which ossicular components never completely ossify?**

Part of the manubrium and the vestibular portion of the stapes footplate.

○   **Which part of the malleus articulates with the incus?**

Head.

O   **When do ossicles reach adult size and shape?**

At the 16th week gestation, they are adult-sized, and by birth, they are adult-shaped.

O   **Where in the ossicular chain does the tensor tympani muscle insert?**

Manubrium of the malleus.

O   **Which part of the malleus creates the malleolar prominence of the TM?**

Lateral process.

O   **Which part of the malleus does the anterior ligament attach to?**

The neck, near the anterior process.

O   **Which part of the incus articulates with the stapes?**

Lenticular process (medial side of long process).

O   **What ligament supports the stapes?**

Annular ligament.

O   **Where does most movement of the stapes occur?**

Anterior-superior portion of the footplate.

O   **Where in the ossicular chain does the stapedius muscle insert?**

Posterior neck of the stapes.

O   **Between which ossicles does the chorda tympani run?**

Manubrium of the malleus and long process of the incus.

O   **What is the function of the chorda tympani nerve?**

Parasympathetic innervation to the submandibular and sublingual glands, and taste to the anterior 2/3 of the tongue.

O   **What is Körner's septum?**

Otherwise known as the "false bottom," it represents the suture line between the petrous and squamous portions of the temporal bone.

O   **Which planes are the oval and round windows oriented in?**

Oval window is in the sagittal plane; round window is in the transverse plane.

O   **At what age is the mastoid process completely pneumatized?**

2.

○ **What is meant by a "diploic mastoid"?**

Occupied by bone marrow instead of air cells.

○ **What structure is situated just medial to the tip of the cochleariform process?**

Geniculate ganglion of the facial nerve.

○ **Describe the path of the facial nerve in the temporal bone.**

Enters the **IAC**; travels laterally for a short distance, then, just superior to the promontory, it makes a sharp turn to run posteriorly (at the **external/first genu** and the **geniculate ganglion**). Nerve continues posteriorly, with a slight infero-lateral inclination (forming the prominence of the facial canal in the medial wall of tympanic cavity). Behind the base of the pyramidal eminence, the nerve makes a broad turn to descend vertically and somewhat laterally (**2nd genu**) through the mastoid cavity.

○ **What is the function of the greater superficial petrosal nerve?**

Lacrimation.

○ **Why is the development of the bony otic capsule unique?**

It is formed from 14 centers of ossification that fuse and leave no suture lines; the centers are formed from cartilage, but retain no areas of chondral growth. The bone retains its fetal character, with Haversian canals.

○ **What is the last part of the otic capsule to ossify?**

Fissula ante fenestrum.

○ **What is the name of the central bony core of the cochlea through which nerves and vessels travel?**

Modiolus.

○ **What structure ends blindly at the round window?**

Scala tympani (lower compartment of the cochlea).

○ **What does the vestibular aqueduct carry?**

Endolymphatic duct and accompanying vein.

○ **What is the name of the area of communication between the scala vestibuli and the scala tympani?**

Helicotrema.

○ **What fluid surrounds the membranous labyrinth?**

Perilymph.

○ **How does perilymph differ from endolymph?**

Perilymph has a pH of 7.2, is high in sodium, low in potassium, and does not contain chloride; endolymph has a pH of 7.5, is low in sodium, and relatively high in potassium and chloride.

○   **T/F: The membranous labyrinth is a self-contained system.**

True.

○   **What are the main structures of the vestibular portion of the membranous labyrinth?**

Utricle, saccule, and semicircular canals.

○   **Which of these receives the crura from the three semicircular canals?**

Utricle.

○   **What structures house the crista?**

Ampulla.

○   **What structure produces endolymph?**

Stria vascularis.

○   **What is the blood supply to the inner ear?**

Labyrinthine artery (branch of anterior inferior cerebellar artery).

○   **What does the superior vestibular nerve innervate?**

Superior and lateral SCCs, utricle, saccule.

○   **What does the inferior vestibular nerve innervate?**

Posterior SCC and macula of the saccule.

○   **What structure forms the arcuate eminence?**

Superior SCC.

○   **How does the course of the facial nerve differ between adults and children?**

At birth, the nerve is located superficially within the poorly formed mastoid; with maturation, the nerve is displaced medially and inferiorly.

○   **What is the last structure of the inner ear to develop?**

Endolymphatic sac.

○   **When does the otic capsule begin formation?**

At 8 weeks, the precursors of the otic capsule are present; at 15 weeks, the ossification centers are present.

○   **When does the otic capsule finish developing?**

By 21 – 24 weeks, it is adult size.

O   T/F: The position of the cochlear duct is always inferior to the lowest border of the stapes footplate.

True.

O   Where is the safest place to create an opening in the stapes footplate?

Central area.

O   What are the average dimensions of the stapes footplate?

1.41 x 2.99 mm.

O   What is the minimum distance from the center of the stapes footplate to the utricle and saccule?

1.2 and 1.4 mm, respectively.

O   What three nuclei supply fibers to the facial nerve?

Motor nucleus in caudal aspect of the pons, superior salivatory nucleus (dorsal to the motor nucleus), and nucleus of the solitary tract in medulla.

O   Which of these nuclei sends parasympathetic fibers to salivary glands?

Superior salivatory nucleus.

O   Which of these nuclei receives taste, proprioceptive, and cutaneous sensory information?

Nucleus of the solitary tract.

O   What are the limits of the fallopian canal?

Fundus of the IAC to the stylomastoid foramen.

O   What are the six segments of the facial nerve?

Intracranial, internal auditory canal, labyrinthine, tympanic, mastoid/vertical, extratemporal.

O   Which segment is shortest?

Labyrinthine.

O   Which segment has the most narrow passageway?

Labyrinthine.

O   Where is the second genu of the facial nerve?

Just distal to the geniculate ganglion, at the sinus tympani between the tympanic and mastoid segments.

O   In its tympanic segment, between which structures does the facial nerve travel?

Superiorly, the lateral SCC; inferiorly, the oval window.

O   **What % of people have a dehiscence of the facial nerve in either the tympanic or mastoid segments?**

50 – 55%.

O   **Where is the most common site of dehiscence?**

Tympanic segment superior to the oval window.

O   **What are some clinical clues to an aberrant facial nerve?**

Congenitally malformed auricle, ossicular abnormalities, craniofacial anomalies, conductive hearing loss.

O   **Where do most facial nerve injuries occur during middle ear surgery?**

Tympanic segment.

O   **What is the most common site of facial nerve injury during mastoid surgery?**

At the pyramidal turn posterolateral to the horizontal SCC.

O   **How does facial nerve innervation to the upper face differ from that to the lower face?**

Upper motor neurons sending information to the upper face cross twice in the pons; upper motor neurons sending information to the lower face cross only once in the pons. Therefore, lesions proximal to the nucleus only affect the lower face.

O   **What is Trautmann's triangle?**

Triangle between the external prominence of the lateral and posterior SCCs and the posterosuperior corner of the mastoid.

O   **What % of preauricular cysts are bilateral?**

20%.

O   **What is Hyrtl's fissure?**

Connection between the subarachnoid space near the IXth ganglion and the hypotympanum that allows middle ear infections to spread to the brain; normally closes with maturation.

O   **What is the facial hiatus?**

Dehiscence of variable size in petrous portion of the temporal bone in the floor of the middle cranial fossa, which marks the entrance of the greater superficial petrosal nerve into the middle cranial fossa.

O   **How is the facial hiatus clinically significant?**

The geniculate ganglion usually lies deep to the hiatus, but in 5 – 10% of patients, it lies under the dura within the hiatus and without a bony covering.

O   **What three branches of the facial nerve are given off in its course through the temporal bone?**

Greater superficial petrosal nerve, nerve to the stapedius muscle, chorda tympani.

O   **Where in the tympanic and mastoid segments of the facial nerve are the sensory fibers located?**

Anterolaterally in the tympanic segment, posterolaterally in the mastoid segment.

O   **Where does the chorda tympani arise in relation to the stylomastoid foramen?**

Usually 4 – 7 mm superior.

O   **What artery accompanies the chorda tympani?**

Posterior tympanic artery.

O   **What is Arnold's nerve?**

Auricular branch of the vagus that innervates skin of the external auditory canal and auricle.

O   **What is the blood supply to the geniculate ganglion?**

Greater superficial petrosal artery (branch of the middle meningeal artery).

O   **What structure bisects the internal auditory canal in the vertical direction? Horizontal direction?**

Bill's bar; transverse/falciform crest.

O   **Adenocarcinoma of the endolymphatic sac is more common in patients with what disease?**

Von Hippel-Lindau disease.

O   **What portion of the facial nerve is closest to the cochlea?**

Labyrinthine.

O   **How can one discern fibrous dysplasia from Paget's disease of the temporal bone on CT scan?**

Paget's disease involves the otic capsule while fibrous dysplasia does not.

O   **What embryologic structures is the auricle developed from?**

The Hillocks of His.

O   **How many are there and which branchial arches do they arise from?**

Six... the first three arise from the first arch and the last three arise from the second arch.

O   **What does each Hillock become?**

1 – tragus
2 – helical crus
3 – helix
4 – antihelix
5 – antitragus

6 – lobule and lower helix

O   **When does development of the external auditory canal begin?**

The channel begins to develop at 28 weeks.

O   **At what age is the EAC adult size?**

Age 9.

O   **What does the eustachian tube develop from?**

From the 1st pouch, between the 2nd arch and the pharynx.

O   **How long is the tube at birth? in adulthood?**

17 mm, 35 mm.

O   **T/F: The tympanic membrane is derived from ectoderm.**

False; it is derived from ecto-, meso-, and endoderm.

O   **What is the significance of a congenitally malformed auricle?**

The auricle develops early, making malformations of the middle ear, mastoid, and VII more likely.

O   **What is the significance of a normal auricle with canal atresia?**

The EAC begins formation late (28th week), so the middle ear and ossicles are more likely to be normal.

O   **How does a preauricular sinus tract form?**

From improper fusion of the 1st and 2nd branchial arches.

O   **What nerve innervates the palatopharyngeus and palatoglossus muscles?**

Vagus.

O   **What are the nuclei of the vagus nerve?**

Nucleus ambiguus, dorsal motor nucleus, and the nucleus of the solitary tract.

O   **Which of these controls voluntary motor information?**

Nucleus ambiguus.

O   **Which of these receives sensory information?**

Nucleus of the solitary tract.

O   **What are the 2 ganglia of the vagus nerve?**

Superior (jugular) ganglion and inferior (nodose) ganglion.

○   **What information is relayed through the superior ganglion?**

Sensation from the EAC and posterior auricle via Arnold's nerve.

○   **What information is relayed through the inferior ganglion?**

Sensation from the epiglottis and larynx.

○   **What is the function of the glossopharyngeal nerve?**

Motor to the stylopharyngeus; taste to posterior 1/3 tongue; parotid gland stimulation; sensation of postauricular skin, pharynx, soft palate, tympanic cavity, and eustachian tube.

○   **Which cranial nerve has the longest intracranial course?**

VI.

○   **Does the foramen rotundum lie lateral or medial to the pterygoid canal?**

Lateral.

○   **What is the largest artery in the pterygopalatine fossa?**

Sphenopalatine.

○   **What opening in the medial wall of the pterygopalatine fossa permits the passage of neurovascular structures into the nasal passages?**

Sphenopalatine foramen.

○   **Where does most of the resorption of endolymph occur?**

Endolymphatic sac.

○   **Which 3 cranial nerves are found beneath the floor of the middle ear cavity?**

IX, X, XI.

○   **Which branchial arch does the tensor tympani muscle arise from?**

I.

○   **What is the name for the entrance to the fallopian canal?**

Fundus.

○   **What is the average diameter of the IAC?**

6.8 mm.

○   **What is the first branch of the facial nerve?**

Greater superficial petrosal nerve.

O   **Where along the course of the facial nerve does this nerve branch off?**

Geniculate ganglion.

O   **What is the last branch of the facial nerve before it passes through the stylomastoid foramen?**

Chorda tympani nerve.

O   **What nerve carries taste fibers supplying taste buds on the palate?**

Greater superficial petrosal nerve.

O   **What is the name of the opening through which the chorda tympani nerve enters the infratemporal fossa?**

Petrotympanic fissure (canal of Huguier).

O   **What produces CSF?**

Choroid plexus.

O   **How much CSF is produced per minute?**

0.35 – 0.37 cc.

O   **What problem results from rupture of the middle meningeal artery?**

Epidural hematoma.

O   **What structures facilitate passage of CSF into the dural venous sinuses?**

Arachnoid villi.

O   **What is Donaldson's line?**

Imaginary line in the plane of the horizontal SCC back to the sigmoid sinus marking the top of the endolymphatic sac.

GENERAL HEAD AND NECK ANATOMY

O   **What structures form the common facial vein?**

Anterior retromandibular and facial veins.

O   **What structures form the external jugular vein?**

Posterior retromandibular and posterior auricular veins.

O   **What is the terminal branch of V2?**

Infraorbital nerve.

○   **What is another term for "inion?"**

External occipital protuberance.

○   **What is the name of the space between the cheeks and the teeth?**

Vestibule.

○   **What is the only sensory nerve arising from the anterior division of V3?**

Buccal nerve.

○   **What structures pass through the mandibular foramen?**

Inferior alveolar artery and nerve.

○   **Where are the cell bodies of the motor fibers of the chorda tympani nerve?**

Superior salivatory nucleus.

○   **What muscle protracts the mandible?**

Lateral pterygoid muscle.

○   **What type of joint is the TMJ?**

Ginglymoarthrodial (hinge/sliding) joint.

○   **What muscle inserts on the disk of the TMJ?**

Superior part of the lateral pterygoid muscle.

○   **What is the blood supply to the upper molars?**

Posterior superior alveolar artery.

○   **What is the name of the opening through which the maxillary artery passes after giving rise to infraorbital and posterior superior alveolar branches?**

Pterygomaxillary fissure.

○   **What is the name of the maxillary artery after it passes through the pterygomaxillary fissure?**

Sphenopalatine artery.

○   **What nerve and vessel pass through the foramen spinosum?**

Middle meningeal artery and meningeal branch of V3.

○   **What passes through the foramen rotundum?**

V2.

○   **The pterygoid plates are part of which bone?**

Sphenoid.

O   **Name the foramen through which the structure passes:**

Meningeal branch of V3	Foramen spinosum.
Terminal branch of V2	Infraorbital foramen.
V3 and accessory meningeal artery	Foramen ovale.
Sphenopalatine artery	Sphenopalatine foramen.
III, IV, VI, V1	Superior orbital fissure.
V2	Foramen rotundum.

O   **What nerve usually passes from lateral to medial over the optic nerve?**

Nasociliary.

O   **What are the layers of the eyelid from superficial to deep?**

Skin, subcutaneous tissue, voluntary muscle, orbital septum, tarsal plate, smooth muscle, and conjunctiva.

O   **What is the name of the fleshy, pink mound of tissue in the medial canthus?**

Lacrimal caruncle.

O   **What glands are contained within the tarsal plates?**

Tarsal glands (Meibomian).

O   **What problem results from blockage of the Meibomian glands?**

Chalazion.

O   **What is a stye?**

Blockage of the sebaceous or sweat glands surrounding the eyelashes.

O   **Which muscles are innervated by the superior division of III?**

Superior rectus and levator palpebrae superioris muscles.

O   **Which skeletal muscles are innervated by the inferior division of III?**

Inferior oblique, inferior rectus, medial rectus muscles.

O   **Periosteum and periorbita meet at the orbital margin and continue into the eyelids as what?**

Orbital septum.

O   **What is the origin of the superior tarsal muscle (of Muller)?**

Deep side of the levator palpebrae superioris.

O   **What structures pass through the superior orbital fissure?**

III, IV, VI, V1, superior ophthalmic vein.

O   **From what nerve do the anterior and posterior ethmoidal nerves arise?**

Nasociliary nerve.

O   **What are the boundaries of the parotid compartment?**

Superiorly, the zygoma; posteriorly, the external auditory canal; anteriorly, the masseter muscle; inferiorly, the styloid process, carotid artery, jugular vessels, styloid muscles.

O   **What structures are found in the prestyloid compartment of the parapharyngeal space?**

Muscles (stylopharyngeus, styloglossus, and stylohyoid), fat.

O   **What structures are found in the poststyloid compartment of the parapharyngeal space?**

Internal jugular vein, internal carotid artery, IX, X, XI, XII.

O   **Where does Stenson's duct arise from in relation to the zygoma?**

1.5 cm inferior to the zygoma.

O   **What muscle does Stenson's duct pierce?**

Buccinator.

O   **Where does Stenson's duct open intraorally?**

Just opposite the 2nd upper molar.

O   **What branch of the facial nerve travels with Stenson's duct?**

Buccal.

O   **What membrane separates the parotid gland from the submandibular gland?**

Stylomandibular membrane.

O   **What three motor branches does the facial nerve give off just after exiting the stylomastoid foramen?**

Nerve to posterior belly of the digastric, nerve to the stylohyoid, nerve to the postauricular muscle.

m How much saliva is produced per day?

500 – 1500 cc.

O   **T/F: Saliva promotes the calcification of teeth.**

True.

O   **How does the saliva produced from the parotid gland differ from that of the sublingual gland?**

The saliva from the parotid is serous, high in enzymes and low in mucin; that from the sublingual gland is primarily composed of mucin.

O   **What is the most consistent landmark for identification of the facial nerve trunk?**

Tympanomastoid suture line.

O   **Where is the facial nerve trunk located in relation to the tympanomastoid suture line?**

6 – 8 mm anteroinferior (between the suture line and the styloid process).

O   **What is the name of the point at which the facial nerve divides into the upper and lower divisions?**

Pes anserinus.

O   **How far is the pes anserinus from the stylomastoid foramen?**

Approximately 1.3 cm.

O   **What nerve parallels the superficial temporal vessels?**

Auriculotemporal nerve.

O   **What is the function of the auriculotemporal nerve?**

Sensation of the scalp, auricle and carries postganglionic parasympathetic nerves from the otic ganglion to the parotid gland to stimulate secretions.

O   **What is the blood supply to the parotid gland?**

Transverse facial artery, a branch of the superficial temporal artery.

O   **What is the major venous drainage of the parotid gland?**

Posterior facial vein.

O   **What is unique about the lymphatic drainage of the parotid gland?**

The lymph nodes are contained within the gland, and it is the only salivary gland with two layers of lymph nodes.

O   **Which layer of lymph nodes has the most nodes (superficial or deep)?**

Superficial.

O   **What is Frey's syndrome?**

Gustatory sweating, secondary to cross-reinnervation of the divided auriculotemporal nerve with cutaneous nerves, after parotidectomy.

O   **What are the treatment options for Frey's syndrome?**

3% scopolamine cream, section Jacobson's nerve, sternocleidomastoid muscle flap, interpose fascia lata between skin and gland.

O   **Describe the pathway of parasympathetic innervation to the parotid gland.**

Preganglionic parasympathetic fibers leave the inferior salivatory nucleus via the glossopharyngeal nerve, pass through the jugular foramen, travel through the middle ear (as Jacobson's nerve), then travel along the floor of the middle cranial fossa (as the lesser petrosal nerve) to the otic ganglion; postganglionic parasympathetic fibers leave the otic ganglion via the auriculotemporal branch of V3 and travel to the parotid gland.

O   **Where does the retromandibular vein lie in relation to the facial nerve?**

In most people, it courses deep to both trunks of the facial nerve. In up to 10% of people, the vein crosses either trunk laterally.

O   **T/F: Enlargement of the preauricular lymph nodes is indicative of parotid pathology.**

False…these nodes enlarge from inflammation or metastasizing tumors from the scalp.

O   **Which lymph nodes drain tumors from the parotid gland?**

Nodes just inferior to the gland adjacent to the sternocleidomastoid muscle and the external jugular vein.

O   **Where does the stylomastoid foramen lie in relation to the origin of the posterior belly of the digastric muscle?**

Anterior.

O   **What is the plane of dissection for raising flaps during parotidectomy and how can one identify this more easily?**

Between the SMAS and the superficial layer of the deep fascia… identify the platysma first and work superiorly.

O   **What are 6 ways to identify the facial nerve trunk during parotidectomy?**

Identification of the tympanomastoid suture line, tragal pointer, posterior belly of the digastric, or styloid process; tracing a distal branch retrograde or tracing the proximal portion forward by drilling out the mastoid segment.

O   **What 2 structures pass between the superior and middle pharyngeal constrictors?**

Stylopharyngeus muscle and IX.

O   **With one exception, all the muscles of the pharynx are innervated by what nerve?**

X.

O   **How much of the blood supply to the brain is normally provided by the internal carotid arteries?**

80%.

O   **What artery provides most of the blood supply to the palatine tonsil?**

Tonsillar branch of the facial artery.

O   **What is the common insertion of the three pharyngeal constrictors?**

Median pharyngeal raphe.

○   **What structures define the thoracic inlet?**

Manubrium, 1st ribs, and the body of C1.

○   **What are the 3 areas of esophageal narrowing?**

Superiorly, from the cricopharyngeus; inferiorly, where the esophagus enters the cardia; and in the middle, where the left mainstem bronchus and the aorta cross anteriorly.

○   **How does the musculature of the upper 1/3 esophagus differ from the lower 2/3?**

Upper 1/3 is striated; lower 2/3 is smooth.

○   **Where is Auerbach's plexus in the esophagus?**

Between the longitudinal and circular muscle fibers.

○   **Where is Meissner's plexus in the esophagus?**

Submucosa.

○   **T/F: The esophagus does not have a serosa.**

True.

○   **What are the 3 layers of the esophageal mucosa?**

Muscularis mucosa, lamina propria, epithelium.

○   **In what directions are the muscle fibers of the inferior constrictor oriented?**

Superiorly, in an oblique fashion; inferiorly, in a transverse fashion.

○   **What are the 2 types of diverticula?**

Pulsion and traction.

○   **Which of these is associated with high intraluminal pressure?**

Pulsion.

○   **Which of these is Zenker's diverticulum?**

Pulsion.

○   **Where do pharyngoesophageal/Zenker's diverticula occur?**

Between the oblique and transverse fibers of the inferior constrictor (Killian's dehiscence), most commonly on the left, and between the cricopharyngeus and the esophagus (Killian-Jamieson area).

○   **What is the blood supply to the esophagus?**

Inferior thyroid artery (branch of the thyrocervical trunk), 2 – 3 branches directly from the thoracic aorta, and the esophageal branch of the left gastric artery.

O   **What is the venous drainage of the esophagus?**

Inferior thyroid vein, azygous and hemiazygous veins (into the IVC), and esophageal veins (into the coronary vein and eventually the portal vein).

O   **What is the normal resting pressure of the upper esophageal sphincter (UES)?**

100 mm Hg in the anteroposterior orientation; <50 mm Hg in the lateral orientation.

O   **What is the normal resting pressure of the lower esophageal sphincter (LES)?**

10 – 40 mm Hg.

O   **What is the effect of beta-adrenergic blockers on LES?**

Increase LES pressure.

O   **Where are the left and right vagus nerves in relation to the esophagus?**

The left is anterior and the right is posterior.

O   **What is the efficacy of ranitidine 150 mg BID compared to proton pump inhibitors in the healing of esophagitis?**

Ranitidine: 35 – 65% efficacy.
Proton pump inhibitors: 95% efficacy.

O   **What finding on barium swallow is classic for cricopharyngeal dysfunction?**

Cricopharyngeal bar.

O   **What is the most common cause of esophageal perforation?**

Surgical instrumentation.

O   **What is the distance from the incisor teeth to the cardia of the stomach in adults?**

40 cm.

O   **What is the distance from the incisor teeth to the cricopharyngeus in adults?**

16 cm.

O   **What test is used to diagnose a Mallory-Weiss tear?**

Endoscopy (contrast studies are not beneficial as the tear is only mucosal).

O   **Where is the tear most commonly located?**

Lower esophagus or cardia of the stomach.

O   **What test is used to diagnose Boerhaave syndrome?**

Water-soluble contrast esophagram (tear is transmural).

O   **What is the only complete cartilage ring of the respiratory tract?**

Cricoid.

O   **T/F: The incidence of foreign body aspiration is equal between the right and left bronchus in children.**

True; the left bronchus is not as obliquely angled as in the adult.

O   **What vessels are in direct contact with the anterior trachea?**

Brachiocephalic artery and the left brachiocephalic vein.

O   **What % of the population has a thyroidea ima artery?**

10%.

O   **Which branchial arches is the larynx derived from?**

III, IV, VI.

O   **What are the nine cartilages of the larynx?**

3 unpaired: thyroid, cricoid, epiglottis.
3 paired: arytenoids, corniculates, cuneiforms.

O   **What are the 2 branches of the superior laryngeal nerve?**

Internal and external.

O   **Which of these supplies sensation to the larynx above the glottis?**

Internal branch.

O   **What membrane must the internal branch penetrate?**

Thyrohyoid.

O . **What blood vessel travels with the internal branch?**

Superior laryngeal artery.

O   **What does the external branch innervate?**

Cricothyroid muscle.

O   **What is the function of the cricothyroid muscle?**

To lengthen the vocal fold and increase pitch.

O   **What separates the two valleculae associated with the tongue and the epiglottis?**

Median glosso-epiglottic fold.

O   **What nerve provides sensory innervation to the pyriform recess of the larynx?**

Internal laryngeal branch of the superior laryngeal nerve.

O   **What nerve provides sensory innervation to the infraglottic space?**

Recurrent laryngeal nerve.

O   **What is the name of the upper free margin of the conus elasticus?**

Vocal ligament.

O   **What is the name of the lower free margin of the quadrangular membrane?**

Vestibular fold.

O   **What is the vertebral level of the hyoid in adults?**

C3.

O   **What is the vertebral level of the cricoid in adults?**

C6.

O   **What is the vertebral level of the carina in adults?**

T4 – T5.

O   **What muscle descends to insert upon the hyoid?**

Geniohyoid.

O   **From which branchial arch does the stylohyoid muscle arise?**

II.

O   **What is the membrane between the cricoid cartilage and the first tracheal ring?**

Cricotracheal membrane.

O   **What part of the thyroid cartilage articulates with the cricoid cartilage?**

Inferior cornu.

O   **What is the only unpaired muscle of the larynx?**

Transverse arytenoid muscle.

O   **What is the only abductor of the vocal cords?**

Posterior cricoarytenoid muscle.

O   **Which muscle comprises part of the vocal fold?**

Thyroarytenoid muscle.

O   **Which muscles anchor and elevate the larynx?**

Omohyoid, sternohyoid, sternothyroid muscles.

O   **Which muscles does the anterior branch of the recurrent laryngeal nerve innervate?**

Lateral cricoarytenoid, thyroarytenoid, vocalis muscles.

O   **Where does the superior laryngeal artery lie in relation to the superior laryngeal nerve?**

Inferior.

O   **What defines the anterior-posterior glottic diameter?**

Distance from the anterior commissure to the posterior border of the cricoid cartilage.

O   **What is the angle of the thyroid cartilage at the anterior commissure in men and women?**

90 degrees in men; 120 degrees in women.

O   **How do the vocal folds move during quiet respiration?**

Adduct during expiration and abduct during inspiration.

O   **What are the layers of the vocal fold from superior to deep?**

Squamous epithelium, Reinke's space (superior layer of lamina propria), intermediate and deep layers of the lamina propria (comprising the vocal ligament), thyroarytenoid muscle.

O   **What are the 2 types of squamous epithelium lining the TVCs?**

Pseudostratified columnar (superiorly and inferiorly) and stratified nonkeratinizing squamous (at the contact points of the TVCs).

O   **Which layers of the vocal cord are primarily responsible for TVC vibration?**

Epithelium and superficial layer of the lamina propria.

O   **What are the anatomic correlations to hoarseness and breathiness?**

Mucosal irregularity causes hoarseness; incomplete glottic closure causes breathiness.

O   **What are the 3 phases of speech?**

Pulmonary, laryngeal, oral.

O   **What are the three primary parameters of voice?**

Quality, loudness, pitch.

○ **What factors determine voice loudness?**

Subglottic air pressure, glottal resistance, rate of airflow, amplitude of vibration.

○ **What factors determine pitch?**

Length, tension, and cross-sectional mass of vocal folds; frequency of vibration.

○ **What is damping?**

Elevation of pitch by narrowing the glottic aperture.

○ **What determines voice quality?**

Symmetry of vocal fold vibration.

○ **What is *dysphonia plicae ventricularis*?**

Muffled hoarseness secondary to approximation of false vocal folds during phonation.

○ **What is "donkey breathing?"**

Vocalization during inspiration.

○ **What is the threshold for the laryngeal adductor reflex response in normal patients?**

Air pulse stimulus less than 4 mm Hg.

○ **What is shimmer?**

Cycle-to-cycle variation in the amplitude of the glottal pulse.

○ **What is jitter?**

Cycle-to-cycle variation in the frequency of the glottal pulse.

PATHOLOGY

O **What is the bilateral benign cystic lymphoepithelial lesion shown below?**

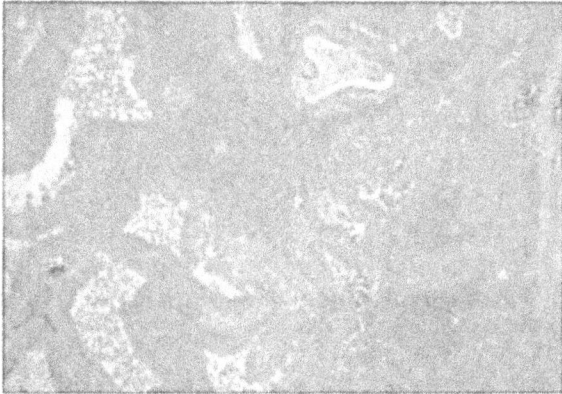

Warthin's tumor.

O **15-year-old boy presented with nasal obstruction and the polypoid mass shown above was resected and bled extensively. What is your diagnosis?**

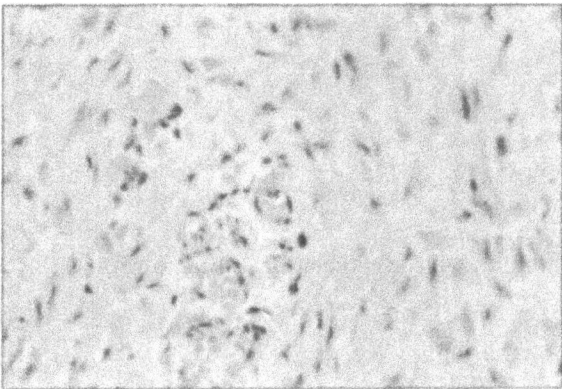

Juvenile nasopharyngeal angiofibroma.

O   **This soft, polypoid nasal mass was resected from a young child. What is your diagnosis?**

Glial heterotopia (nasal glioma).

O   **This lesion is from the mandible of a 19-year-old female near the mental foramen, what is the diagnosis?**

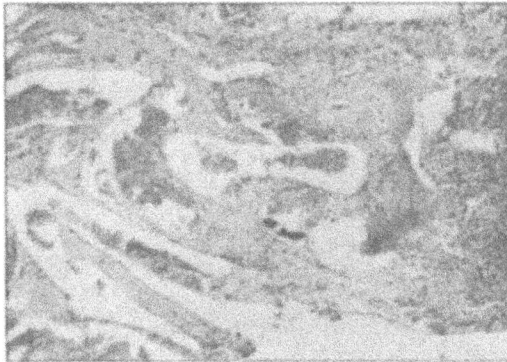

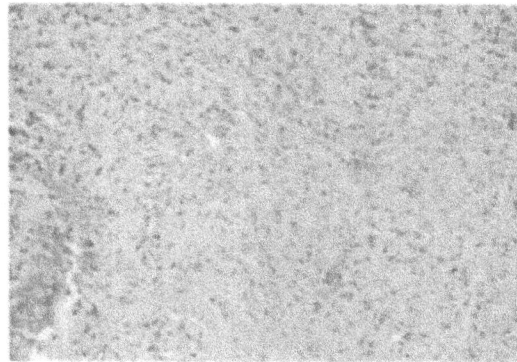

Central giant cell granuloma.

O   **The tumor depicted below is most commonly found near the eyelid and is associated with a poor prognosis. What is your diagnosis?**

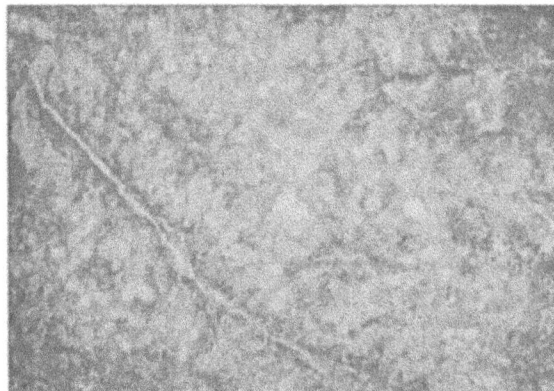

Sebaceous carcinoma.

❍   **The tumor shown below most commonly arises in the parotid gland of older males and is highly aggressive. What is your diagnosis?**

Salivary duct carcinoma.

❍   **Which histologic growth pattern of the tumor shown below is associated with the highest recurrence rate?**

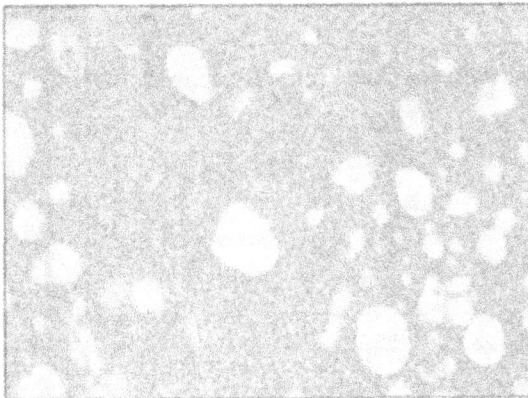

The three growth patterns of adenoid cystic carcinoma are tubular, cribiform, and solid. The solid pattern is associated with essentially 100% recurrence, the cribiform is characterized by a 90% recurrence rate, while the tubular pattern is associated with a 60% recurrence rate.

❍   **The tumor shown below is shown ultrastructurally to be composed of tumor cells filled with abundant mitochondria. What is your diagnosis?**

Oncocytoma.

O   **The tumor shown below occurs most frequently in the parotid gland, is slightly more common in females, is benign and shows a number of histologic patterns. What is your diagnosis?**

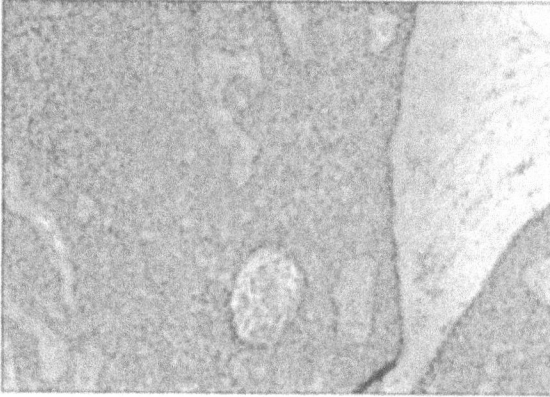

Basal cell adenoma.

O   **Which genus is responsible for the infection shown below, sometimes referred to as "lumpy jaw"?**

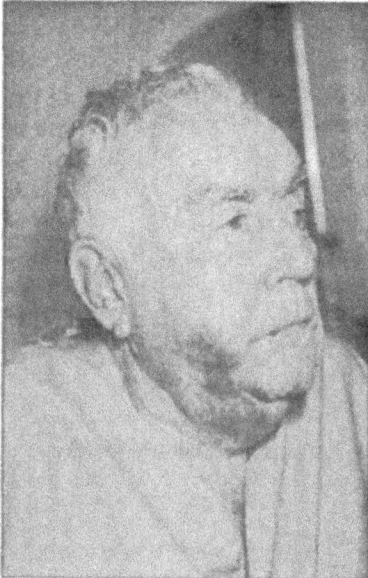

Patient with lumpy jaw

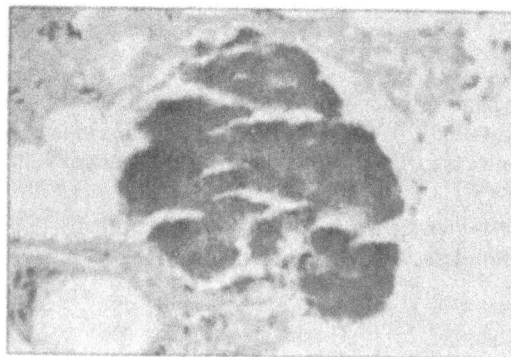

Actinomyces.

RADIOLOGY

○ **What are the contraindications to MRI?**

Cardiac pacemaker, cochlear implant, pacer wires, Swan-Gantz catheter, metallic intraocular foreign body, intracranial aneurysm clips.

○ **What is a flow void?**

Complete lack of signal after contrast due to moderate to high blood flow.

○ **What is the advantage of multidetector CT imaging over conventional CT imaging?**

Extremely fast, thin slices with high resolution.

○ **Why is speed important in head and neck imaging?**

Breathing and swallowing can limit resolution.

○ **On CT scan with axial cuts, what structures are seen in the same plane as the porus acousticus (mouth of the IAC)?**

Head of the malleus, horizontal SCC, and epitympanic recess.

○ **On CT scan with axial cuts, what structures are seen in the same plane as the stapes?**

Sinus tympani, handle of the malleus, vestibule, cochlea, and pyramidal eminence.

○ **What is the Mondini deformity?**

Absence of the anterior 1 1/2 turns of the cochlea in the presence of a normally developed basal turn.

○ **How does it appear on CT scan?**

Wide vestibular aqueduct, plumb-deformed vestibule, and "empty cochlea".

○ **How does otosclerosis appear on CT scan?**

Early on, areas of deossification, in particular, a double low attenuation ring paralleling the cochlear turns and lucencies along the margins of the oval window are present. As the disease progresses, foci of denser bone develop, eventually resulting in obliteration.

○ **What other diseases can mimic otosclerosis radiographically?**

Paget's disease and osteogenesis imperfecta.

○ **What distinguishes otosclerosis from Paget's disease radiographically?**

The radiographic changes are more extensive and pronounced with Paget's disease; they also are more likely to be bilateral and may include narrowing of the IAC.

O   **What is in the differential diagnosis of a soft tissue mass on the promontory?**

Congenital cholesteatoma, paraganglioma, aberrant carotid artery, persistent stapedial artery, and glomus tympanicum.

O   **What is the signal intensity produced by fat on T1 and T2-weighted MRI?**

T1 – high signal; T2 – low signal.

O   **What is the signal intensity produced by water on T1 and T2-weighted MRI?**

T1 – low signal; T2 – high signal.

O   **Which temporal bone structures are best visualized with T1-weighted MRI?**

Nerves within the IAC.

O   **Which temporal bone structures are best visualized with T2-weighted MRI?**

Fluid-filled compartments.

O   **An asymptomatic patient has an incidental finding of a high signal in the left petrous apex on T1-weighted images. What is the significance of this finding?**

Asymmetric pneumatization of the petrous tip is present in 4% of patients; the high signal is from the bone marrow.

O   **How does cholesterol granuloma appear on MRI?**

High signal on both T1 and T2-weighted images.

O   **How does a cholesteatoma appear on MRI?**

Intermediate signal on T1 and high signal on T2-weighted images.

O   **T/F: Cholesteatomas enhance with gadolinium.**

False.

O   **How does a glomus jugulare tumor appear on MRI?**

"Salt and pepper" appearance on T1-weighted images with gadolinium.

O   **What are the typical findings of a meningioma on MRI?**

Broad-based with "dural tail sign" on MRI with gadolinium.

O   **What problems can occur with MRI fat suppression at the skull base?**

Artifact, secondary to air meeting soft tissue, can obscure important anatomical details (i.e. foramina).

O   **What is the alternative method used to image the skull base?**

Comparison of pre- and post-gadolinium images.

○   **How do PET/SPECT work?**

Radionuclide metabolic substrates are injected IV and detected by either production of positrons (PET) or by a directionally sensitive gamma camera (SPECT)... metabolically active tissues light up.

○   **What are the problems with using PET in the head and neck?**

Poor resolution (a focus of SCCA needs to be several mm to be detected) and difficult to correlate with exact anatomy.

○   **What substrate is used in lymph node functioning imaging?**

Superparamagnetic iron oxide coated dextran.

○   **What scan can be used for diagnosis of malignant otitis externa?**

Technetium[99].

○   **What scan can be used for monitoring the progress of malignant otitis externa?**

Gallium citrate scan.

○   **In patients with an unknown primary of the head and neck, how useful is a PET scan in detecting the primary tumour site?**

PET scan will identify the primary in approximately 35% of cases of unknown primary.

○   **Why should radionuclide scanning precede CT scan imaging of the thyroid gland?**

CT scan contrast will linger in the thyroid gland for up to 6 months and interfere with radionuclide scanning.

○   **What is the accuracy of CT imaging in detecting bony erosion?**

85%.

○   **What is the main problem with using CT imaging to evaluate sinonasal tumors?**

Limited accuracy in differentiating soft tissue masses from secretions.

○   **What is the accuracy of MRI in detecting sinonasal tumors?**

94%, 98% if done with gadolinium.

○   **Using MRI, how can one distinguish inflammation from tumor in the sinuses?**

Tumor will be isointense on both T1 and T2 weighted images, while inflammation will be hyperintense on T2 weighted images.

○   **What is the Steeple sign?**

Narrowing of the airway 5 – 10 mm below the true vocal cords on an AP neck film; seen in 50 – 60% of children with croup.

O   **What are the criteria of abnormal swelling of the retropharynx on a lateral neck film?**

At the level of C2, 7mm or greater thickness of the retropharynx is abnormal; at the level of C6, 22mm or greater thickness of the retropharynx is abnormal.

ANESTHESIA

○ **What is the mechanism of action of local anesthetics?**

Prevent increases in the permeability of nerve membranes to sodium ions.

○ **What are the 2 main classes of local anesthetics?**

Those with an ester linkage and those with an amide linkage.

○ **How do these classes differ in metabolism?**

Those with an ester linkage are metabolized in the plasma by cholinesterase; those with an amide linkage are metabolized in the liver by the p-450 system.

○ **Which local anesthetics are amide compounds?**

Lidocaine, ropivacaine, and bupivacaine.

○ **Which antihypertensive medication prolongs the effect of regional anesthesia with amide anesthetics?**

Clonidine.

○ **What are the toxic side effects of local anesthetics?**

CNS excitability or depression, myocardial depression, peripheral vasodilation, methemoglobinemia, allergic reactions.

○ **Which local anesthetic produces toxicity at the lowest dose?**

Tetracaine.

○ **T/F: All local anesthetics are weak bases and produce vasodilation.**

False. Cocaine and ropivacaine are the exceptions.

○ **Which topical anesthetics have been shown to induce methemoglobinemia?**

Prilocaine, benzocaine, lidocaine and procaine.

○ **What is the treatment for methemoglobinemia?**

Slow intravenous infusion of 1% methylene blue solution (total dose 1 – 2 mg/kg).

○ **What is the maximum recommended dose of cocaine?**

2 – 3 mg/kg.

○ **In which patients should the use of topical cocaine be avoided?**

Patients with hypertension and those taking adrenergic modifying drugs such as reserpine, tricyclic antidepressants and monoamine oxidase inhibitors.

O   **What is the maximum recommended dose of bupivacaine?**

2 – 3 mg/kg.

O   **What is the duration of action of bupivacaine?**

3 – 10 hours.

O   **T/F: Bupivacaine has a depressant effect on cardiac contractility 4 times that of lidocaine.**

True.

O   **How does ropivacaine differ from bupivacaine?**

Ropivacaine is also a long-acting amide with equivalent anesthetic properties to bupivacaine but has less potential to cause serious cardiotoxic reactions and has intrinsic vasoconstrictive properties.

O   **What is the maximum recommended dose of lidocaine?**

5 mg/kg without epinephrine; 7 mg/kg with epinephrine.

O   **How much epinephrine is contained in 1 cc of 1:100,000 epinephrine?**

10 micrograms.

O   **Where should local anesthetic be injected to block the superior laryngeal nerve?**

Half-way between the hyoid and thyroid cartilages.

O   **Where should local anesthetic be injected to anesthetize the subglottis? Preepiglottic space?**

Cricothyroid membrane, thyroid notch, respectively.

O   **What surgical prep solution is contraindicated for use on the face?**

Hibiclens as it is caustic to the eyes.

O   **Which nasal spray has less cardiac toxicity… oxymetazoline or neosynephrine?**

Oxymetazoline.

O   **What are the adverse side effects of succinylcholine?**

Cardiac dysrhythmias, fasciculations, hyperkalemia, myalgia, myoglobinuria, increased pressures (ocular, gastric and cranial), trismus, allergic reactions; it can also trigger malignant hyperthermia.

O   **Which patients are more likely to have adverse reactions to succinylcholine?**

Those with closed-angle glaucoma, space-occupying intracranial lesions, or severe crush injuries of the lower extremity

O   **What are the signs of malignant hyperthermia?**

Masseter spasm, sustained muscle rigidity, myoglobinuria, rapid rise in core body temperature, PVCs, and an erythematous flush.

O   **What is the mechanism of action behind malignant hyperthermia?**

Inhibition of calcium reuptake into the sarcoplasmic reticulum of skeletal muscle.

O   **What is the treatment for malignant hyperthermia?**

Total body cooling, vigorous hydration, dantrolene.

O   **What medication is used to reverse opioids?**

Naloxone, in 20 – 40 microgram increments.

O   **What is a complication of rapid administration of naloxone?**

Flash pulmonary edema.

O   **What medication is used to reverse benzodiazepines?**

Flumazenil, 200 micrograms IV over 15 seconds, repeated every 15 seconds up to 1 mg.

O   **Which anesthetic should be discontinued 15 minutes prior to placing a tympanic membrane graft?**

Nitrous oxide.

O   **What is the primary disadvantage of the laryngeal mask airway (LMA) compared to endotracheal intubation?**

Easier to displace than a secured endotracheal tube (ETT).

O   **What are contraindications to LMA?**

Upper airway obstruction, preexisting pulmonary aspiration, and conditions that restrict pulmonary compliance.

O   **How is the gum bougie introducer for endotracheal intubation of the "difficult airway" patient used?**

Any part of the laryngeal airway, usually the posterior glottis, is visualized with the anterior commissure laryngoscope, the bougie is passed through the scope into the larynx, and the ETT is passed over the bougie.

O   **What are the best options for the "can't intubate, can't ventilate" situations after induction of general anesthesia?**

LMA, transtracheal needle jet ventilation, Combitube, or surgical airway.

O   **What situations are best for the use of the lightwand during endotracheal intubation?**

For patients with cervical spine injury, for children with mandibular hypoplasia, or when copious secretions are present.

○   **What is the esophagotracheal Combitube?**

A twin-lumen device with upper and lower balloons that is inserted blindly into the hypopharynx.

○   **What is Poiseuille's law?**

Resistance to airflow is directly proportional to the density of inhaled gases.

○   **What is the minimum effective concentration of helium in heliox administration in children with airway obstruction?**

60%.

○   **What are the advantages of using heliox during laser surgery on the airway?**

It reduces the amount of inspired oxygen concentration and thus the chance of tube ignition, and it facilitates rapid dissipation of heat.

○   **Which medication has been shown to decrease the catecholamine response during suspension laryngoscopy?**

Fentanyl.

○   **Which laryngoscope exposes the vocal folds best?**

Kleinsasser.

○   **Which laryngoscopes are best for visualizing the anterior commissure or the subglottis?**

Holinger and Benjamin.

○   **What is the preferred anesthetic technique for bronchoscopy in adults?**

A modified endotracheal tube or a jetting system used with a relaxant and controlled ventilation.

○   **What is the preferred anesthetic technique for bronchoscopy in infants and children?**

Spontaneous respiration with inhalation anesthesia.

○   **Which hypertensive medications classically cause withdrawal hypertension and, therefore, should not be stopped prior to surgery?**

Beta-blockers and clonidine.

○   **When is the risk of rebound hypertension from propranolol withdrawal the greatest?**

4 to 7 days after the drug is discontinued.

○   **Of Goldmann's risk factors, which has been shown to be the most significant?**

Congestive heart failure (CHF).

O   **What is the appropriate preoperative work-up for a young patient with frequent premature ventricular contractions (PVCs)?**

An ECG, holter monitor and a cardiac stress test.

O   **When should a patient quit smoking to have the greatest decrease in perioperative pulmonary complications?**

8 weeks before the planned procedure.

O   **What is the accepted stress dose of corticosteroids for patients undergoing major procedures?**

Hydrocortisone, 100 mg, the night before the procedure with repeat administration every 8 hours until the stress has passed.

O   **When should oral hypoglycemics be discontinued prior to surgery?**

24 hours.

O   **When should warfarin therapy be discontinued prior to surgery?**

96 to 115 hours (4 doses).

O   **What factors increase the risk of postoperative pulmonary embolism (PE)?**

Age > 40 years, history of lower extremity venous disease, malignancy, CHF, trauma and paraplegia.

O   **What are the advantages of a thallium stress test over an exercise stress test?**

The thallium stress test can better identify the location and extent of myocardial ischemia.

O   **Children may have unlimited clear liquids up to how many hours prior to scheduled anesthetic induction?**

2 to 3 hours.

O   **T/F: Individuals who take clear liquids close to their time of surgery are at greater risk of aspiration than those who remain NPO.**

False.

O   **What is the risk of perioperative MI in patients undergoing surgery within 3 to 6 months of an MI?**

16%.

O   **What is the most common site of perforation of the surgeon's glove during surgery?**

The nondominant index finger.

O   **What is the death rate from anesthesia in patients with an ASA class I or II?**

1 in 200,000.

○ **What is the cause of most anesthetic-related deaths?**

Human error (50 to 75%).

○ **What are the most common problems associated with adverse anesthetic outcomes?**

Those related to the airway (i.e., inadequate ventilation, unrecognized esophageal intubation and unrecognized disconnection from the ventilator).

○ **What is the inheritance pattern and incidence of pseudocholinesterase deficiency?**

Autosomal recessive with an incidence of about 1 in 3000.

○ **What patient population might have a decreased amount of pseudocholinesterase?**

Patients taking anticholinesterase medications for glaucoma or myasthenia gravis, chemotherapeutic drugs and patients with a genetically atypical enzyme.

○ **T/F: Beta-blocker eye drops can cause bronchoconstriction in patients under anesthesia.**

True.

○ **Patients requiring an emergency tracheostomy for an obstructed airway may develop what postoperative pulmonary complication?**

Pulmonary edema.

○ **What makes midazolam particularly useful in the outpatient setting?**

It has a relatively short onset of action and an elimination half-life of 2 to 4 hours.

○ **What role might oral clonidine play in the preoperative period?**

As an alpha-2 adrenergic agonist, it can reduce anesthetic requirements and has been used to provide sedation and anxiolysis while maintaining hemodynamic stability.

○ **What is the standard endocarditis prophylaxis for dental, oral or upper airway procedures in adult patients at risk?**

Amoxicillin 2 gm orally, 1 hour before the procedure.

○ **How does the presence of an upper respiratory infection (URI) in an infant influence the perioperative risk of respiratory complications?**

Intubation results in edema and a greater reduction in cross-sectional area of the trachea.

○ **What factors predispose children with viral URIs to airway hyperactivity?**

Age less than 5 years; family history of allergic disease; infections secondary to respiratory syncytial virus; parainfluenza rhinovirus, influenza or M. pneumonia, coexisting malaise; rhinorrhea and excess mucus production; male sex, and preexisting airway reactivity.

○ **What respiratory symptoms are considered contraindications to elective surgery by most anesthesiologists?**

Fever, rhinorrhea and productive cough.

○ **What is the single most important factor predicting postoperative cardiac morbidity?**

History of congestive heart failure (CHF).

○ **What is the single most important factor that determines the length of stay after general anesthesia in ambulatory patients?**

Post-anesthesia nausea.

○ **What are the advantages of propofol over volatile agents in pediatric ambulatory patients?**

Decreased postoperative nausea and vomiting and decreased incidence of airway obstruction.

○ **What is a reliable alternative induction technique in a 5-year-old struggling child who refuses the mask and cannot be managed by intravenous induction because of lack of accessible veins?**

A sedating intramuscular injection of ketamine (3 mg/kg).

○ **What are the most common anesthetic complications seen in the PACU?**

Nausea, vomiting and airway compromise.

○ **What anesthetic considerations must be taken into account in a patient with sickle cell disease?**

Adequate hydration and oxygenation. Spinal or local anesthesia should be used whenever possible.

○ **T/F: All opioids cause bradycardia.**

False; meperidine is the exception.

○ **What comorbid factor provides the greatest risk of perioperative myocardial infarction during major elective noncardiac surgery?**

Coronary artery disease.

○ **Acute renal failure after major ablative head and neck cancer surgery increases the mortality risk by how much?**

10%.

○ **What factors are responsible for transfusion-induced immunosuppression?**

Serum factors, and fragmented debris from white blood cells and platelets.

○ **What should be given to cancer patients who need a blood transfusion to minimize the immunosuppression?**

Washed RBCs.

○ **Allergy to what substance is a contraindiaction to use of propofol?**

Soy.

ANTIBIOTICS

❍ **In emergency surgery following trauma, which organisms are most likely to cause serious sepsis?**

Gram-negative bacteria.

❍ **Wound infections that occur in clean operations are most commonly caused by what organisms?**

Staphylococci.

❍ **Why do hematomas increase the risk of infection?**

They prevent fibroblast migration and capillary formation.

❍ **What perioperative factors are associated with an increased risk of postoperative wound infection?**

Long preoperative hospitalization; no preoperative shower; early shaving of the operative site; hair removal; and prior antibiotic therapy.

❍ **Which antibiotic agents are bacteriostatic?**

Chloramphenicol, clindamycin, erythromycin, sulfonamides, tetracyclines and trimethoprim.

❍ **Why are iodine solutions superior to chlorhexidine as a surgical antiseptic?**

Chlorhexidine is not effective against viruses and fungi.

❍ **What is the best time to begin prophylactic antibiotic therapy for elective surgery?**

1 hour prior to the operation.

❍ **What is the incidence of wound infections in clean, clean-contaminated, contaminated and dirty cases?**

Less than 2%, 10%, 20% and 40%, respectively.

❍ **T/F: Closed suction drainage decreases the incidence of wound infection in clean cases.**

False.

❍ **In patients with postoperative pneumonia, empiric monotherapy should cover which organisms?**

Gram negative organisms.

❍ **Vancomycin is effective against which bacteria?**

Gram-positive cocci, including methicillin-resistant *Staphylococcus aureus* (MRSA), *Staphylococcus epidermidis*, enterococci, diphtheroids and *Clostridium difficile*.

○ **What is Red Man's Syndrome?**

Flushing of the face and neck, pruritus and hypotension associated with rapid infusion of vancomycin and subsequent release of histamine.

○ **What problem has arisen with the increase use of vancomycin?**

Development of vancomycin resistant enterococci (VRE).

○ **What characteristic is common to clavulanate, sulbactam and tazobactam?**

They are all beta-lactamase inhibitors.

○ **T/F: The dose of metronidazole must be modified for patients with significant liver disease.**

True.

○ **What organisms do penicillin G and V cover?**

Streptococcal pyogenes, *Streptococcal pneumococcus*, *Actinomyces*, oral anaerobes.

○ **How do organisms inactivate penicillin?**

Produce beta-lactamase.

○ **Which organisms can produce beta-lactamase?**

Staphylococcus aureus, *Haemophilus influenzae*, *Moraxella catarrhalis*, oral anaerobes.

○ **What is the incidence of rash after taking penicillin?**

5%.

○ **What % of these patients will develop a rash the next time they take penicillin?**

50%.

○ **Which penicillins are most active against *Staphylococcus aureus*?**

Methicillin, oxacillin, dicloxacillin, nafcillin.

○ **Which of these attains the highest blood levels?**

Dicloxacillin.

○ **Which of these is best for patients with renal failure?**

Nafcillin.

○ **Which of these is not active against *Streptococcus pneumoniae*?**

Methicillin.

O **What organisms are covered by amoxicillin and ampicillin that are not covered by penicillin?**

Proteus, *E. Coli*, *Haemophilus influenzae*.

O **What % of patients with mononucleosis will develop a rash after taking amoxicillin ?**

50%.

O **Which penicillin derivatives are active against *Pseudomonas*?**

Ticarcillin-clavulanate (Timentin), piperacillin-tazobactam (Zosyn).

O **What % of patients with penicillin allergy will have a cephalosporin allergy?**

16%.

O **Which 1st generation cephalosporin has the longest half-life?**

Cefazolin (Ancef or Kefzol).

O **Which 3rd generation cephalosporin is associated with possible clotting impairment?**

Cefoperazone (Cefobid).

O **Which penicillin analogue can be given to patients with a history of anaphylaxis after taking penicillin?**

Aztreonam.

O **Which macrolide does not cover *Haemophilus influenzae*?**

Erythromycin.

O **What is the mechanism of action of quinolones?**

They inhibit DNA gyrase, which is needed to package DNA into dividing bacteria.

O **How do the general antimicrobial spectra differ between 1st, 2nd, 3rd, and 4th generation quinolones?**

1st generation (nalidixic acid): only gram negative, no Pseudomonas coverage.
2nd generation (ciprofloxacin, ofloxacin): gram negative, including Pseudomonas; Staph aureus but not pneumococcus; some atypicals.
3rd generation (levofloxacin): gram negative, including Pseudomonas; gram positive, including Staph aureus and pneumococcus; expanded atypical coverage.
4th generation (gatifloxacin, moxifloxacin): same as 3rd generation with enhanced coverage of pneumococcus; decreased activity against Pseudomonas.

O **Which medications can be used to treat people exposed to meningococcus?**

Rifampin, ciprofloxacin, or ceftriaxone.

O   **What is the best medication to eradicate nasal colonization with methicillin-resistant _Staphylococcus aureus_?**

Mupirocin.

O   **How long may the onset of pseudomembranous enterocolitis begin after initiation of antibiotics?**

6 weeks.

O   **What % of cases of antibiotic-associated diarrhea are due to _Clostridium difficile_?**

10 – 20%.

O   **Which antibiotics are most commonly associated with development of _Clostridium difficile_?**

Clindamycin, cephalosporins, and penicillins.

O   **Aminoglycosides are effective against what bacteria?**

Aerobic gram negative bacilli (including _Pseudomonas aeruginosa_), enterococci, staphylococci and streptococci.

O   **What risks are associated with the use of aminoglycosides?**

Prolonged neuromuscular blockade, ototoxicity and nephrotoxicity.

O   **Why is the mg/kg dosage of gentamicin given to infants higher than that given to older children?**

Infants have a higher extracellular fluid volume per weight.

O   **Which antibiotics potentiate muscle blockade induced by curare?**

Aminoglycosides.

O   **What is the mechanism of action of aminoglycoside ototoxicity?**

Primarily damage to the outer hair cells, first to the basal turn of the cochlea.

O   **What is the most important factor determining risk of ototoxicity with use of aminoglycosides?**

Duration of therapy >10days.

O   **What is the incidence of bone marrow suppression with chloramphenicol?**

1:24,000.

MEDICAL TOPICS

○ **What are the most common causes of hypothyroidism?**

Hashimoto's thyroiditis, pituitary tumor, and radioactive I^{131} treatment for thyrotoxicosis.

○ **What are the most common causes of hyperthyroidism?**

Graves' disease, autonomous toxic nodule, subacute thyroiditis, pituitary tumor.

○ **What is the treatment of choice for patients over 40 with Graves' disease?**

Radioactive I^{131}.

○ **What medications are used for the routine treatment of hyperthyroidism?**

PTU and methimazole.

○ **What infectious diseases can cause chronic thyroiditis?**

Actinomycosis, TB, and syphilis.

○ **What thyroid disorder is characterized by replacement of the thyroid gland with fibrous tissue?**

Reidel's struma (invasive fibrous thyroiditis, woody thyroiditis).

○ **What is the most common type of autoimmune thyroiditis?**

Hashimoto's.

○ **Which cardiovascular medication will interfere with radioiodine scanning?**

Amiodarone.

○ **Which fungal infection is endemic to the Mississippi and Ohio River valleys?**

Histoplasma capsulatum.

○ **What are the ENT manifestations of *Histoplasma capsulatum*?**

Dysphagia, sore throat, hoarseness, painful mastication, gingival irritation; granulomatous lesions on the lips, gingiva, tongue, pharynx, larynx.

○ **What is the typical appearance of the lesions caused by *Histoplasma capsulatum*?**

Firm, painful ulcers with heaped-up margins, often with a verrucous appearance.

○ **What % of adults with disseminated disease present with oropharyngeal involvement?**

40 – 75%.

O   **What % of children with disseminated disease present with oropharyngeal involvement?**

18%.

O   **How is *Histoplasma capsulatum* diagnosed?**

Biopsy or swab is taken from the center of a lesion and cultured on Sabouraud's medium.

O   **What are the ENT manifestations of *Blastomycosis dermatitidis*?**

Erythematous hyperplasia of the mucosa in the larynx and hypopharynx, fibrosis of the vocal cords, pharyngocutaneous fistula.

O   **What disease is characterized by the presence of black eschar on the middle turbinate?**

Invasive fungal sinusitis.

O   **What are the ENT manifestations of non-invasive *Aspergillus fumigatus* infection?**

Single sinus cavity involvement with thick, dark nasal secretions and facial fullness.

O   **What is the appearance of the *Aspergillus fumigatus* on microscopic exam?**

Septate, bifurcating hyphae.

O   **Which fungal disease is endemic to Southern India and Sri Lanka?**

Rhinosporidium seeberi.

O   **What are the ENT manifestations of *Rhinosporidium seeberi*?**

Painless, polypoid, friable lesions on the mucous membranes of the nose, conjunctiva, and palate ("strawberry lesions").

O   **Which parasitic infection is transmitted to humans by the sandfly?**

Leishmaniasis.

O   **What is the most common ENT manifestation of toxoplasmosis?**

Persistent neck mass.

O   **What is the most common ENT manifestation of tuberculosis?**

Scrofula.

O   **Where is scrofula most commonly located in children?**

Submandibular triangle.

O   **Where is scrofula most commonly located in adults?**

Posterior cervical triangle.

O   **Which area is most commonly involved when TB spreads to the larynx?**

Arytenoids.

O   **Which area is most commonly involved when TB spreads to the oral cavity?**

Tongue.

O   **How does TB involvement of the ear most commonly present?**

Multiple TM perforations with thin, watery otorrhea.

O   **What is the risk of performing FNA on scrofula?**

May lead to a chronically draining cutaneous fistula.

O   **What are the ENT manifestations of leprosy?**

Mucosal nodules at the anterior inferior turbinates, septal perforation, lateral loss of eyebrows, leonine facies.

O   **Which organisms can cause cat-scratch disease?**

Rochalimaea henselae or *Afipia felis.*

O   **What % of patients with cat-scratch disease are under 18?**

90%.

O   **What are the typical histologic findings of biopsied lymph nodes from patients with cat-scratch disease?**

Suppurative and necrotizing granulomatous lymphadenitis with stellate abscesses.

O   **What are the 4 diagnostic criteria for cat-scratch disease?**

1. History of contact with a cat or presence of a scratch.
2. Positive skin test or serologic antibody test.
3. Positive gram stain or culture.
4. Characteristic histopathology.

O   **What is bacillary angiomatosis?**

Caused by the same organisms of cat-scratch disease with similar manifestations but occurs in immunocompromised patients and is progressive and fatal if left untreated.

O   **What is the treatment for cat-scratch disease and bacillary angiomatosis?**

Erythromycin, doxycycline, rifampin; incision and drainage of necrotic lymph nodes if abscess occurs.

O   **What is the most common ENT manifestation of actinomycosis?**

A red, indurated, non-tender, subcutaneous mass in the submandibular triangle with the overlying skin having a purplish discoloration.

O   **What is the characteristic appearance of actinomycosis on microscopic exam?**

Sulfur granules.

O   **What is the treatment for actinomycosis?**

Oral penicillin or tetracycline for 2 – 4 months or 6 weeks of parental penicillin (for severe cases).

O   **What are the ENT manifestations of primary syphilis?**

Painless ulcer (chancre) of the lips, tongue, or tonsils with reactive lymphadenopathy.

O   **What are the ENT manifestations of secondary syphilis?**

Widespread mucocutaneous maculopapular lesions, acute rhinitis, pharyngitis, laryngitis, otitis media, loss of eyelashes, localized alopecia.

O   **What are the ENT manifestations of tertiary syphilis?**

Gumma formation can result in septal and hard palate perforations, laryngeal ulcerations, hearing loss, vertigo, osteomyelitis of the temporal bone.

O   **What are the ENT manifestations of congenitally acquired syphilis?**

Saddle nose deformity, frontal bossing, short maxilla, Hutchinson's incisors, mulberry molars, mental retardation, SNHL.

O   **What test is used to screen for syphilis?**

VDRL.

O   **T/F: FTA-ABS becomes negative once a patient has been adequately treated for syphilis.**

False.

O   **What disease is characterized by Mikulicz's cells and causes stenosis of the nose, larynx, and tracheobronchial tree?**

Klebsiella rhinoscleromatis (rhinoscleroma).

O   **What is the treatment for rhinoscleroma?**

Streptomycin or tetracycline.

O   **What is the term for a painless, soft lesion found along the gingival mucosa composed of granulation tissue?**

Pyogenic granuloma.

O   **Where are reparative granulomas most commonly located?**

The peripheral form is most commonly located on the anterior aspect of the mandible; the central form is most commonly located anterior to the first molar within the bone of the mandible.

O **Where is gout most commonly located in the head and neck?**

Helix or antihelix of the ear.

O **What are Langerhans cells?**

Mononuclear cells normally found in the skin that play a role in various immune functions.

O **What structures are unique to Langerhans cells and are used to diagnose Langerhans cell histiocytosis (LCH)?**

Birbeck granules, or cytoplasmic inclusion bodies.

O **What is the term for the localized form of LCH?**

Eosinophilic granuloma.

O **Where are eosinophilic granulomas most commonly located?**

Flat bones of the skull.

O **What is the acute, disseminated form of LCH?**

Letterer-Siwe disease.

O **What is the chronic, disseminated form of LCH?**

Hand-Schuller-Christian disease.

O **What triad of diseases is commonly seen in patients with Hand-Schuller-Christian disease?**

Multiple calvarial osteolytic lesions (geographic skull), exophthalmos, and diabetes insipidus.

O **Where is necrotizing sialometaplasia most commonly found?**

Junction of hard and soft palate.

O **What is the typical histologic appearance of necrotizing sialometaplasia?**

Metaplastic epithelial cells lining salivary ducts with preservation of lobular architecture.

O **What diseases are commonly mistaken for necrotizing sialometaplasia?**

Squamous cell and mucoepidermoid carcinoma.

O **T/F: Most lesions of necrotizing sialometaplasia resolve spontaneously within two to three months and do not require excision.**

True.

O   **What disease closely resembles Wegener's granulomatosis and lymphoma clinically but is characterized by angiocentric infiltration of atypical polymorphonuclear cells on histologic exam?**

Polymorphic reticulosis (a.k.a. lethal midline granuloma, lymphomatoid granulomatosis, angiocentric lymphoma).

O   **What are the ENT manifestations of polymorphic reticulosis?**

Rapid necrosis of the external nose, nasal cavity, soft and hard palates, and nasopharynx.

O   **What is the treatment for polymorphic reticulosis?**

Radiation.

O   **How is amyloidosis diagnosed?**

Can only be diagnosed by biopsy; amyloid is highly refractile with an affinity for Congo red dye and shows green birefringence with polarized light.

O   **What tumors is amyloidosis associated with?**

Multiple myeloma and Hodgkin's lymphoma.

O   **What is the most common site of involvement of amyloidosis in the larynx?**

Ventricle.

O   **What is lupus pernio?**

A cutaneous manifestation of sarcoidosis most commonly occurring on the nose, cheeks, or ears that appears as an indurated blue-purple, shiny, swollen lesion.

O   **What % of patients with sarcoidosis have parotid gland involvement?**

10%.

O   **What % of patients with sarcoidosis have laryngeal involvement?**

5%.

O   **What are some common laboratory findings in patients with sarcoidosis?**

Hypergammaglobulinemia, elevated LFTs, calcium, ESR, and angiotensin converting enzyme (ACE).

O   **What % of patients with sarcoidosis will have an elevated ACE?**

80 – 90%.

O   **What % of patients with hilar adenopathy will have histologic findings consistent with sarcoidosis on lower lip minor salivary gland biopsy?**

2/3.

O   **What histologic finding is the hallmark of sarcoidosis?**

Noncaseating granulomas.

O   **What finding is typical of laryngeal involvement of sarcoidosis?**

Edema of the supraglottis.

O   **What is the treatment for insulin-dependent diabetic patients with sarcoidosis?**

Methotrexate.

O   **What are the ENT manifestations of systemic lupus erythematosus (SLE)?**

Malar rash, oral ulceration, arthritis of the cricoarytenoid or cricothyroid joints, vocal cord thickening, anterior septal perforations, acute parotid gland enlargement, cranial nerve neuropathy.

O   **Which drugs may precipitate a lupus-like reaction?**

Procainamide, hydralazine, pencillin, sulfonamides, and hydantoins.

O   **What is the most common cause of arthritis of the cricoarytenoid joint?**

Rheumatoid arthritis.

O   **What are the head and neck manifestations of rheumatoid arthritis?**

Arthritis of the temporomandibular and cricoarytenoid joints, recurrent laryngeal nerve paresis/paralysis, conductive hearing loss, SNHL.

O   **What are the differences between primary and secondary Sjögren's syndrome?**

Primary (a.k.a. sicca syndrome) is isolated to the lacrimal and salivary glands; secondary (a.k.a. sicca complex) is associated with other connective tissue diseases.

O   **What are the ENT manifestations of Sjögren's syndrome?**

Xerostomia, dental caries, oral candidiasis, recurrent salivary gland enlargement, keratoconjunctivitis sicca, nasal crusting/epistaxis.

O   **What is an abnormal Schirmer test?**

Less than 5 mm wetting after 5 minutes; less than 10 mm wetting after stimulation with 10% ammonia.

O   **What are the systemic manifestations of Sjögren's syndrome?**

Glomerulonephritis, vasculitis, sensory polyneuropathy, interstitial pneumonitis, thyroid disease resembling Hashimoto's thyroiditis.

O   **What tests are use to diagnose Sjögren's syndrome?**

Minor salivary gland biopsy showing mononuclear cell infiltration, SS-A, SS-B, and ANA, RF.

O   **What malignancy is associated with Sjögren's syndrome?**

Non-Hodgkin's lymphoma.

O   **What laboratory test is associated with lymphoproliferative malignancy in patients with Sjögren's syndrome?**

Decreased level of serum IgM.

O   **How is Sjögren's syndrome distinguished from malignant lymphoma?**

By the presence of myoepithelial islands.

O   **What are the head and neck manifestations of scleroderma?**

Dysphagia, hiatal hernia, trismus, thin lips and vertical perioral furrows, gingivitis, xerostomia, hoarseness, Raynaud's phenomenon of the tongue, trigeminal neuralgia, facial nerve palsy.

O   **What are the head and neck manifestations of polymyositis and dermatomyositis?**

Weakness of neck muscles, dysphagia, skin rash on the eyelids, nose, and cheeks.

O   **What head and neck malignancies are more common in patients with polymyositis/dermatomyositis?**

Tumors of the parotid gland and tonsil; nasopharyngeal cancer in endemic areas.

O   **What are the diagnostic features of relapsing polychondritis?**

Recurrent chondritis of the auricles, nonerosive inflammatory polyarthritis, chondritis of the nasal cartilages, inflammation of ocular structures, chondritis of laryngeal or tracheal cartilages, cochlear or vestibular damage.

O   **What % of patients with relapsing polychondritis have airway involvement?**

53%.

O   **What are the typical laboratory findings in patients with relapsing polychondritis?**

Elevated ESR, moderate leukocytosis, mild to moderate anemia.

O   **What are the diagnostic criteria for mixed connective tissue disease?**

Elevated titers of anti-U1 RNP (ribonucleoprotein antibody) and three of either hand edema, synovitis, myositis, Raynaud's phenomenon, or acrosclerosis.

O   **What are the head and neck manifestations of mixed connective tissue disease?**

Mucocutaneous changes, malar rash, discoid lupus, sclerodermatous skin changes, septal perforations, esophageal dysfunction.

O   **What vasculitic disease is characterized by a prodromal stage of allergic rhinitis, nasal polyposis, and asthma?**

Churg-Strauss syndrome.

O   **What is the 5-year survival rate of patients with Churg-Strauss syndrome?**

50%.

О **What are the head and neck manifestations of hypersensitivity vasculitis?**

Petechiae and purpura of oral and nasal mucosa, angioedema, serous otitis media.

О **What are the head and neck manifestations of polyarteritis nodosa?**

Sudden bilateral SHNL, and vestibular problems; ulceration of nasal, buccal, or soft palate mucosa; facial nerve palsy.

О **What are the typical features of Wegener's granulomatosis?**

Necrotizing granulomas of the upper airway and lungs, focal necrotizing glomerulonephritis, and disseminated vasculitis

О **What are the most common ENT complaints of patients with Wegener's?**

Nasal obstruction, bloody rhinorrhea, nasal crusting, and nasal pain.

О **What are the most common laryngeal manifestations of Wegener's?**

Laryngeal ulceration, subglottic stenosis.

О **What are the most common otologic manifestations of Wegener's?**

Serous otitis media, SNHL.

О **What test is most specific for Wegener's?**

c-ANCA.

О **What is the significance of a rising c-ANCA titer in a patient with Wegener's?**

Usually indicates a relapse of active disease.

О **What antibiotic is effective for treatment of Wegener's?**

Trimethoprim/sulfamethoxazole.

О **What are the head and neck manifestations of temporal arteritis?**

Tender and erythematous temporal artery, jaw claudication, lingual claudication, vertigo and hearing loss, blindness, cranial nerve deficits.

О **How is temporal arteritis diagnosed?**

Temporal artery biopsy (ESR for screening).

О **What % of these patients have involvement of the ophthalmic artery?**

1/3.

О **What disease is characterized by uveitis and oral and genital ulcers?**

Behçet's disease.

○   **What are the characteristics of Cogan's syndrome?**

Vestibuloauditory dysfunction and interstitial keratitis.

○   **What are the specific otologic manifestations of Cogan's syndrome?**

Similar to Menière's (fluctuating hearing loss, vertigo, tinnitus, aural fullness) but bilateral.

○   **What are the most common presenting symptoms in patients with Kawasaki's disease?**

Oral cavity erythema and cervical lymphadenopathy.

○   **What antibodies are most commonly seen in patients with rheumatoid arthritis?**

HLA-DW4 antibodies.

○   **What is the most specific test for the diagnosis of autoimmune sensorineural hearing loss?**

Western blot assay for 68 kD inner ear antigen (Otoblot) (95% specific).

○   **What is the most specific test for the diagnosis of Cogan's syndrome?**

Western blot assay for 55 kD inner ear antigen.

○   **Patient with Cogan's syndrome usually have elevated titers to what organism?**

Chlamydia.

○   **T/F: Patients with Cogan's syndrome who are not treated promptly with high-dose corticosteroids will have total permanent hearing loss.**

True.

○   **Can patients with total hearing loss secondary to Cogan's syndrome have a cochlear implant?**

Yes.

○   **In which ethnic group is Kawasaki's disease most common?**

Japanese.

○   **What is the appearance of the rash in patients with Kawasaki's disease?**

Non-vesicular polymorphous rash starting in the perineal area and spreading to the trunk.

○   **What is the treatment for Kawasaki's disease?**

High-dose aspirin and a single dose of IVIG 2 g/kg.

○   **How long should a patient with Kawasaki's disease remain on aspirin?**

For at least 6-8 weeks; ECHO is then performed, and if negative, can discontinue.

○   **What % of patients with Kawasaki's disease will develop coronary aneurysms?**

Up to 30%.

○   **What is the drug of choice for the prophylaxis of *Pneumocystis carinii* infections in patients with HIV?**

TMP-SMX.

○   **What is the alternate therapy and when should it be initiated?**

Dapsone should be used when severe reactions (e.g., skin blistering, mucosal involvement, or anaphylaxis) to TMP-SMX occur.

○   **What factors significantly increase the risk of *Staphylococcus aureus* infection in patients with HIV?**

Presence of a vascular catheter, CD4 count < 100, nasal carriage of *S. aureus*, neutropenia.

○   **What 2 factors are associated with a higher prevalence of rhinosinusitis in patients with HIV?**

Low CD4 count and bilateral absence of maxillary infundibular patency.

○   **What is the most common oral manifestation of AIDS?**

Candidiasis.

○   **What are the 2 most common AIDS-related neoplasms?**

Kaposi's sarcoma and non-Hodgkin's lymphoma.

○   **What is the significance of oral hairy leukoplakia in patients with HIV?**

50% of patients with HIV and hairy leukoplakia will develop AIDS within 16 months and up to 80% will develop HIV within 30 months.

○   **What is the most appropriate treatment for a patient with AIDS who develops bilateral progressive SNHL secondary to otosyphilis?**

Penicillin G, 24 million U daily for 3 weeks.

○   **What is the latency period for developing antibodies to hepatitis C?**

Up to 4 months.

○   **Which body fluids were involved in all reported HIV seroconversions in health care workers?**

Blood and sanguinous fluids.

○   **What is the latency period for seroconversion following exposure to the HIV virus?**

6 to 12 months.

○   **What is the risk of seroconversion following percutaneous exposure to HIV?**

0.31%.

O   **How is the risk of seroconversion altered with AZT prophylaxis after percutaneous exposure to HIV?**

Decreased by 79%.

O   **What is the most common vector-borne disease in the US?**

Lyme disease.

O   **What are the early manifestations of Lyme disease?**

80% will have erythema migrans at the site of the tick bite with flu-like symptoms.

O   **What are the late manifestations of Lyme disease?**

15% of untreated patients will develop neurological problems within weeks of the tick bite.... Meningitis, encephalitis, cranial neuropathy, radiculoneuritis, mononeuritis multiplex, cerebellar ataxia, myelitis. 60% of untreated patients will develop large joint swelling and pain within months of the tick bite. 5% of untreated patients will develop chronic neuroborreliosis with spinal radicular pain or distal paresthesias or acute cardiac problems with AV block, acute myopericarditis or mild LV dysfunction.

O   **What disease is characterized by significant painless, posterior triangle cervical lymphadenopathy that typically resolves without treatment within 6 months?**

Kikuchi's disease.

PEDIATRIC OTOLARYNGOLOGY

○ **What are the clinical differences between a hemangioma and a vascular malformation?**

Vascular malformations are present at birth, grow proportionately with the child, and are associated with distortion or destruction of surrounding bone or cartilage; hemangiomas generally emerge after birth, proliferate and then regress, and do not affect surrounding bone or cartilage.

○ **What are the histologic differences between a hemangioma and a vascular malformation?**

Cellular proliferation is characteristic of hemangiomas; vessel dilatation is characteristic of vascular malformations.

○ **What % of infants have a hemangioma by age 1?**

12%.

○ **What is the incidence of hemangiomas in premature infants weighing less than 1000 grams?**

23%.

○ **Between what ages do hemangiomas grow most rapidly?**

8 to 18 months.

○ **What % of hemangiomas regress by age 7?**

70%.

○ **Where exactly are most subglottic hemangiomas located?**

Posterolaterally and submucosally.

○ **What % of patients with a subglottic hemangioma have an associated cutaneous hemangioma?**

50%.

○ **What are the typical MRI findings of hemangiomas?**

Serpentine high-volume flow voids surrounded by nonvascular soft tissue.

○ **What is the most common treatment for hemangiomas?**

Observation, parental reassurance.

○ **When is intervention warranted?**

For massive, ulcerative, disfiguring lesions; for those that produce hematologic, cardiovascular, or upper aerodigestive tract compromise; and for large periorbital lesions that obstruct vision.

O   **What syndrome is characterized by profound thrombocytopenia associated with a hemangioma?**

Kasabach-Merritt syndrome.

O   **What medications can be used to treat hemangiomas?**

High-dose corticosteroids (2 – 3 mg/kg/day) and interferon alpha-2a or 2b.

O   **Which of these is more likely to result in rebound growth with discontinuance?**

Corticosteroids.

O   **What is the mechanism of action of steroids in the treatment of hemangiomas?**

Block the estradiol-17 receptor.

O   **What are the mechanisms of action of interferon alpha-2b?**

Inhibit epithelial cell migration and proliferation and inhibit growth factor.

O   **What are the potential side effects of interferon alpha-2b?**

Fever, weight loss, liver enzyme elevation, DIC.

O   **What are the 4 main types of vascular malformations?**

Capillary, venous, lymphatic, and arteriovenous malformations.

O   **What is the most common vascular malformation?**

Port wine stain.

O   **Which type of vascular malformation is a port wine stain?**

Capillary.

O   **What syndrome is characterized by capillary hemangiomas along the distribution of V1 with concomitant capillary, venous, and arteriovenous malformations of the leptomeninges?**

Sturge-Weber syndrome.

O   **What is the optimal treatment for port wine stains?**

Argon laser in darker-skinned adults; flashlamp pulsed tunable dye laser in children and lighter-skinned adults.

O   **Which lesions respond best to pulsed dye laser?**

Lesions less than 20 cm^2 in children <1 year of age.

O   **What are the histologic features of venous malformations?**

Dilated, ectatic vascular channels with a normal endothelial lining and areas of thrombosis.

O **What are the typical clinical features of venous malformations?**

Soft, compressible, nonpulsatile masses most commonly found on the lip or cheek within the head and neck; also can be found within the masseter muscle or mandible.

O **When found in the mandible, how do these lesions appear radiographically?**

Have a honeycomb or soap bubble appearance.

O **What are the typical histologic characteristics of lymphatic malformations?**

Multiple dilated lymphatic channels lined by a single layer of epithelium.

O **What are the 4 categories of lymphatic malformations?**

Capillary, cavernous, cystic (hygroma), and lymphangiohemangioma.

O **Which of these is associated with episodic bleeding?**

Lymphangiohemangioma.

O **Which of these is most commonly found on the tongue or floor of mouth?**

Capillary.

O **Which of these is associated with location in the posterior triangle of the neck?**

Cystic hygroma.

O **Which of these is more likely to rapidly enlarge during a URI?**

Lymphangiohemangioma.

O **What are the indications for definitive treatment of lymphatic malformations?**

When vital structures are endangered, when episodic hemorrhage occurs, or if macroglossia is present.

O **Which lesions are less likely to respond to sclerosis with OK-432 (Picibanil)?**

Microcystic, previously operated-on, and those with massive craniofacial involvement.

O **What is an absolute contraindication to treatment with OK-432?**

Penicillin allergy.

O **What is the imaging modality of choice for lymphatic malformations?**

MRI. CXR should also be performed to rule out mediastinal extension or pleural effusion.

O **How do lymphatic malformations appear on MRI?**

Hypointense on T1, hyperintense on T2.

O **What are the clinical features of arteriovenous malformations?**

Brightly erythematous lesions of the skin with an associated thrill and bruit.

○   **After benign lymphoid hyperplasia, what is the most common benign nasopharyngeal tumor?**

Juvenile nasopharyngeal angiofibroma (JNA).

○   **In which countries does this tumor most often occur?**

India and Egypt.

○   **From which site in the nasopharynx does this tumor develop?**

Trifurcation of the palatine bone, horizontal ala of the vomer, and the root of the pterygoid process.

○   **What finding on CT scan is pathognomonic for JNA?**

Anterior bowing of the posterior wall of the maxillary antrum (Holman-Miller sign).

○   **What hormone receptors are present in JNAs?**

Dihydrotestosterone and testosterone.

○   **What adjunctive test should be performed in a female with suspected JNA?**

Chromosome analysis.

○   **What is the histologic appearance of these tumors?**

Unencapsulated admixture of vascular tissue and fibrous stroma; vessel walls lack elastic fibers and have decreased or no smooth muscle; mast cells are abundant in the stroma.

○   **Using the system of Session et al, what is the stage of a JNA involving the posterior nares and the sphenoid sinus?**

IB.

○   **What is the stage of a JNA eroding the skull base with minimal intracranial extension?**

IIIA.

○   **Where does the main blood supply to these tumors most often come from?**

Internal maxillary artery or the ascending pharyngeal artery.

○   **What are the contraindications to surgical resection of JNAs?**

Poor surgical risk, recurrent tumor that has proved refractory to previous excisions, and involvement of vital structures.

○   **What is the best surgical approach to resection of JNAs?**

Medial maxillectomy via lateral rhinotomy or midface degloving approach.

○ **What condition is seen in adolescent patients with severe, frequently recurring epistaxis and pulmonary arteriovenous malformations?**

Hereditary hemorrhagic telangiectasia.

○ **What are the advantages of using argon plasma coagulation for the treatment of hereditary hemorrhagic telangiectasia (HHT)?**

Noncontact application, limited and controlled tissue penetration with low risk of septal perforation, no safety measures required (ie, for lasers), low thermal damage to adjacent tissue, inexpensive.

○ **What effect do estrogens have on nasal mucosa?**

Induce metaplasia of nasal mucosa from ciliated columnar epithelium to stratified keratinizing squamous epithelium.

○ **What is the surgical treatment of choice for giant congenital melanocytic nevi?**

Tissue expansion followed by total excision.

○ **How does the position of the larynx differ between neonates and adults?**

In the neonate, the larynx is positioned more anterosuperiorly, lying at the level of C2-C3, with the cricoid lying at C3-C4. In the adult, the larynx lies at the level of C5 and the cricoid at C7.

○ **T/F: Compared to the gag reflex, the cough reflex correlates better with a newborn's ability to eat safely.**

True.

○ **What % of neonates less than 5 days old have a functioning cough reflex?**

25%.

○ **What prevents air from escaping through the glottis during the cough reflex?**

Adduction and turning down of the false vocal cords (FVC).

○ **What is the sequence of events during the glottic closure reflex?**

Closure of the true vocal cords (TVC), followed by closure of the FVC, followed by adduction of the aryepiglottic folds.

○ **What muscle adducts the FVC and aryepiglottic folds?**

Thyroarytenoid muscle.

○ **What is laryngospasm?**

Maladaptive and exaggerated glottic closure reflex .

○ **Unlike the glottic closure reflex, laryngospasm is mediated solely by stimulation of what nerve?**

Superior laryngeal nerve.

O   **At what age gestation can an infant suckle feed?**

34 weeks.

O   **How does infant swallowing differ from adult swallowing?**

The pharyngeal phase of swallowing in infants is faster and more frequent.

O   **What is the sequence of events during a normal swallow?**

1.   Oral phase: food is chewed and mixed with saliva.
2.   Oropharyngeal phase: the food bolus is propelled posteriorly.
3.   Pharyngeal phase: the soft palate elevates, glottis closes, pharyngeal constrictors contract, and the cricopharyngeus relaxes.
4.   Esophageal phase: the bolus is propelled into the stomach by peristaltic waves.

O   **What is aspiration?**

Penetration of secretions below the TVC.

O   **What are the 2 types of aspiration?**

Primary or direct from oral substances and secondary or indirect from gastric substances.

O   **Why are infants more prone to aspiration than adults?**

Compared to adults, infants have a relatively lax epiglottis, large arytenoids, and wide aryepiglottic folds.

O   **What is the most common cause of GERD in children?**

Transient lower esophageal sphincter relaxation.

O   **What other factors can predispose an infant to aspirate?**

CNS disease, prematurity, mechanical barriers (NG tube, ET tube, tracheostomy), anatomic barriers (esophageal atresia/stricture, vascular rings, T-E fistula), scoliosis.

O   **What is the most common sign of GERD in infants?**

Regurgitation.

O   **What is the most common complication of GERD in infants?**

Distal esophagitis.

O   **What are other signs or complications of GERD in infants?**

Failure to thrive, vomiting, recurrent aspiration pneumonia, acute life-threatening events .

O   **What is the sensitivity of an upper GI for detecting aspiration?**

69%.

O   **What is the best test to evaluate swallowing?**

Videofluoroscopic barium swallow.

○   **What information does esophageal manometry provide?**

Upper esophageal sphincter responsiveness and pharyngeal peristalsis.

○   **What is the sensitivity of the 24 hour pH probe for GERD?**

92 – 94%.

○   **What is the Euler-Byrne formula?**

$X + 4Y$ where X = # episodes pH<4 and Y = # episodes pH<4 for >5 minutes; a score of 50+ is clinically significant for GERD.

○   **What is the lipid laden alveolar macrophage index?**

Secretions are collected during bronchoscopy and stained with oil red O (which detects lipids). 100 macrophages are counted and scored from 0 – 4 according to the amount of staining. A score of >70 is significant for aspiration.

○   **What is the sensitivity and specificity of this test?**

85% sensitivity; 80% specificity.

○   **What are the problems with this test?**

Invasive; false positives possible from breakdown of endogenous lipids or toxic response to certain medications; clearance time of lipids from the lungs is unknown.

○   **What % of infants with GERD will spontaneously resolve by 18 months?**

85%.

○   **What is the best initial approach for management of mild GERD with no adverse clinical consequences in an infant?**

Parental reassurance; reverse Trendelenburg, prone positioning after feeding.

○   **What are the indications for antireflux surgery in children?**

Mild to moderate symptoms that fail medical therapy; severe GERD with life-threatening symptoms.

○   **T/F: Thickening formula decreases the amount of reflux in children.**

False; no studies have proven any benefit of this. It may decrease the amount of visible regurgitation, but it does not improve reflux.

○   **What is the difference between a Nissen and a Thal fundoplication?**

Nissen is a 270 degree wrap; Thal is a 360 degree, or complete, wrap.

○   **What is intractable aspiration?**

Persistent aspiration despite maximum medical management and minor surgery.

O   **What are the surgical options for treatment of intractable aspiration?**

Narrow-field laryngectomy, endolaryngeal stent, laryngeal closure, and tracheoesophageal diversion (TED) or laryngotracheal separation (LTS).

O   **What are the 3 laryngeal closure procedures?**

Epiglottic flap, glottic closure, and vertical laryngoplasty.

O   **What are the primary disadvantages of glottic closure?**

It does not allow speech, is difficult to reverse, and rarely works unless the larynx is bilaterally denervated.

O   **Of TED and LTS, which is technically easier?**

LTS.

O   **Which is easier to reverse?**

TED.

O   **Which is preferred if the patient has or has had a tracheostomy?**

LTS.

O   **Can these patients talk?**

Potentially, via esophageal speech.

O   **What is the most common cause of cough in children?**

URI.

O   **What organism is the most common cause of bacterial tracheitis in children?**

Staphylococcus aureus.

O   **What is the most common cause of laryngotracheobronchitis (croup) in children?**

Parainfluenza virus.

O   **Other than URI, what are the most common causes of cough in infants up to 18 months?**

Aberrant innominate artery, cough-variant asthma, and GERD.

O   **In children 18 months to 6 years?**

Sinusitis (50%), cough-variant asthma (27%).

O   **In children 6 to 16 years?**

Cough-variant asthma (45%), psychogenic (32%), and sinusitis (27%).

O   **What disease is characterized by a seal-like barking cough?**

Croup.

O   **How is croup managed?**

Humidification, dexamethasone and racemic epinephrine.

O   **What disease is characterized by a staccato cough?**

Chlamydial pneumonia.

O   **What diseases may present with hemoptysis in children?**

Bronchiectasis, cystic fibrosis, foreign body, pulmonary hemosiderosis, TB.

O   **What is the most common notifiable and vaccine-preventable disease in children under age 5?**

Pertussis.

O   **What test is used to diagnose pertussis?**

Culture from the nasopharynx using a Dacron or calcium alginate swab placed on a Regan-Lowe or Bordet-Gengou agar plate.

O   **What is the sensitivity of this test?**

80% (less if already on antibiotics).

O   **How should contacts be treated?**

14 days of erythromycin.

O   **What tests are most sensitive and specific for diagnosing the etiology of cough in infants up to 18 months of age?**

Endoscopy, barium esophagram, and empiric treatment with bronchodilators.

O   **In children 18 months to 6 years?**

Paranasal sinus films, endoscopy, and empiric treatment with bronchodilators.

O   **In children 6 to 16 years?**

Pulmonary function tests (PFT) with methacholine challenge, paranasal sinus films.

O   **What is the sensitivity and specificity of inspiratory/expiratory and lateral decubitus films for foreign body aspiration?**

67% sensitive, 67% specific.

O   **What are the 3 most common causes of stridor in children?**

Laryngomalacia, vocal cord paralysis, and congenital subglottic stenosis.

○   **What is stertor?**

Inspiratory low-pitched sound resulting from turbulent airflow through the nasal cavity and nasopharynx.

○   **What is the first sign of respiratory distress in children?**

Tachypnea.

○   **Stridor that increases in intensity with crying, agitation, or straining is characteristic of what disorders?**

Laryngomalacia and subglottic hemangioma.

○   **After 2 weeks of intubation for ventilatory support, a 32-week premature infant is extubated and severe upper airway obstruction results. What is the most likely cause?**

Subglottic edema.

○   **What is the typical appearance of a type 1 posterior laryngeal cleft?**

A soft tissue defect in the interarytenoid musculature without a defect in the cricoid cartilage.

○   **What is the typical presentation of child with a laryngeal cleft type 2 or greater?**

History of aspiration pneumonia, choking, coughing during feeds, and symptoms of airway obstruction.

○   **What are the 3 modes of supraglottic obstruction causing laryngomalacia?**

Prolapse of the mucosa overlying the arytenoids, foreshortened aryepiglottic folds, and posterior displacement of the epiglottis.

○   **What is the test of choice for diagnosing laryngomalacia?**

Flexible fiberoptic laryngoscopy in the office.

○   **What are the indications for rigid bronchoscopy in children with laryngomalacia?**

Severe or atypical stridor, an abnormal high kilovolt cervical radiograph, or a high degree of suspicion for a synchronous airway lesion.

○   **What is the incidence of synchronous airway lesions in children with laryngomalacia?**

18 – 20%.

○   **What % of these require surgical intervention?**

<5%.

○   **What is the only clinical sign that is strongly associated with a synchronous airway lesion?**

Cyanosis.

○   **What are the indications for surgical treatment of laryngomalacia?**

Dyspnea at rest or during effort, feeding difficulties and failure to thrive.

O   **What % of infants with laryngomalacia require surgical treatment?**

10%.

O   **What is the relationship between laryngomalacia and GERD?**

Essentially all children with laryngomalacia have GERD.

O   **How can one diagnose exercise-induced laryngomalacia?**

With exercise flow-volume spirometry.

O   **What % of children with choanal atresia have other congenital anomalies?**

50%.

O   **What % of cases of choanal atresia are bilateral?**

40%.

O   **Persistence of what membrane results in choanal atresia?**

Buccopharyngeal.

O   **What % of cases of choanal atresia involve only a mucosal diaphragm or membrane?**

10%.

O   **What approach is used to for revisions of failed choanal atresia repairs?**

Transpalatal.

O   **What is the best treatment for nasal pyriform aperture stenosis?**

Sublabial medial maxillectomy.

O   **What common cause of congenital airway obstruction is characterized by inspiratory stridor at birth that decreases when placed on the side of the lesion?**

Unilateral vocal cord paralysis.

O   **What % of cases of congenital vocal cord paralysis are bilateral?**

20%.

O   **What % of theses patients require tracheotomy?**

90%.

O   **What is the most common neurologic condition causing vocal cord paralysis in children?**

Arnold-Chiari malformation.

O   **What effect does the timing of treatment for Arnold-Chiari have on the outcome of vocal cord paralysis?**

If the ICP is normalized within 24 hours, vocal cord function will recover within 2 weeks in most patients.

O   **What is the recovery rate for idiopathic vocal cord paralysis in children?**

20%.

O   **Birth trauma accounts for what % of vocal cord paralysis in children?**

20% (associated with forceps use and C-section).

O   **What surgical procedure is the most common cause of iatrogenic vocal cord paralysis in children?**

Tracheo-esophageal fistula repair.

O   **Where do most laryngeal webs occur?**

At the anterior glottis (75%).

O   **When is the typical onset of symptoms in patients with subglottic hemangioma?**

Usually asymptomatic at birth and symptomatic by 6 months of age.

O   **What kind of stridor is heard in patients with tracheomalacia?**

Expiratory.

O   **What test has the highest yield for diagnosis of vascular rings?**

Direct laryngoscopy and bronchoscopy.

O   **What is the most common vascular ring?**

Innominate artery compression.

O   **What is the typical endoscopic appearance of innominate artery compression?**

Pulsatile compression of the anterior tracheal wall in the distal trachea.

O   **What is the "Waterson sign"?**

Obliteration of the right radial pulse by compressing the anterior tracheal indentation with the tip of the bronchoscope.

O   **What is the most likely cause of stridor after ligation of a patent ductus arteriosus?**

Iatrogenic injury of the left recurrent laryngeal nerve.

O   **What is the earliest gestational age that complete glottic atresia could be detected on ultrasound?**

22 weeks.

O   **What would the ultrasound show in a fetus with complete glottic atresia?**

Distension of the airway and lung parenchyma; flattening of the diaphragm; edema of the placenta; compression of the heart, great vessels, and thoracic duct.

O   **T/F: Airway foreign bodies are more common than esophageal foreign bodies.**

False.

O   **What is the most common esophageal foreign body in children <5?**

Coins.

O   **What is the most common diagnosis given inappropriately to a child with an airway foreign body?**

Asthma.

O   **What is the term for the treatment of airway obstruction in children with craniofacial abnormalities where the mandible is gradually elongated?**

Distraction osteogenesis.

O   **What % of premature infants develops subglottic stenosis (SGS)?**

4%.

O   **What is Cotton's grading system for SGS?**

Grade 1: less than 50% laryngeal lumen obstruction.
Grade 2: 51 – 70% laryngeal lumen obstruction.
Grade 3: 71 – 99% laryngeal lumen obstruction.
Grade 4: complete obstruction.

O   **What is the biggest risk factor for acquired SGS?**

Prolonged endotracheal intubation.

O   **What are other etiologies of SGS?**

Congenital anomalies, increased infant activity, autoimmune mechanisms (antibodies to type II collagen, anti-neutrophil cytoplasmic antibodies), infection, GERD, caustic injury, high tracheostomy.

O   **What are the treatment options for SGS?**

Dilation, steroid injection, lathyrogenic agents, cryotherapy, laser therapy, anterior cricoid split, one-stage laryngotracheoplasty, autogenous cartilage grafts, four-quadrant cartilage division, end-to-end tracheal anastomosis, flaps.

O   **What are the advantages of serial bouginage for the treatment of SGS?**

Non-invasive, growth may take care of the stenosis, avoids concerns regarding the potential for laryngeal growth inhibition with open procedures.

O   **What are the disadvantages of serial bouginage?**

Multiple treatment applications over a prolonged period of time, lack of stabilization if cartilaginous destruction or instability has occurred, generally requires a tracheotomy.

O   **What are some predictors of failure for endoscopic CO_2 laser treatment of SGS?**

Circumferential scarring, scarring longer than 1 cm, tracheomalacia and loss of cartilage support, history of severe bacterial infection associated with tracheostomy, posterior laryngeal inlet scarring with arytenoid fixation, multiple stenotic sites.

O   **What effects do multiple laser procedures have on the airway?**

Increased scarring, ossification of the cricoid cartilage.

O   **What are lathyrogenic agents?**

Compounds that inhibit collagen cross-linking, such as penicillamine and N-acetyl-L-cysteine.

O   **What is mitomycin C?**

Substance produced by *Streptomyces caespitosus* that inhibits DNA synthesis and fibroblast proliferation.

O   **What criteria should be met before performing single-stage LTR in neonates?**

At least 2 failed attempts at extubation, documentation of stenosis endoscopically, weight >1500 g, spontaneous ventilation with F_{IO2} <35%, no evidence of lower respiratory tract infection or congestive heart failure within 30 days of the operation, no hypertension.

O   **What must be done prior to single-stage laryngotracheoplasty?**

Assess for adequate vocal cord mobility and treat GERD.

O   **What are the advantages of single-stage laryngotracheoplasty?**

Avoidance of prolonged indwelling stents with associated danger of displacement or breakage, no need for tracheotomy care, single procedure, long term antibiotic therapy (such as with stenting) is not required.

O   **How long should the patient remain intubated after single-stage LTR?**

3 – 7 days with anterior graft only; 12 – 15 days with anterior and posterior grafts.

O   **What are the contraindications to single-stage LTR?**

Abnormal pulmonary function, co-existent medical problems that require a tracheostomy, and severe grade 4 stenosis.

O   **What is the overall decannulation rate after single-stage LTR?**

83% (Cotton).

O   **What is the most important factor associated with successful and permanent decannulation after LTR?**

Age >24 months at the time of LTR.

O   **T/F: Children with congenital laryngotracheal stenosis have a better voice outcome after surgical correction compared to children with acquired stenosis.**

True.

O   **After open repair of subglottic stenosis, what adjuvant treatment is necessary postoperatively?**

Speech therapy.

O   **What is the primary advantage of early laryngotracheal reconstruction?**

Better speech acquisition.

O   **What is the best approach for the treatment of the funnel-like morphologic variant of congenital long-segment tracheal stenosis?**

Single-stage anterior LTR with cartilage or pericardium grafting.

O   **What are the indications for four-quadrant cartilage division?**

Congenital elliptical cricoid cartilage, severe congenital or acquired SGS, calcification of the cricoid cartilage from failed LTRs.

O   **What is the primary disadvantage of this technique?**

Requires long-term stenting (1 – 12 months).

O   **Why is end-to-end tracheal anastomosis rarely used in children?**

Difficult to perform in the subglottic region without damaging the vocal cords.

O   **T/F: Division of the cricoid cartilage has not been shown to inhibit its further growth.**

True.

O   **In placing an autogenous cartilage graft, where does the surface bearing perichondrium face?**

Toward the lumen of the larynx.

O   **How does one identify the anterior commissure during laryngofissure?**

By identifying Montgomery's aperture, a small hole just inferior to the anterior commissure or through direct laryngoscopy.

O   **What is the procedure of choice for reconstruction of the anterior commissure?**

Epiglottopexy laryngoplasty.

O   **What is the microtrapdoor flap used for?**

To correct posterior glottic stenosis.

O   **What is the most common etiology of posterior glottic stenosis?**

Endotracheal intubation.

O   **What is Grillo's rule?**

Any patient who develops symptoms of airway obstruction, who has been intubated and ventilated in the recent past, must be considered to have an airway lesion until proven otherwise.

O   **What is the most common anomaly associated with congenital tracheal stenosis?**

Aberrant left pulmonary artery (pulmonary artery sling complex).

O   **What is the mortality in children with congenital tracheal stenosis treated conservatively with tracheotomy and intensive respiratory care?**

35%.

O   **What factors increase the risk of postintubation tracheal stenosis?**

Difficult intubation, an overinflated cuff, repeated reintubations, poorly performed tracheostomy.

O   **What is the treatment for acute airway obstruction secondary to postintubation tracheal stenosis?**

Dilatation with rigid ventilating bronchoscopes; tracheostomy is only performed if a prolonged period is needed prior to definitive treatment of the stenosis.

O   **Why is jet ventilation contraindicated in patients with tracheal stenosis?**

Expiration of air is more difficult than inspiration during jet ventilation in patients with tracheal stenosis and can result in air trapping and pneumothoraces.

O   **How does one avoid postoperative hemorrhage from the innominate artery after repair of tracheal stenosis?**

Dissect immediately on the trachea without disrupting the artery or its investments; if the artery has been previously dissected or the lesion is fixed to it, interpose a pedicled strap muscle between the anastomosis and the artery.

O   **How does one avoid injury to the recurrent laryngeal nerves during repair of tracheal stenosis?**

Avoid dissecting out the nerves and carry out dissection immediately on the trachea.

O   **Why is it important to avoid dissection of the trachea for more than 1 – 1.5 cm proximal or distal to the anastomotic site?**

To protect the blood supply to the trachea.

O   **When is hilar release contraindicated?**

In patients with poor pulmonary reserve.

O   **What is the primary advantage of slide tracheoplasty compared to end-to-end anastomosis for the repair of tracheal stenosis?**

Ability to span longer segments.

○ **Slide tracheoplasty increases the cross-sectional airway area by how much?**

4-fold.

○ **What is the primary disadvantage of augmentation tracheoplasty for the treatment of tracheal stenosis?**

Need for multiple bronchoscopies due to recurrent granulation tissue formation at cartilage graft sites (thought to be secondary to the need for prolonged intubation postoperatively).

○ **After pericardial patch augmentation tracheoplasty, what factors significantly increase the likelihood of fatal outcome?**

Tracheal involvement within 1 cm of the carina or involvement of either mainstem bronchus.

○ **What are the contraindications to tracheal sleeve resection?**

Involvement of the glottis or subglottis, stenosis longer than 6 cm, temporary or chronic respiratory failure or neurological deficit.

○ **What are the treatment options when sleeve resection is contraindicated?**

Endotracheal prosthesis, tracheostomy with a cannula or a Montgomery T tube.

○ **What has been shown to decrease the incidence of postoperative granulomas after LTR?**

Use of absorbable suture.

○ **What is the significance of hemoptysis after tracheal sleeve resection?**

May portend rupture of the innominate artery.

○ **How much trachea can be resected without using a release technique?**

3 cm (possibly 4 cm with the patient's head in extreme flexion).

○ **What techniques are available to gain additional tracheal length in resection cases (10)?**

Extreme flexion, suprahyoid release, infrahyoid release, inferior constrictor release, peritracheal mobilization, intercartilaginous incisions, dissection and mobilization of the right hilum, release of the inferior pulmonary ligament, dissection of the pulmonary vasculature, and transsection and reimplantation of the left main stem bronchus.

○ **Which of these is most likely to result in prolonged postoperative dysphagia?**

Combined infrahyoid and inferior constrictor release.

○ **Which of these allows the greatest amount of mobilization?**

Mobilization of the right hilum with release of the inferior pulmonary ligament, dissection of the pulmonary vasculature, and transection and reimplantation of the left main stem bronchus allows up to 6 cm of superior mobilization.

○ **How much mobilization can be achieved with peritracheal mobilization (dissection of the annular ligaments)?**

Up to 1.5 cm.

O   **How much mobilization can be achieved with the suprahyoid release?**

Up to 5 cm.

O   **What structures are removed or transected with the suprahyoid release?**

Stylohyoid, mylohyoid, geniohyoid, and genioglossus muscles are transected, and the body of the hyoid bone is transected at its attachments to the greater and lesser cornus.

O   **What is a Grillo stitch?**

Non-absorbable suture extending from the periosteum of the mentum to the sternum used to keep the neck flexed after tracheal resection.

O   **What is Gerlach's tonsil?**

Lymphoid tissue arising from the fossa of Rosenmüller that extends into the eustachian tube.

O   **Which muscles form the anterior and posterior tonsillar pillars?**

Palatoglossus and palatopharyngeus, respectively.

O   **What is the plica triangularis?**

Point at which the palatine and lingual tonsils meet.

O   **In what % of the population does the carotid artery lie deep to the floor of the tonsillar fossa?**

1%.

O   **What syndrome is characterized by hypernasal speech, cardiac malformations, cleft palate, and medial displacement of the carotid arteries?**

Velocardiofacial syndrome.

O   **What immunoglobulin is produced by the tonsils?**

Antigen-specific secretory IgA.

O   **What % of acute tonsillar infections are bacterial?**

5 – 30%.

O   **What % of cultured organisms in patients with recurrent tonsillitis produce beta-lactamase?**

39%.

O   **In what age group is tonsillitis from group A streptococci most common?**

Ages 6 – 12.

O   **What tests confirm the diagnosis of infectious mononucleosis?**

Blood smear showing atypical mononuclear cells and a positive Paul-Bunnell test (elevated heterophile titer of Epstein-Barr virus).

O   **What is the initial treatment for patients with adenotonsillar hypertrophy and infectious mononucleosis?**

Corticosteroids.

O   **Why should general anesthesia be avoided in patients with mononucleosis?**

They are at a heightened risk of suffering hepatotoxicity from the anesthetics.

O   **What is the most common presenting complaint of patients with rheumatic fever?**

Migratory joint pain (75%) that is out of proportion to physical findings.

O   **What is the most common valvular problem resulting from rheumatic fever?**

Mitral valve stenosis.

O   **What is Eagle's syndrome?**

Elongation of the styloid process or ossification of the stylohyoid ligament resulting in nonspecific throat pain, foreign body sensation, and increased salivation.

O   **What is the incidence of submucous cleft palate?**

1 in 1200.

O   **What are the physical signs associated with submucous cleft palate?**

Bifid uvula, abnormal palatal motion, midline diastasis of the palatal muscles, V-shaped notch of the hard palate.

O   **What syndrome, characterized by deletion of band 11 on the long arm of chromosome 22, is a contraindication to adenoidectomy?**

Velocardiofacial syndrome (VCFS).

O   **What is platybasia?**

Phenotypic characteristic of VCFS where the cranial base is angled obtusely, resulting in expanded velopharyngeal volume and incomplete velopharyngeal closure.

O   **By what age is the adenoid pad mostly atrophied?**

Age 7 or 8.

O   **T/F: Nasal steroids given twice daily for 6 months are likely to reduce adenoidal size.**

True.

O   **According to the Paradise study from 1984, what are the criteria for adenotonsillectomy for recurrent tonsillitis?**

At least 3 episodes in each of 3 years or 5 episodes in each of 2 years or 7 episodes in 1 year… with each episode documented by a physician.

O   **What are the indications for polysomnography prior to adenotonsillectomy for obstructive sleep apnea?**

If history and physical exam are not in agreement or if the child is at an unusually high risk for perioperative complications.

O   **When is a post-treatment culture indicated in a child with group A streptococcal pharyngitis?**

If the child is at an unusually high risk for rheumatic fever, remains symptomatic, or develops recurring symptoms.

O   **When should an asymptomatic patient with a positive post-treatment culture for group A streptococci be treated?**

If the patient or someone in his family has a history of rheumatic fever.

O   **Which patients are at risk for atlantoaxial subluxation?**

Patients with Down syndrome, achondroplasia, Arnold-Chiari, and rheumatoid arthritis.

O   **What % of patients with Down syndrome have an unstable transverse ligament of the atlas?**

10%.

O   **What test should be performed prior to operating on these children?**

Flexion and extension lateral neck films

O   **When should aspirin be discontinued prior to surgery? Naproxen? All other NSAIDS?**

2 weeks, 4 days, 3 days, respectively.

O   **Disorders of which clotting factors can cause prolongation of the PTT?**

VIII, IX, XI, XII, and lupus anticoagulant.

O   **Which subtype of von Willebrand's disease responds to treatment with desmopressin?**

Type I, the most common, where qualitatively normal von Willebrand factor is present in subnormal levels.

O   **What tests confirm the diagnosis of von Willebrand's disease?**

Elevated PTT and bleeding time, decreased or absent von Willebrand factor serum levels.

O   **How are children with von Willebrand's disease managed perioperatively?**

IV administration of desmopressin (0.3 microgram/kg) preoperatively, 12 hours postoperatively, and every morning until the fossae are completely healed; aminocaproic acid pre- and postoperatively. Alternatively, Factor VIII concentrate can be given perioperatively.

O   **When do serum levels peak after administration of IV desmopressin?**

45 – 60 minutes.

○   **What is the function of aminocaproic acid?**

Counteracts the high concentration of fibrinolytic enzymes in the oral cavity.

○   **What are the adverse effects of desmopressin?**

Hyponatremia , seizures, and tachyphylaxis.

○   **How are children with ITP managed perioperatively?**

CBC is drawn 1 week prior to the procedure, and if thrombocytopenia is present, IVIG is administered preoperatively (400 mg/kg for 4 days).

○   **How are children with sickle cell disease managed perioperatively?**

Preoperative transfusion to decrease the hemoglobin S ratio to less than 40% and preoperative intravenous hydration are recommended.

○   **What are the guidelines set by the AAO-HNS for 23-hour admission after adenotonsillectomy?**

Poor oral intake, vomiting, hemorrhage, age younger than 3, home more than 45 minutes from the nearest hospital, poor socioeconomic situation with possible neglect, and other medical problems.

○   **Which patients are at greatest risk for respiratory problems after adenotonsillectomy?**

Those with PSG-proven OSA, Down syndrome, cerebral palsy, or congenital defects.

○   **Why are children under 3 routinely admitted after adenotonsillectomy?**

Less likely to cooperate with oral intake and more likely to have surgery for airway obstruction.

○   **What is the incidence of hemorrhage after adenotonsillectomy?**

0.1 – 8.1%.

○   **What is the most cost-effective predictor of post-tonsillectomy hemorrhage?**

Personal and family history of bleeding.

○   **What group of patients is at increased risk for hemorrhage?**

Age >20 who have surgery during the winter.

○   **T/F: The mortality rate is highest in patients who bleed within 24 hours after adenotonsillectomy.**

True.

○   **Why is pulmonary edema a potential complication after adenotonsillectomy?**

Long-standing partial airway obstruction from enlarged tonsils serves as a natural PEEP. Sudden relief of the obstruction/PEEP can result in transudation of fluid into the interstitial and alveolar spaces.

O   **What is the initial management of post-tonsillectomy pulmonary edema?**

Reintubation and administration of PEEP, gentle diuresis.

O   **What factors affect pain after adenotonsillectomy?**

Older age, use of electrocautery are associated with greater pain; postoperative administration of antibiotics has been shown to decrease pain.

O   **What is the advantage of using ibuprofen over acetaminophen with codeine for postoperative tonsillectomy pain?**

Less postoperative nausea.

O   **T/F: Electrocautery tonsillectomy reduces intraoperative bleeding but has the same postoperative bleeding rate as the cold technique.**

True.

O   **What has been shown to accelerate the return to a normal diet after tonsillectomy?**

A single intraoperative dose of steroids.

O   **What is the incidence of clinically significant VPI after adenoidectomy?**

1:1500 – 3000.

O   **What is the treatment for post-adenoidectomy VPI?**

If it persists beyond 2 months, speech therapy; beyond 6 – 12 months, palatal pushback, pharyngeal flap surgery, or sphincter pharyngoplasty.

O   **Which of these procedures is best for patients with poor palate movement and good lateral wall movement?**

Superior pharyngeal flap.

O   **Which of these procedures is best for patients with poor lateral wall movement and good palate movement?**

Sphincter pharyngoplasty.

O   **Which of these procedures creates lateral ports through the nasopharynx for breathing?**

Superior pharyngeal flap.

O   **Why is tonsillectomy recommended prior to or in conjunction with these procedures?**

Hypertrophied tonsils may tether the palate and contribute to the VPI; raising the flaps is more difficult in the presence of tonsils; keeping the tonsils increases the risk of obstructive sleep apnea postoperatively.

O   **What are the most common complications of pharyngeal flap surgery?**

Bleeding, airway obstruction, obstructive sleep apnea.

○   **What disease increases the risk of nasopharyngeal stenosis after adenotonsillectomy?**

Syphilis.

○   **What is Grisel's syndrome?**

Vertebral body decalcification and laxity of the anterior transverse ligament secondary to infection in the nasopharynx.

○   **How is adenoidectomy related to Grisel's syndrome?**

Traumatic adenoidectomy can result in Grisel's syndrome.

○   **How is atlantoaxial subluxation diagnosed?**

Neck pain and torticollis with an atlas-dens interval of >4 mm in children and >3 mm in adults.

○   **What proportion of children will have had at least one episode of OM by age 1?**

2/3.

○   **What age group has the highest incidence of OM?**

6 – 18 months.

○   **What is the mean duration of otitis media with effusion after AOM?**

40 days.

○   **What % of children with an episode of AOM will still have an effusion present 3 months later?**

10%.

○   **What is the significance of day care on the risk of developing OM?**

Children in group day care are more likely to develop OM after URI compared to those in home care. The rate of tympanostomies and adenoidectomies is 59 – 67% higher in children <3 who attend day care.

○   **What is the significance of the seasons on the risk of developing OM?**

OM is most common in the winter and lasts longer when it occurs in the winter.

○   **What is the significance of genetics on the risk of developing OM?**

Risk of OM is higher if a sibling has a history of recurrent OM.

○   **What is the significance of breast feeding on the risk of developing OM?**

The duration of breast-feeding is inversely related to the incidence of OM.

○   **What is the significance of passive smoke exposure on the risk of developing OM?**

A higher incidence of tympanostomy tubes, chronic and recurrent OM, and otorrhea is seen in children whose mothers smoke. High concentrations of serum cotinine (marker for tobacco exposure) are associated with an increased incidence of AOM and persistent middle ear effusion following AOM.

O   **What medical conditions predispose a child to OM?**

Cleft palate, craniofacial anomalies, congenital or acquired immune deficiencies, ciliary dysfunction, enlarged adenoids, sinusitis, Down syndrome.

O   **At what angle does the eustachian tube lie in adults? In children?**

45 degrees in relation to the horizontal plane; 10 degrees in children.

O   **Where does the nasopharyngeal orifice of the eustachian tube lie in relation to the hard palate in adults? In children?**

Orifice is situated 10 mm above the plane of the hard palate in adults; at the level of the hard palate in children.

O   **What is the only muscle related to active opening of the eustachian tube?**

Tensor veli palatini.

O   **Which muscles constrict the eustachian tube?**

None.

O   **How does the composition of gas in the middle ear differ from that of room air?**

Lower oxygen level and higher carbon dioxide and nitrogen levels.

O   **Decreased levels of which immunoglobulin are common in children who are prone to otitis media?**

IgG2.

O   **What organisms most frequently cause AOM?**

Streptococcus pneumoniae (30 – 35%), nontypeable strains of *Haemophilus influenzae* (20 – 25%), and *Moraxella catarrhalis* (10 – 15%).

O   **Which organisms more frequently cause AOM in infants younger than 6 weeks?**

Escherichia coli, *Klebsiella*, and *Pseudomonas aeruginosa*.

O   **What % of middle ear fluid cultures are negative for bacteria?**

25 – 30%.

O   **T/F: The 23-valent pneumococcal vaccine is not effective in children <2.**

True.

O   **How many serotypes of pneumococcus are responsible for 83% of invasive disease in children <4?**

7.

O   **What is the reduction in total invasive pneumococcal disease in children who receive one or more doses of the heptavalent pneumococcal vaccine?**

89.1%.

O   **What is the reduction in the need for myringotomy tubes in children who receive the heptavalent pneumococcal vaccine?**

20.1%.

O   **Vaccination against what virus had been shown to decrease the incidence of acute otitis media in infants and children?**

Influenza.

O   **What are the 3 most commonly identified viruses in middle ear fluid?**

RSV (74%), parainfluenza, and influenza.

O   **What is the mechanism of resistance for *S. pneumoniae*?**

Altered penicillin-binding proteins.

O   **What organisms most frequently cause chronic suppurative OM?**

P. aeruginosa(most common), *S. aureus*, *Corynebacterium*, and *Klebsiella*.

O   **What finding on pneumatic otoscopy is most specific for OM?**

Immobility of the tympanic membrane.

O   **What are the AAO-HNS indications for myringotomy and tympanostomy tubes?**

3 or more episodes of OM in 6 months; 4 or more episodes in 12 months.
Hearing loss >30 dB from OME.
OME >3 months.
Chronic TM retraction.
Impending mastoiditis or other complication of OM.
Autophony secondary to patulous eustachian tube.
ET dysfunction secondary to craniofacial anomalies or head and neck radiation.

O   **What is the significance of adenoidectomy on OM?**

Data by Gates showed a 47% reduction in recurrent effusion in children who received adenoidectomy and myringotomy tubes compared to a 29% reduction in recurrent effusion in children who received only myringotomy tubes.

O   **What is the differential diagnosis of a midline neck mass in a child?**

Thyroglossal duct cyst, dermoid cyst, ectopic thyroid tissue, lymphadenopathy, lipoma, hemangioma, fibroma.

O   **Which of these is most common?**

Thyroglossal duct cyst.

○   **What is the etiology of thyroglossal duct cysts (TGDC)?**

Persistence of the connection between the base of tongue (foramen cecum) and the descended thyroid gland.

○   **Why do some people recommend radioisotope scanning or ultrasound of the thyroid gland prior to removal of a TGDC?**

To prevent inadvertent removal of the only functioning thyroid tissue.

○   **What % of TGDC contains thyroid tissue?**

20%.

○   **What is the standard surgical approach for removal of TGDCs?**

Sistrunk procedure.

○   **What is the recurrence rate following the Sistrunk procedure?**

1 – 4%.

○   **What is the recurrence rate following excision of a TGDC without removal of the midportion of the hyoid and the ductal remnant?**

38%.

○   **What is the incidence of carcinoma arising in a TGDC?**

<1%.

○   **What is the etiology of a preauricular pit?**

Failure of fusion between Hillocks of His 1 and 2.

○   **What is the etiology of a type 1 first branchial cleft cyst?**

Duplication error of the ectodermal elements of the external auditory canal (EAC).

○   **What is the etiology of a type 2 first branchial cleft cyst?**

Duplication error of the ectodermal and mesodermal elements of the EAC.

○   **Where are most type 1 cysts located?**

In the periauricular region, lateral to VII, connecting the skin to the EAC.

○   **Where are most type 2 cysts located?**

Just inferior or posterior to the angle of the mandible with variable relationship to VII.

○   **Where are most 2nd branchial cleft cysts located?**

Below the angle of the mandible and anterior to the sternocleidomastoid muscle.

○   **What is the typical course of the tract of 2nd branchial cleft cysts?**

Pass superiorly and laterally to IX, XII; turn medially to pass between the internal and external carotid arteries; terminate close to the middle constrictor muscle or may open into the tonsillar fossa.

○   **What is the typical course of the tract of 3rd branchial cleft cysts?**

Ascend lateral to the common carotid artery, pass posterior to the internal carotid artery, superior to XII and inferior to IX; course medially to pierce the thyrohyoid membrane superior to the internal branch of the superior laryngeal nerve

○   **What is the typical course of the tract of left-sided 4th branchial cleft cysts?**

Begin at the apex of the pyriform sinus, descend lateral to the recurrent laryngeal nerve into the thorax, loop around the aortic arch, ascend to the neck posterior to the common carotid artery, cross XII, descend to open into the skin at the anterior-inferior aspect of the sternocleidomastoid muscle.

○   **What is the typical course of the tract of right-sided 4th branchial cleft cysts?**

As above, except they loop around the subclavian artery instead of the aorta.

○   **What inflammatory disease is associated with 3rd and 4th branchial anomalies in children?**

Recurrent acute suppurative thyroiditis.

○   **What organisms are most commonly cultured from this disorder?**

E. Coli, *Klebsiella*, *Proteus*, and *Clostridium*.

○   **What are the 3 types of laryngoceles?**

Internal, external, and combined.

○   **Through which membrane do external laryngoceles protrude?**

Thyrohyoid.

○   **What are the 4 types of germ cell tumors?**

Dermoid cyst, teratoid cyst, teratoma, and epignathi.

○   **Which of these are composed only of mesoderm and ectoderm?**

Dermoid cysts.

○   **Where are dermoid cysts most commonly found in the head and neck?**

Submental area.

○   **How can one differentiate a dermoid cyst from a thyroglossal duct cyst?**

Dermoid cyst will not elevate with tongue protrusion.

O   **What is the characteristic feature of a teratoid cyst?**

Very poor differentiation of all three germ layers.

O   **What differentiates a teratoid cyst from a teratoma?**

The germ layers are well-differentiated in teratomas such that recognizable organs may be found within the masses.

O   **What % of teratomas become malignant?**

20%.

O   **What prenatal condition is associated with a higher incidence of cervical teratomas?**

Maternal polyhydramnios.

O   **Which branchial pouch is the thymus derived from?**

3rd.

O   **What is the term for the connection of the 3rd branchial pouch to the thymus gland as the gland descends into the thorax?**

Thymopharyngeal duct.

O   **What is the etiology of cervical thymic cysts?**

Persistence of the thymopharyngeal duct.

O   **What is a Thornwaldt's cyst?**

Cyst in the nasopharyngeal bursa secondary to persistent embryonic communication between the anterior tip of the notochord and the nasopharyngeal epithelium.

O   **What is the most useful study of nontuberculous mycobacterial adenitis of the head and neck region in children?**

Culture.

O   **What is the 2nd leading cause of death among children ages 1 to 14?**

Cancer.

O   **What is the most common solid malignant tumor in infants <1 year?**

Neuroblastoma.

O   **What are the precursor cells of neuroblastoma?**

Neural crest cells.

O   **What is the most common head and neck manifestation of neuroblastoma?**

Cervical metastatic disease.

○   **What is the survival rate after complete excision of lesions in children <1?**

90%.

○   **What is the most common head and neck tumor of children?**

Lymphoma.

○   **In what age groups is Hodgkin's lymphoma most common?**

Bimodal peak incidence, with one peak in the 15 – 34 year old age group and another in later adulthood.

○   **What % of Hodgkin's lymphoma cases are associated with EBV?**

40%.

○   **T/F: Axillary, inguinal, and Waldeyer's ring involvement is uncommon in patients with Hodgkin's lymphoma.**

True.

○   **What cells are unique to Hodgkin's lymphoma?**

Reed-Sternberg cells.

○   **Involvement of 2 or more lymph node sites on the same side of the diaphragm is designated as which stage according to the Ann Arbor system?**

Stage II.

○   **Which lymphoma accounts for 50% of childhood malignancies in equatorial Africa?**

Burkitt's lymphoma.

○   **What is the most common soft tissue sarcoma of the head and neck in children?**

Rhabdomyosarcoma.

○   **In what age groups is rhabdomyosarcoma most common?**

Ages 2 – 5 and 15 – 19.

○   **What are the 3 main histologic types of rhabdomyosarcoma?**

Embryonal, alveolar, and pleomorphic.

○   **Which is most common in the head and neck?**

Embryonal.

○   **What is the treatment for rhabdomyosarcoma?**

Multimodality; primary chemoradiation followed by surgery for recurrent or residual disease.

○   **Involvement in which area of the head and neck by rhabdomyosarcoma has the best prognosis?**

Orbit.

○   **What is the most common type of well-differentiated thyroid carcinoma in children?**

Papillary.

○   **What is the most common benign neoplasm of the larynx in children?**

Papillomas.

○   **What is the incidence of laryngeal papillomas in children?**

4.3 per 100,000 children per year.

○   **What % of patients with recurrent respiratory papillomatosis (RRP) develop distal tracheal and pulmonary spread of papillomas?**

5%.

○   **High expression of which nuclear antigen is significantly associated with distal tracheobronchial spread and increased frequency of recurrences?**

Ki-67.

○   **What % of patients with RRP require tracheostomy?**

15%.

○   **What % of patients with distal spread have had a previous tracheostomy?**

95%.

○   **What is the incidence of stomal papilloma recurrence rate after tracheostomy for RRP?**

>50%.

○   **What are the most common subtypes of HPV isolated from RRP?**

6 and 11 (found in >95%).

○   **Which of these subtypes is associated with a more aggressive disease course?**

11.

○   **What are the most common respiratory complications of distal RRP?**

Pneumatocele, abscess, tracheal stenosis.

○   **What are the characteristic histologic findings of RRP?**

Exophytic papillary fronds of multilayered benign squamous epithelium containing fibrovascular cores; cytologic atypia, in particular koilocytotic atypia, is not unusual.

O   **What is the most common complication after repeated laser treatments for RRP?**

Anterior glottic webs.

O   **When airway stenosis occurs after repeated laser treatments for RRP, what part of the glottis is most commonly involved?**

Posterior glottis.

O   **When is open repair of posterior glottic stenosis in a patient with RRP possible?**

When there has been no papilloma regrowth 8 or more weeks after ablation.

O   **What are the 3 most common congenital midline nasal masses?**

Encephaloceles, gliomas, and dermoid cysts.

O   **Which of these has an intracerebral connection?**

Encepholoceles.

O   **What % of gliomas have a fibrous tract connecting to the subarachnoid space?**

15%.

O   **What findings on CT scan are diagnostic for encephalocele?**

Enlarged foramen cecum, crista galli erosion, increased interorbital distance, and a mixed soft tissue and fluid density mass.

O   **Which chromosome carries the gene responsible for cystic fibrosis?**

Long arm of chromosome 7.

O   **T/F: Frontal sinus hypoplasia is common in patients with cystic fibrosis.**

True.

O   **What % of Caucasians carry the gene defect for cystic fibrosis?**

5%.

O   **What is the leading cause of chronic cervical lymphadenopathy in young children?**

Nontuberculous mycobacterium or atypical TB.

O   **What are the most common organisms causing nontuberculous mycobacterium?**

Mycobacterium avium-intracellulare complex and *Mycobacterium scrofulaceum.*

O   **What are the clinical features of cervical nontuberculous mycobacterium?**

Typically affects children ages 1 – 5 years, unilateral, upper cervicofacial lymph nodes, negative or weakly positive PPD, normal CXR.

O   **What the clinical features of cervical tuberculosis?**

Affects all ages, bilateral supraclavicular lymph nodes, positive PPD, positive CXR, respond to curretage and macrolide antibiotics.

O   **What are the typical presenting features of ankyloglossia?**

Infant has difficulty latching-on during breast feeding and mother experiences prolonged nipple pain.

O   **What are the 2 most common inflammatory salivary diseases of childhood?**

Mumps parotitis and recurrent parotitis of childhood.

O   **What are the clinical features of recurrent parotitis of childhood?**

Typically presents at age 5 – 7, more common in males, unilateral, gets less severe with time, 55% will resolve spontaneously, and frank pus is rarely seen.

SYNDROMES

○ **What is a syndrome?**

Pattern of multiple anomalies pathogenetically related.

○ **What is a sequence?**

Multiple defects arising from a single structural anomaly (ie Pierre Robin).

○ **What is an association?**

Nonrandom occurrence of a group of anomalies not known to be a sequence or a syndrome (ie CHARGE, VATER).

Name the syndrome/sequence/association:

Epicanthal folds, macroglossia, short neck, occipito-atlanto-axial instability:

Down.

Short, webbed neck, congenital hearing loss, cervical and/or thoracic fusion:

Klippel-Feil.

Craniosynostosis, beak nose, stapedial fixation, hypoplastic midface with relative mandibular prognathism, syndactyly, cervical fusion, foramen magnum stenosis:

Apert's (acrocephalosyndactyly).

Craniosynostosis, maxillary hypoplasia, shallow orbits, proptosis, cervical fusion:

Crouzon's (craniofacial dysostosis).

Pterygium colli, epicanthal folds, cervical cystic hygromas, cervical hypoplasia:

Turner's.

Hemifacial microsomia, epibulbar dermoids, colobomas, microtia, micrognathia, cleft lip/palate, facial nerve anomalies:

Goldenhar's (oculo-auriculo-vertebral spectrum).

Tracheoesophageal fistula with esophageal atresia, cervical segmentation defects, imperforate anus:

VATER.

Klippel-Feil anomaly with SNHL, VI nerve palsy, retracted globe, fused ribs:

Wildervanck (cervico-oculo-acoustic).

Large calvaria with frontal bossing, low nasal bridge, midface hypoplasia, congenital hearing loss:

Achondroplasia.

Midface retrusion, depressed and broad nasal bridge, congenital joint dislocations, congenital hearing loss, cervical instability:

Larsen's.

Coarse facial features, prominent frontal bones, mandibular prognathism, vertebral anomalies:

Mucopolysaccharidoses.

Nevoid basal cell carcinomas, odontogenic keratocysts, palmar pits, bifid ribs:

Gorlin.

Congenital hearing loss, blue sclerae, scoliosis:

Osteogenesis imperfecta.

Hyperextensible skin, joint hypermobility, easy bruising, cervical ligament instability:

Ehlers-Danlos.

Microcephaly, short palpebral fissures, epicanthal folds, long and smooth philtrum, thin upper lip vermilion border, congenital hearing loss, midface hypoplasia, C2-C3 fusion:

Fetal alcohol.

Cardiac malformations, hypernasal speech, clefting of the secondary palate, slender hands, learning disabilities:

Velocardiofacial syndrome.

White forelock, hearing loss, irridial chromic heterogeneity, dystopia of medial canthi:

Waardenburg's syndrome.

Uveitis, parotid enlargement, VIIth nerve paralysis:

Heerfordt's syndrome.

Cleft palate, micrognathia, glossoptosis.

Pierre Robin sequence.

Multiple telangiectasias of the skin and mucous membranes:

Osler-Weber-Rendu syndrome (hereditary hemorrhagic telangiectasia).

Multiple cavernous hemangiomas, dyschondroplasia, and propensity for development of chondrosarcoma:

Maffucci syndrome.

Hemangiomas of the cerebellum and retina and cysts of the pancreas and kidney:

Von Hippel-Lindau disease.

Port-wine stain, AV fistula, extremity angiomatosis, and skeletal hypertrophy:

Klippel-Trenaunay-Weber syndrome

Multiple blue, compressible, cutaneous angiomas and visceral angiomatosis:

Blue rubber bleb nevus syndrome.

O   **What other syndromes is blue rubber bleb nevus syndrome associated with?**

Maffucci's and Klippel-Trenaunay-Weber syndromes.

Facial port-wine stain, macroglossia, hypertrophy of pancreatic islet cells with hyperinsulinemia and hypoglycemia, and hypertrophy of the renal medulla and liver:

Beckwith-Wiedemann syndrome.

Paralysis of IX, X, and XI from a lesion in the jugular foramen:

Vernet's syndrome.

Ipsilateral tongue paralysis and fasciculations along with manifestations of Vernet's syndrome secondary to a lesion in the jugular foramen extending below the skull base:

Collet's syndrome.

Sympathetic trunk compromise in addition to IX-XII paralysis secondary to a lesion extending out of the jugular foramen:

Villaret's syndrome.

O   **What are the characteristics of Crouzon's syndrome?**

Hypoplasia of the orbits, zygomas and maxilla and variable craniosynostoses.

O   **What is the most frequently involved cranial suture in Crouzon's syndrome?**

The coronal suture.

O   **What are the differences between Apert's syndrome and Crouzon's syndrome?**

Children with Apert's syndrome also have syndactyly of the hands, a significant incidence of cleft palate and more serious facial deformities.

O   **Treacher Collins syndrome (mandibulofacial dysostosis) is characterized by hypoplasia of what embryologic structures?**

Those derived from the first and second brachial arches.

O   **What syndromes are associated with well-differentiated thyroid carcinoma in children?**

Gardner's syndrome and Cowden syndrome.

CLEFT LIP AND PALATE

○   **What is the most common facial cleft?**

A cleft uvula.

○   **Which ethnic group has the highest incidence of cleft lip?**

Native Americans.

○   **Which ethnic group has the highest incidence of isolated cleft palate?**

Equal incidence among racial groups.

○   **What is the male:female ratio for cleft lip, with or without cleft palate?**

2:1.

○   **What is the male:female ratio for isolated cleft palate?**

1:2.

○   **What is the incidence of cleft lip, with or without cleft palate, in term newborns?**

1 in 1000.

○   **What is the incidence of isolated cleft palate in term newborns?**

1 in 2000.

○   **What is the chance of producing a cleft-lipped child when one parent is affected?**

4%.

○   **What is the most common single gene transmission error causing clefts?**

Trisomy 21.

○   **What are the most common environmental causes for clefts?**

Poorly controlled maternal diabetes and amniotic band syndrome.

○   **What divides the palate into the primary and secondary palates?**

Incisive foramen.

○   **What artery runs through the incisive foramen?**

Lesser palatine artery.

○   **What structures form the hard palate?**

Maxilla, horizontal process of the palatine bone, and the pterygoid plates.

O   **What muscles form the soft palate?**

Palatopharyngeus, salpingopharyngeus, levator and tensor veli palatini, muscular uvula, palatoglossus, and superior constrictor muscles.

O   **At which points is the normal vermillion the widest?**

At the peaks of Cupid's bow.

O   **When does the primary palate develop?**

4 – 5 weeks gestation.

O   **When does the secondary palate develop?**

8 – 9 weeks gestation.

O   **How does the secondary palate develop?**

As a medial ingrowth of the lateral maxillae with fusion in the midline.

O   **How does the primary palate develop?**

As a mesodermal and ectodermal proliferation of the frontonasal and maxillary processes.

O   **T/F: At no time in the development of the normal primary palate is there a separation.**

True.

O   **T/F: A cleft lip is always associated with a cleft alveolus.**

False; but a cleft alveolus is always associated with a cleft lip.

O   **During embryologic development, what causes a cleft lip?**

Lack of mesodermal proliferation results in an incomplete epithelial bridge.

O   **What is the characteristic nasal deformity in a child with a unilateral cleft lip?**

Inferior and posterior displacement of the alar cartilage on the cleft side.

O   **What happens to the orbicularis oris muscle in a complete cleft lip?**

Muscle fibers follow the cleft margins and terminate at the alar base.

O   **What happens to the orbicularis oris muscle in an incomplete cleft lip?**

Muscle fibers remain continuous but are hypoplastic across the cleft.

O   **What is Simonart's band?**

The bridge of tissue connecting the central and lateral lip in an incomplete cleft lip.

O **What is the difference between a complete cleft of the primary palate and that of the secondary palate?**

A complete cleft of the primary palate extends into the nose, is always associated with a cleft lip, and does not expose the vomer. A complete cleft of the secondary palate involves both the hard and soft palates, extends into the nose, and exposes the vomer.

O **What is an incomplete cleft?**

A varying amount of midline mucosal attachment is preserved with an underlying muscular deficiency.

O **What type of cleft is a submucous cleft palate?**

Incomplete cleft of the secondary palate.

O **What happens to the soft palate muscles in a secondary cleft palate?**

Muscle fibers follow the cleft margins and insert into the posterior edge of the remaining soft palate.

O **What are the boundaries of a unilateral cleft of the primary palate?**

From the incisive foramen anteriorly, between the canine and adjacent incisor to the lip.

O **What are the 2 most commonly used classification systems for clefts?**

Veau and Iowa classifications.

O **Feeding difficulties are most severe with which type of cleft?**

Secondary palate clefts (either isolated or in combination with clefts of the lip and primary palate).

O **What strategies can be used to assist feeding with a cleft palate?**

Specialized nipples, upright feeding to minimize nasal regurgitation, palatal plates.

O **What % of children with cleft palate do not require tympanostomy tubes?**

8 – 10%.

O **What further facial deformities often occur as a child with a cleft palate grows?**

Collapse of the alveolar arch, midface retrusion, and malocclusion.

O **What is the role of palatal plates in the treatment of cleft palates?**

A palatal plate, when worn for 3 months prior to surgery and adjusted weekly to bring the palate and alveolus into a more normal shape, has been shown to lessen closure tension during surgery.

O **What was the first approach described for cleft lip repair?**

Straight line closure.

O **What is lip adhesion?**

A preliminary step in cleft lip repair where a complete cleft lip is converted into an incomplete cleft.

O   **What is the purpose of lip adhesion?**

To facilitate definitive repair by decreasing the tension across the wound.

O   **When is lip adhesion performed?**

2 – 4 weeks of age.

O   **What is the primary disadvantage of lip adhesion?**

Creates scar tissue that can interfere with definitive repair.

O   **What is the most important factor in the aesthetic outcome of lip reconstruction?**

Alignment of the vermillion border.

O   **When is a cleft lip normally repaired?**

When the child is 10 weeks old, weighs 10 lbs, and has a hemoglobin of 10 ("rule of 10's"); this is delayed 4 months if lip adhesion is first performed.

O   **When is cleft palate repair performed?**

>6 months.

O   **What is the significance of the timing of palatal repair on midfacial growth and speech?**

Earlier repair is associated with better speech but midface retrusion; later repair is associated with worse speech but minimal midface retrusion. More evidence exists to support the importance of timing on speech than on midface retrusion.

O   **What sounds are most difficult for patients with cleft palate?**

Consonants, as they require full palatal lift.

O   **What muscle is primarily responsible for preventing velopharyngeal insufficiency?**

Superior constrictor muscle.

O   **What % of patients eventually require pharyngoplasty to reduce VPI?**

Up to 20%.

O   **At what age is pharyngoplasty typically performed?**

4 years.

O   **What are the indications for pharyngoplasty after cleft palate repair?**

Intractable VPI not responsive to speech therapy.

O   **When is alveolar bone grafting typically performed?**

Between ages 9 and 11.

○ **What disorder should be suspected in children with cleft palate who fall below the 5th percentile in growth?**

Growth hormone deficiency, as it is 40 times more common in this population.

○ **When does midface retrusion present in children with cleft palate?**

In the teenage years when the growth spurt occurs.

○ **How is midface retrusion treated?**

Maxillary advancement through LeFort osteotomies.

○ **What is usually the last surgery performed in children with clefts?**

Rhinoplasty.

○ **What are the 3 techniques most often used for unilateral cleft lip repair?**

Straight line repair, Tennison triangular flap repair, and Millard rotation advancement flap.

○ **What are the key features of the Millard cleft lip repair?**

A medial rotation flap to align the vermillion, a triangular C flap to lengthen the columella and an advancement flap to close the upper lip and nostril sill.

○ **In a Millard repair, which part of the lip is rotated and which is advanced?**

The medial segment is rotated inferiorly, and the lateral segment is then advanced medially.

○ **What are the major advantages of the Millard repair?**

It preserves cupid's bow and the philtral dimple, and by placing the tension of closure under the alar base, it reduces flare and promotes improved molding of the underlying alveolar process.

○ **What is the most common repair for complete unilateral cleft palate?**

Two flap palatoplasty, described by Bardach and Slayer.

○ **What is the term for repair of the levator veli palatini muscle during cleft palate repair?**

Intravelar veloplasty.

○ **What are the 2 most common methods of secondary cleft palate repair?**

The V-Y advancement and the double reversing Z-plasty.

○ **Which is best for clefts extending into the hard palate?**

The V-Y advancement.

○ **For which types of clefts is the double reversing Z-plasty best?**

For narrow soft palate clefts and submucous clefts.

O   **What are 2 techniques for pharyngoplasty?**

Superior based pharyngeal flap and sphincter pharyngoplasty.

ALLERGY AND SINUS

○ **What congenital disease is associated with a relatively high incidence of latex allergy?**

Spina bifida.

○ **What is the incidence of latex allergy?**

1 – 6% among the general population; 5 – 17% among health care workers; 20 – 60% among those with spina bifida.

○ **A patient who is to undergo surgery reports a positive result on a latex-specific RAST test as part of a job screening process but denies any symptoms of latex allergies. Should any precautions be taken during surgery?**

Yes, the procedure should be performed under latex-free conditions.

○ **A patient develops erythematous, eczematous lesions on her arm 48 hours after having her blood drawn. This reaction is characteristic of which Gell and Coombs reaction?**

Type IV, delayed hypersensitivity.

○ **What effect does zinc have on viral URIs?**

Decreases the duration of symptoms.

○ **T/F: Prolonged use of high-dose nasal steroids has been found to cause ocular hypertension.**

False. This association was found with high-dose *orally inhaled* steroids only.

○ **When do the maximum effects of fluticasone used once a day occur?**

3 weeks.

○ **What effect does daily use of fluticasone have on nasal mucous?**

Decreases the number of eosinophils in the mucous.

○ **What is a rare, but devastating, complication of steroid injection into the inferior turbinates?**

Blindness secondary to embolization to the ophthalmic artery.

○ **How do corticosteroids diminish IgE hypersensitivity reactions?**

Diminish capillary permeability, block migratory inhibiting factor, stabilize lysosomal membranes, and inhibit edema formation.

○ **What is the mechanism of action of nasal cromolyn sodium?**

Inhibits degranulation of mast cells.

O   **What is the only nonsedating antihistamine that is eliminated primarily through the kidneys?**

Cetirizine.

O   **Which group of papillae on the tongue lack taste buds?**

Filiform.

O   **What nerve mediates taste sensation from the circumvallate papillae?**

IX.

O   **What nerve mediates taste sensation from the taste buds on the palate?**

Greater superficial petrosal nerve (VII).

O   **What portion of patients after total laryngectomy will report loss of olfaction?**

2/3.

O   **What maneuvers help facilitate preservation of olfaction after total laryngectomy?**

Rapid facial or buccal movements, "clicking" of the palate, and movement of the olfactory source.

O   **What is the most common cause of taste loss?**

Olfactory dysfunction.

O   **What is dysosmia?**

Perception of an unpleasant odor.

O   **What is phantosmia?**

Perception of an odor in the absence of a stimulus.

O   **What is parosmia?**

Distorted perception of an odor.

O   **What study confirms the diagnosis of primary ciliary dyskinesia?**

Electron microscopic study of cilia from nasal respiratory mucosa.

O   **What is the ciliary defect in patients with Kartagener's syndrome?**

Absence of dynein side arms on A-tubules.

O   **What is the early-phase allergic response?**

Initial sensitization to an allergen results in cross-linking of IgE antibodies on mast cells upon subsequent exposure. Mast cells then degenerate and release chemical mediators like histamine. Histamine stimulates dilatation of the blood vessels in the nose, mucus glands to produce mucin, and leakage of plasma from capillaries and venules. Resulting symptoms include sneezing, itching, rhinorrhea, and nasal congestion.

○   **What is the late-phase allergic response?**

Approximately 50% of allergic patients will have a late-phase response 3 – 12 hours after the early-phase response. Mediators released from mast cells cause infiltration of eosinophils and neutrophils to the exposure site. Nasal congestion is the primary symptom. Nasal mucosa becomes more sensitive to subsequent allergen exposure (priming) and to nonspecific environmental stimuli (nonspecific hyperresponsiveness).

○   **What do the 3 valleys on acoustic rhinometry represent?**

1st valley – nasal valve; 2nd valley – anterior portion of the middle turbinate; 3rd valley – middle portion of the middle turbinate.

○   **What is the most narrow portion of the nasal cavity?**

Nasal valve.

○   **Topical decongestants have a statistically significant different response between normal and allergic subjects for which valley on acoustic rhinometry?**

1st valley.

○   **Acoustic rhinometry showing decreased cross-sectional area and nasal volume that does not improve with a topical decongestant suggests what disorder?**

Septal deviation.

○   **What effect do nasal dilator strips have on nasal airflow as measured by spirometry?**

Increase peak inspiratory flow rates.

○   **What is the most common organism found in patients with atrophic rhinitis?**

Klebsiella ozaenae.

○   **What are the diagnostic criteria for allergic fungal sinusitis (AFS) as described by Bent and Kuhn?**

Allergic mucin.
Nasal polyposis.
CT scan findings consistent with chronic rhinosinusitis.
Positive fungal histology or culture.
Type I hypersensitivity diagnosed by history, positive skin test, or serology.

○   **What is allergic mucin?**

Clusters of eosinophils and their by-products (eg, Charcot-Leyden crystals and major basic protein).

○   **What are Charcot-Leyden crystals?**

Degraded eosinophils.

○   **T/F: Calcifications on sinus CT scans are common to both invasive and noninvasive fungal sinusitis.**

True.

O   **What organism is most commonly involved in fungal sinusitis?**

Aspergillus species.

O   **What is the incidence of AFS in cases of chronic rhinosinusitis treated surgically?**

6 – 7%.

O   **What test should be performed in a patient with suspected AFS who does not have classic findings on CT scan or positive middle meatal cultures?**

Aspergillus skin test and precipitins.

O   **What test is used to diagnose invasive fungal sinusitis?**

Tissue biopsy.

O   **What are the histologic findings of invasive fungal sinusitis?**

Hyphae with tissue invasion and noncaseating granulomas.

O   **What is the cure rate of invasive fungal sinusitis treated with surgery and antifungals?**

30 – 80%.

O   **T/F: Fluid collections are rare in all forms of fungal disease.**

True.

O   **How does allergic fungal sinusitis appear on CT?**

Peripheral rim of low-density edematous mucosa surrounding homogeneous, high-attenuation material often with scattered calcifications and sinus wall expansion or destruction.

O   **How does nasal polyposis appear radiographically?**

Hypodense on CT, hyperintense on T-1 and T-2 weighted MRI.

O   **In which sinus are mucoceles most commonly found?**

Frontal.

O   **How do mucoceles appear radiographically?**

Hypodense on CT and do not enhance; variable on MRI.

O   **What condition is characterized by nasal eosinophils, rhinorrhea, normal IgE levels, and negative skin tests for allergens?**

Nonallergic rhinitis with eosinophilia syndrome (NARES).

O   **What is the basic method of skin endpoint titration (SET)?**

Antigen testing is initiated with a strength predicted to be non-reacting and continued with progressively stronger extracts until a positive wheal is noted. Treatment begins with the endpoint strength and progresses to the maximally tolerated strength that relieves symptoms.

○ **What is the basic method of skin prick testing?**

Testing begins with a prick test and proceeds to intradermal testing (with a single antigen strength of 1:500 or 1:1000) if prick testing is negative or equivocal. Treatment begins at 1:100,000 strength and progresses to 1:20, regardless of the size of skin test reactions.

○ **What is the basic difference between SET and prick testing?**

SET is a quantifying test; prick testing is a qualitative test.

○ **What are the advantages of SET over other allergy testing methods?**

Standardized, safe for co-seasonal testing, potency of each antigen is adjusted to match patient's sensitivity, and starting dose is usually more potent than the arbitrary dose chosen after single dilution testing.

○ **What are the advantages of skin testing over RAST?**

Skin testing is more sensitive and unlike RAST, allows for assessment of immediate, delayed, and late-phase reactions.

○ **What are the relative contraindications to immunotherapy?**

Pregnancy, HIV, autoimmune disease, use of beta blockers.

○ **The wheal and flare response is which type of Gell and Coombs reaction?**

Type I.

○ **How is a positive wheal defined?**

A positive wheal will enlarge at least an additional 2 mm beyond the size of the "negative" (5 mm) wheal within 10 minutes.

○ **How is the endpoint defined in SET testing?**

The endpoint is the antigen strength that produces the first positive wheal and is followed by a larger positive wheal with the next highest antigen concentration.

○ **What is a variant whealing response?**

When the size of the positive wheal is more than 2 mm larger than the preceding one.

○ **What is a flash response?**

When a series of negative responses is suddenly followed by a large positive wheal.

○ **What is the significance of a flash response?**

Usually signifies a concomitant food allergy.

○ **What should you do if a flash response is obtained?**

Return the patient for retesting the next day.

○   **What is a plateau response?**

When 2 or more positive wheals (in succession) are the same size.

○   **What is an hourglass response?**

Wheals of decreasing size are followed by a clear zone, after which the usual progression occurs.

○   **What is the significance of an hourglass response?**

Usually occurs when testing begins at a very dilute level.

○   **What is the significance of the endpoint?**

Serves to identify the relative degree of sensitivity to the antigen and indicates the strength of antigen that can be used to initiate immunotherapy.

○   **What factors affect skin reactivity?**

1.   Location (back and upper arm are more reactive than forearm and wrist).
2.   Time of day (skin is 2 times more reactive between 7 – 11 pm).
3.   Previous immunotherapy.
3.   Season (more reactive if carried out during the season of the offending pollen).
4.   Dermatographism (wheal and flare response to trauma).
6.   Concomitant food allergies.
7.   Medications.

○   **What medications need to be discontinued at least 36 hours prior to skin testing?**

Antihistamines, tricyclic antidepressants.

○   **Before administering immunotherapy, what test should be done as a safety precaution?**

0.01 cc intradermal injection of the treatment vial should produce a wheal of 11 mm or less.

○   **How is immunotherapy administered after SET testing?**

Begin with 0.05 cc of the antigen mixture (with the strength of each antigen designated by the endpoint) and advance by 0.05 cc increments weekly or biweekly until symptoms are alleviated or 0.50 cc is attained.

○   **When should subsequent immunotherapy doses be advanced?**

If the local reaction is <25 mm (size of a quarter) and symptoms are still present.

○   **When should subsequent immunotherapy doses be decreased?**

If the local reaction is 30 mm or more (size of a half-dollar), the next dose should be reduced by one-half.

○   **What is the next step when 0.50 cc of the initial treatment vial is reached and tolerated satisfactorily?**

If symptoms are still present, proceed to an antigen mixture 5 times stronger than those in the initial vial.

❍ **What should be done if symptoms worsen after a dose?**

The dose is probably too high and should be decreased.

❍ **How long do most patients require immunotherapy?**

3 – 5 years.

❍ **What effect does immunotherapy have on antigen-specific IgE levels?**

Initially rise, then gradually decline with blunting of seasonal rise.

❍ **What effect does immunotherapy have on IgG blocking antibody?**

Rise is rapid initially, then becomes more gradual; response is dose-dependent.

❍ **What effect does immunotherapy have on white blood cells?**

Basophils become less reactive, lymphocyte antigen-specific responsiveness decreases, and lymphocyte surface markers become altered.

❍ **How do levels of fungal-specific IgE change in response to immunotherapy against fungal antigens?**

Remain stable or increase slightly.

❍ **How do levels of fungal-specific IgG change in response to immunotherapy against fungal antigens?**

No consistent pattern of change has been found.

❍ **What is the prevalence of Type I reactions to food antigens?**

5%.

❍ **How is susceptibility to food-induced type I reactions identified?**

Specific in vitro blood IgE measurement.

❍ **What is the most common form of immune reaction causing food hypersensitivity?**

Type III reactions.

❍ **Why do newborns and infants have an increased incidence of food allergy?**

Their gut mucosa is highly permeable, increasing antigen uptake.

❍ **What is a fixed food allergy?**

Type I, IgE-mediated response occurring seconds to hours after contact with the allergen.

○   **What are the different manifestations of fixed food allergies?**

Atopic dermatitis, asthma, allergic rhinitis, urticaria, angioedema, oral allergy syndrome, gastrointestinal distress, or severe anaphylaxis.

○   **What are the most common IgE-mediated food allergens in infants with atopic dermatitis?**

Cow's milk, fish and eggs.

○   **What are the most common IgE-mediated food allergens causing urticaria and angioedema?**

Shellfish, fish, milk, nuts, beans, potatoes, celery, parsley, spices, peanuts, and soy.

○   **What is oral allergy syndrome?**

IgE-mediated reaction causing immediate swelling of the lips, tingling of the tongue and throat, and blistering of the oral mucosa. Symptoms are commonly associated with the ingestion of various fruits and vegetables that cross-react with their specific allergic rhinitis-inducing pollen.

○   **What is cyclic food allergy?**

Non-IgE-mediated delayed sensitivity to food allergens, primarily the result of type III immune complex disease.

○   **T/F: Cyclic food allergy is not related to dose or frequency of allergen exposure.**

False. Unlike fixed food allergy, cyclic food allergy is dose and frequency dependent.

○   **T/F: Patients with a cyclic food allergy often crave a certain food, feeling better when regularly eating it.**

True. This is known as "masked sensitization."

○   **How are fixed food allergies diagnosed?**

In vitro specific IgE testing, and measurement of basophil histamine release.

○   **What results of IgE testing are considered significant?**

Class III or higher in adults; class II or higher in young children.

○   **What is the main advantage of measuring basophil histamine release over IgE testing?**

May also detect non-IgE-mediated food reactions. It also can be applied to more antigens than are available with IgE testing.

○   **Which type of reactions do patch tests detect?**

Type I and type IV reactions.

○   **What are the primary disadvantages of patch testing?**

Less reproducible than other skin tests and can be difficult to differentiate irritative reactions from true allergic responses.

○ **What is the oral challenge test?**

Gold standard for detection of cyclic food allergies (not recommended for fixed reactions) where a specific food is eliminated for 4-5 days. A positive response occurs when a strong response is provoked by ingestion of large amounts of the specific food after the elimination period.

○ **What is another method of testing for cyclic food allergy?**

Intradermal progressive dilution food test (IPDFT); test has a 20% false-negative rate with provocation of symptoms and 20% false-positive rate with wheal response.

○ **What are the most common causes of anaphylaxis?**

Food (33%), unknown (20%), insect sting (14%), drugs (13%), and exercise(7%).

○ **What is the incidence of major systemic reactions after immunotherapy injections?**

0.005%

○ **Which antigens are known to have the most potential for causing severe reactions?**

Cottonseed, flaxseed, castor bean, peanut, and any allergen the patient suspects of causing serious reactions.

○ **Which patients are at higher risk for severe reactions?**

Young children, patients with a prior history of anaphylaxis, patients with active or uncontrolled asthma, and patients taking a β-adrenergic blocker.

○ **What precautions should be considered in treating these patients with immunotherapy?**

Multiple short diagnostic skin testing sessions, slow treatment buildup, wait in the office longer than the traditional 20 – 30 minutes after allergen injections, obtaining a Medic Alert identification bracelet, avoid home immunotherapy, use antihistamine premedication before treatment injections.

○ **In confusing or fatal cases, what blood tests can confirm that anaphylaxis did occur?**

Serum tryptase, total IgE, and specific IgE values between 45 minutes and 6 hours after the initial symptoms.

○ **What are the 3 types of allergy-related reactions?**

Vasovagal events, delayed allergic reactions, and immediate allergic reactions.

○ **What are the characteristic features of vasovagal reactions?**

Pale skin, cold sweating, slow pulse, and normal recumbent blood pressure. Rarely have itching or respiratory distress.

○ **What are the characteristic features of anaphylactic reactions?**

Red or flushed, warm, dry skin, rapid pulse, and low recumbent blood pressure. Commonly have urticaria, angioedema or pruritus and commonly have respiratory distress. Diaphoresis is uncommon.

○   **What is the incidence of anaphylactoid reactions from contrast agents? During general anesthesia?**

1 in 5000; 1 in 6000 – 20000.

○   **What are the most common type of antigens causing delayed, immune complex- or T-cell-mediated reactions?**

Mold or food antigens.

○   **What is the typical presentation of a delayed allergic reaction?**

The immediate skin reactions fade away then reappear in 6 or more hours, usually peaking at 1 – 2 days. Delayed systemic reactions also may occur, usually in the form of worsening of allergic symptoms.

○   **What are the 4 types of immediate allergic reactions?**

Local, large/severe local, general/systemic, and anaphylaxis.

○   **T/F: A history of prior large local or general reactions is statistically linked with increased risk of anaphylaxis.**

False.

○   **What is the difference between a local reaction and a large local reaction?**

Local reactions are common, are 3 cm or smaller, and do not require treatment other than preinjection oral antihistamine. Large local reactions are at least 4 cm and indicative of an antigen overdose or concomitant exposure to a strong environmental or food allergen. The antigen dose should be lowered if a large local reaction occurs and retesting should be performed if lowering the dose is not effective.

○   **What are the typical features of a general reaction?**

Exacerbation of preexisting allergic symptoms, bronchospasm, urticaria, and angioedema. Symptoms are self-limited and do not progress to anaphylaxis.

○   **What are the early signs and symptoms of anaphylaxis?**

Marked exacerbation of allergic symptoms with nasal, throat, and ocular itching, facial flushing, and throat tightness; tachycardia; bronchospasm and cough, urticaria or pruritus, angioedema, and sense of impending doom; less commonly, diarrhea, cramps, vomiting, and urinary urgency.

○   **T/F: The longer the delay from exposure to onset of anaphylaxis, the less severe the reaction.**

True. The exception is food allergies, where symptoms may not occur until several hours after ingestion.

○   **Why should patients be hospitalized after initial treatment of anaphylaxis?**

Up to 20% may subsequently relapse hours later into protracted late-phase reactions (biphasic reaction).

○   **T/F: Biphasic reactions are more likely to occur when the antigen exposure has been by the oral route and often require greater doses of epinephrine in the initial treatment phase.**

True.

○ **What is the most common reason of death from anaphylaxis?**

Hypoxia (75%) due to upper airway edema or intractable asthma.

○ **How do β-blockers complicate treatment of anaphylaxis?**

β-blockers are pro-allergenic, blocking smooth muscle relaxation and increasing production of anaphylactic mediators. They also may cause hypertensive crisis due to unopposed α-adrenergic effects of epinephrine given to treat the anaphylaxis.

○ **How do tricyclic antidepressants and monoamine oxidase inhibitors complicate treatment of anaphylaxis?**

TCAs block reuptake of catecholamines, causing both hypertension and sensitizing patients to arrhythmias, and also have α-adrenergic blocking effects. MAO inhibitors prevent degradation of catecholamines, thus allowing their buildup to levels that can cause symptoms ranging from severe headache to hypertensive crisis.

○ **How do medications with α-adrenergic blocking activity (some antihypertensives, phenothiazines, TCAs) complicate treatment of anaphylaxis?**

α-blockade can cause refractory hypotension that is not improved with epinephrine (a pure α-agonist, such as phenylephrine, should be used instead).

○ **What is the recommended initial dose of epinephrine for anaphylaxis?**

0.3 – 1.0mg IM in adults; 0.01mg/kg IM in children; 0.2mg in seniors or those on β-blockers.

○ **What is the recommended initial dose of epinephrine for patients on MAO inhibitors?**

0.05mg or less.

○ **How often should epinephrine be given in an anaphylactic reaction?**

Every 3 – 5 minutes until stable in an adult; every 40 minutes until stable in a child.

○ **What are other methods of administering epinephrine?**

Inhalation, IV, subcutaneous, sublingual, intrathecally.

○ **What is the drug of choice of treatment of catecholamine-excess hypertensive crisis?**

Phentolamine in 5- to 10-mg IV increments every 5 – 15 minutes.

○ **What is the drug of choice for ventricular ectopy?**

Lidocaine, 1.0 – 1.5 mg/kg IV bolus; repeat every 3 – 5 minutes to a max of 3 mg/kg; then start IV drip at 2 – 4 mg/minute.

○ **What is the drug of choice for bradyarrhythmias and heart block?**

Atropine, 0.5 – 1.0 mg IV every 5 minutes to a max of 2 – 3 mg.

○   **What is the treatment for patients on β-blockers who are not responding to initial epinephrine treatment?**

Inhalation or IV infusion of a pure β-agonist, isoproterenol or low-dose IV dopamine.

○   **In which patients is isoproterenol contraindicated?**

In those with coronary artery disease.

○   **What adjunctive drugs can be used for anaphylaxis refractory to epinephrine?**

Ipratropium, heparin, H_1 and H_2 antihistamines, corticosteroids, and glucagon.

○   **What is the role of H_1 and H_2 antihistamines in anaphylaxis treatment?**

Reversal of myocardial pump failure; combined H_1 and H_2 blockade has shown to be superior to either one alone.

○   **What is the role of corticosteroids in anaphylaxis treatment?**

Mostly for prevention of late-onset reactions.

○   **Why is heparin a useful drug in anaphylaxis treatment?**

Heparin inactivates histamine, improves anaphylactic-induced coagulopathy, and has anti-inflammatory effects.

○   **What is the usual dose of heparin in patients with anaphylaxis?**

10,000 U IV in adults; 50 – 75 U/kg in children; followed by heparin drip of 1000 U/hr (children 25 U/kg/hr).

○   **What medications should be given for bronchospasm during anaphylaxis?**

Initially, combined inhaled β-agonists and anticholinergic drugs; once IV access is established, IV glucagon, magnesium and vitamin C.

○   **What is the difference between acute, chronic, and recurrent acute sinusitis?**

Acute <4 weeks; chronic >12 weeks; recurrent acute >4 episodes/year with resolution between episodes.

○   **What distinguishes bacterial from viral rhinosinusitis?**

Symptoms that worsen after 5 days, persist longer than 10 days, or are out of proportion to those typical of viral infection are characteristic of bacterial rhinosinusitis.

○   **What % of patients with viral rhinosinusitis develops bacterial rhinosinusitis?**

0.5 – 2.0%.

○   **What are the most common symptoms of chronic rhinosinusitis?**

Nasal congestion and obstruction.

O **What are host risk factors for chronic rhinosinusitis?**

Hypogammaglobulinemia, selective IgA deficiency, AIDS, cystic fibrosis, granulomatous disorders (especially sarcoidosis), primary ciliary dyskinesia, chronic stress, asthma.

O **Patients with perennial allergic rhinitis have a significantly higher rate of nasal carriage of which organism?**

Staphylococcus aureus.

O **What is the mean rate of nasal carriage of *S. aureus* in the general population?**

37.2% (range 19% to 55.1%).

O **T/F: The severity of airway symptoms and the extent of rhinosinusitis is associated with nasal colonization with *S.aureus* in patients with chronic rhinosinusitis.**

False.

O **What local factors predispose to sinusitis?**

Narrow osteomeatal complex, osteomyelitis, polyps, accessory maxillary sinus ostia, nose blowing, dental disease.

O **What is the most common symptom of isolated sphenoid disease?**

Headache.

O **What is Sluder's syndrome?**

Sinonasal headaches secondary to irritation of the sphenopalatine ganglion.

O **What procedure appears to relieve contact-point headaches?**

Lateral displacement of the turbinates.

O **What % of patients with rhinogenic headaches secondary to septal impaction experience relief after surgery?**

50%.

O **What disease should be considered in an adult patient who underwent sinus surgery prior to 18 years of age?**

Cystic fibrosis.

O **What adjuvant to endoscopic sinus surgery has been shown to decrease the need for subsequent surgery in patients with cystic fibrosis?**

Serial antibiotic lavage.

O **What is Sampter's triad?**

Aspirin sensitivity, nasal polyposis, asthma.

O   **What % of patients undergoing surgery for chronic rhinosinusitis have Sampter's triad?**

10%.

O   **What % of patients undergoing surgery for chronic rhinosinusitis have allergic rhinitis?**

41% to 84%, with perennial hypersensitivity predominating.

O   **T/F: The concordance of allergy and chronic rhinosinusitis is higher in the pediatric population.**

True.

O   **What impact does allergic rhinitis have on surgical outcomes in endoscopic sinus surgery?**

The long-term success rate decreases from 90-93% (uncomplicated rhinosinusitis in otherwise healthy patients) to 78-85%.

O   **What is montelukast?**

An antileukotriene, believed to stabilize rhinosinusitis in patients with Sampter's triad.

O   **A limited coronal CT scan of the sinuses is least sensitive for detecting disease in which sinus?**

Frontal sinus.

O   **What % of patients, asymptomatic with regard to their sinuses and undergoing CT scan of the head for other indications, have mucosal thickening of their sinuses?**

24 – 39%.

O   **How well do CT scan findings correlate with patient symptoms and endoscopic findings in patients with chronic rhinosinusitis?**

Positive endoscopic findings correlate well with positive CT scans, but only 71% of patients with negative endoscopic findings will have a negative CT scan. CT scan findings correlate poorly with patient symptoms.

O   **Where does mucosal thickening most often occur on CT scans of the sinuses?**

Osteomeatal complex.

O   **What is the incidence of accessory maxillary sinus ostia in patients with chronic sinusitis?**

10 – 30%.

O   **What problem does an accessory maxillary sinus ostium create?**

Enables mucous to re-circulate back into the sinus.

O   **What are the most common organisms causing acute bacterial rhinosinusitis?**

Streptococcus pneumoniae, Haemophilus influenza, Branhamella catarrhalis, Staphylococcus aureus, anaerobes (<10%), other streptococcal species (7%).

O   **What organisms are commonly cultured from patients with chronic sinusitis but rarely seen in patients with acute sinusitis?**

Gram-negative bacteria.

O   **What organisms are commonly cultured from the middle meatus in healthy patients?**

Coagulase-negative staphylococci (35%), *Corynebacterium* species (23%), and *S.aureus* (8%) in adults. *H. influenzae* (40%), *M. catarrhalis* (34%), and *S. pneumoniae* (50%) in children.

O   **What are the diagnostic criteria for sarcoidosis of the sinuses?**

Radiographic evidence of sinusitis, histopathologic confirmation of noncaseating granulomas in the sinus tissue, negative serologic test for syphilis and C-ANCA, negative stains for fungus and AFB.

O   **Which organism was found, using PCR techniques, to be present in the sinus tissue of most patients with sarcoidosis?**

Propionibacterium granulosum.

O   **What effect does oxymetazoline have on the nasal cilia?**

Paralyzes them.

O   **What is the Pretz maneuver?**

Sinus irrigation where saline is flushed into one nostril and aspirated from the other nostril while the patient is supine with the nasopharynx parallel to the floor.

O   **Which adjuvant therapies have proven to hasten recovery from acute sinusitis?**

No adjuvant therapies (e.g. antihistamines, decongestants, steroids) have proven to hasten recovery from acute sinusitis.

O   **What are the most common intracranial complications of rhinosinusitis?**

Subdural empyema (38%), intracerebral abscess, extradural abscess, meningitis, cavernous and superior sagittal sinus thrombosis (listed in decreasing order of frequency).

O   **Why are infants more prone to meningitis as a complication of rhinosinusitis?**

The arachnoid mater normally serves as a barrier to infection, but in infants, the arachnoid mater is immature.

O   **What % of patients who develop an intracranial complication from rhinosinusitis have a prior history of chronic rhinosinusitis?**

10%

O   **What is the most common organism cultured from an intracerebral abscess resulting from rhinosinusitis?**

Streptococcus milleri (commensal found in the mouth, vagina, and feces).

O   **What are 4 processes of bacterial resistance to antibiotics?**

Inability of the antibiotics to penetrate the bacterial cell, ß - lactamase production, altered penicillin-binding protein affinity, and methicillin-resistance pattern.

○   **What % of *Haemophilus influenzae* and *Branhamella catarrhalis* are ß - lactamase positive?**

63% and 80%, respectively.

○   **Which method is responsible for the resistance of *Pneumococcus* to penicillins?**

Decreased penicillin-binding protein affinity.

○   **What can be done to overcome this method of resistance?**

Increase the concentration of the drug.

○   **Why are anaerobes particularly difficult to treat with antibiotics?**

The presence of an anaerobe indicates decreased blood supply and, hence, decreased delivery of the antibiotic to the organism.

○   **T/F: The incidence of pseudomembranous enterocolitis with clindamycin is comparable to that of other antibiotics, including amoxicillin.**

True.

○   **T/F: Antibiotic prophylaxis for recurrent sinusitis is supported by randomized, controlled trials.**

False.

○   **In patients who fail to respond to medical therapy, what is the outcome after undergoing FESS?**

At 1.5 years postoperatively, >95% feel improved.

○   **What are the indications for surgical intervention in patients with sinusitis?**

Well-documented history, failure of medical management, significant quality of life issues; history confirmed with CT scan and nasal endoscopy.

○   **What are the 2 classic endoscopic approaches for FESS?**

Messerklinger and Wigand.

○   **What is the basic principle of the Messerklinger approach?**

Identify the skull base first then follow it in a posterior to anterior direction.

○   **For which patients are gravity-dependent inferior antrostomies required?**

Patients with dysfunctional cilia (immotile cilia, cystic fibrosis).

○   **How does the orbital anatomy viewed through the endoscope differ on the right and left sides to the surgeon?**

Right nasal meatal anatomy lies visually straight back, whereas on the left, the ethmoids appear to be more medial, especially anteriorly and superiorly.

O   **What is the significance of this difference?**

If the surgeon operating on the left takes the same straight back approach as the right, he or she will contact the lamina papyracea and enter the orbit.

O   **What are the three most important surgical landmarks during endoscopic ethmoidectomy?**

Lamina papyracea, fovea ethmoidalis, anterior ethmoid artery.

O   **What external structure serves as a landmark for the fovea ethmoidalis?**

Medial canthus.

O   **Where does one enter the posterior ethmoids endoscopically?**

At the junction of the oblique and horizontal portions of the basal lamella.

O   **When performing an external ethmoidectomy, where is the anterior ethmoid artery found?**

2.5 cm posterior to the lacrimal crest in the frontoethmoid suture line.

O   **Where is the posterior ethmoid artery in relation to the optic nerve?**

5 mm anterior.

O   **Which is more serious – isolated frontal sinusitis or frontal sinusitis associated with pansinusitis?**

Isolated frontal sinusitis.

O   **What are the indications for surgical treatment of acute frontal sinusitis?**

Isolated frontal sinusitis with no improvement after 48 – 72 hours of IV antibiotics.

O   **What are the 2 most common causes of frontal recess obstruction in the nonoperated patient?**

Medially displaced uncinate process and enlarged agger nasi cell.

O   **What structure forms the anterior border of the frontal recess?**

Superior attachment of the uncinate process to the lamina papyracea, skull base, or posterior-medial wall of an agger nasi cell.

O   **What are the other borders of the frontal recess?**

Lamina papyracea forms the lateral border, middle turbinate forms the medial border, and superior aspect of the ethmoid bulla and the anterior ethmoid artery form the posterior border. Supraorbital cells may also contribute to the posterior border and intersinus frontal cells can contribute to the medial border.

O   **During revision endoscopic frontal sinus surgery, what is the most commonly identified cause of frontal recess obstruction?**

Residual ethmoid bulla or agger nasi cell remnants.

○   **What are frontal recess cells?**

Ethmoid cells situated above the agger nasi that pneumatize into the frontal sinus.

○   **What is a type 1 frontal cell?**

Single anterior ethmoid cell above the agger nasi cell whose posterior wall is a free partition in the frontal recess (not skull base).

○   **Which type of frontal recess cell mimics the shape of a balloon on a string?**

Type 4.

○   **T/F: All frontal recess cells occur above an agger nasi cell.**

True.

○   **A single large anterior ethmoid cell above the agger nasi cell extending far into the true frontal sinus whose superior wall inserts upon the inner aspect of the anterior frontal sinus table is which type of frontal sinus cell?**

Type 3.

○   **Which type of frontal recess cell is very difficult to recognize without both sagittal and coronal CT images?**

Type 4.

○   **What is the primary difference between a suprabullar cell and a frontal bullar cell?**

The frontal bullar cell extends into the frontal sinus but the suprabullar cell does not.

○   **Which type of frontal recess pneumatization pattern is characterized by attachment of the superior uncinate process to the medial orbital wall, below the internal frontal ostium?**

Recessus terminalis.

○   **Where does the frontal sinus drain when this is present?**

Directly into the middle meatus.

○   **Which frontal recess cells are found anteriorly?**

Agger nasi cells and frontal cells (Type 1- 4).

○   **Which frontal recess cells are found posteriorly?**

Frontal bullar cells, suprabullar cells, and supraorbital ethmoid cells.

○   **Which frontal recess cells are found medially?**

Interfrontal sinus septal cells, ostium of the frontal sinus.

O   **Why must all mucosa be removed during frontal sinus obliteration?**

To prevent mucocele formation.

O   **What are the indications for endoscopic frontal sinus drillout?**

Patients with mucoceles or severe frontal sinusitis in whom previous surgery has failed.

O   **Where do most osteoplastic flaps for frontal sinus obliteration fail?**

Frontal recess and upper anterior ethmoids.

O   **What is the significance of purulence from the opening of the nasolacrimal duct?**

Can indicate inflammation of a pneumatized agger nasi.

O   **What is the significance of pus above the eustachian tube orifice?**

Posterior ethmoid or sphenoid sinus disease.

O   **What is the most common intraoperative complication of FESS?**

Bleeding.

O   **What is the most common postoperative complication of FESS?**

Synechiae.

O   **Where does this most commonly occur?**

Between the middle turbinate and lateral nasal wall.

O   **What is bulgarization?**

Technique to incite synechiae formation between the middle turbinate and septum to prevent the middle turbinate from collapsing and obstructing the OMC postoperatively.

O   **What % of patients develop frontal recess stenosis after undergoing surgery in this area?**

12%

O   **What factors increase the likelihood of requiring revision sinus surgery?**

Smoking, severe diffuse disease preoperatively.

O   **What are the potential complications of an inferior antrostomy?**

Injury to the greater palatine artery, synechiae, osteomyelitis, tooth numbness, pain, or injury, particularly in children.

O   **What are the most common complications of middle meatal antrostomy?**

Epiphora secondary to nasolacrimal duct injury, synechiae.

O   **What are the most common complications of osteoplastic frontal sinus surgery?**

Hypoesthesia in the region of the supraorbital nerve, wound infection.

O   **What are some other complications?**

Persistent postoperative pain, cosmetic scarring or forehead abnormalities, dural exposure.

O   **What factors predispose to complications from ethmoidectomy?**

General anesthesia, multiple previous surgeries, advanced disease, long-term chronic or fungal disease, intraoperative hemorrhage, right-handed right-sided surgery, endoscopic right-handed left-sided surgery, surgeon inexperience.

O   **Is an orbital hematoma a pre- or postseptal injury?**

Postseptal.

O   **Orbital hemorrhage occurs most frequently from trauma to which vessels?**

Orbital veins lining the lamina papyracea and anterior ethmoid artery.

O   **How can one differentiate between pre- and postseptal orbital bleeding?**

Preseptal hematoma is darker, more diffuse with more lid edema; proptosis, chemosis, and mydriasis are characteristic of postseptal hematomas.

O   **How long can the retina tolerate high intraocular pressures?**

60 – 90 minutes; 15 – 30 minutes in the presence of an arterial bleed.

O   **If orbital fat is exposed during the operation, why should the nose not be overly packed?**

Packing may press into the periorbita and posterior chamber, increasing pressure and causing proptosis.

O   **If eye changes occur during surgery, what should be done?**

Awaken patient, massage eye, and administer IV mannitol, +/- steroids; if pressure is not reduced, perform lateral canthotomy and cantholysis. Next, perform medial orbital decompression by Lynch external ethmoidectomy. Lastly, periorbital incisions can be made.

O   **Which 2 eye muscles are most prone to damage during FESS?**

Superior oblique and medial rectus muscles.

O   **What is the treatment for subcutaneous emphysema after FESS?**

Observation and reassurance… usually resolves in 7 – 10 days.

O   **How can a CSF fistula be detected intraoperatively?**

Diluted fluorescin injected intrathecally can be detected intranasally after 20 – 30 minutes.

O   **What is the treatment for a CSF fistula detected postoperatively?**

Conservative management initially… if still present after 2 – 3 weeks, surgical closure.

O   **What is one of the most common arteries responsible for profuse intraoperative bleeding during FESS?**

Posterior septal artery running below the sphenoid and feeding into the posterior middle turbinate.

O   **What should be done for an intraoperative arterial hemorrhage that cannot be controlled with packing?**

Compress carotid artery, induce hypotension under general anesthesia, have blood ready for transfusion, call neurosurgery, perform arteriogram with balloon occlusion test; if balloon occlusion is normal, ligate carotid artery. If changes occur, insert Swan-Gantz catheter, administer Hespan and repeat occlusion test. If still abnormal, carotid bypass or barbjturate coma is indicated.

O   **What is the average success rate for endoscopic DCR?**

80%.

O   **What are the 3 transpalatal approaches to the sphenoid sinus?**

Midline palatal split, U-shaped incision, S-shaped incision.

O   **What is the most common space-occupying lesion of the sphenoid sinus?**

Mucocele.

O   **After resection, what is the most important factor in preventing recurrence?**

Providing wide drainage.

O   **What are the causes of septal perforation?**

Trauma, surgery, epistaxis, intranasal cocaine, nasal steroid sprays, SLE, Wegener's.

O   **What are the relative contraindications to transsphenoidal approach to the pituitary gland (TSAP)?**

Active sinus infection, limited air cell development, septal perforation, giant pituitary tumor or vascular tumor that would require wide exposure.

O   **Why is suprasellar tumor extension not a contraindication to TSAP?**

Resection is facilitated by auto decompression of the tumor into the sphenoid cavity.

O   **What is the optimal graft material for sealing the sphenoid cavity?**

Abdominal fat.

O   **Why is this preferred over muscle?**

Improved take rate, less atrophy, increased resistance to infection, better sealing, less donor site morbidity.

O   **If there is no evidence of a CSF leak intraoperatively, is a fat graft still used?**

Yes, if a thin, bulging diaphragma sella is left, the fat will help prevent secondary empty sella syndrome and the potential for delayed CSF leak.

O   **What are the complications of TSAP?**

Numbness of teeth and gums, nasal septal perforation, short-term crusting/dryness of nasal mucosa, CSF leak.

O   **Compared to children with chronic sinusitis, children with recurrent sinusitis are more likely to be what?**

Older.

O   **What is the incidence of incidental ethmoid mucosal thickening on CT scan in children?**

30%.

O   **What is the most common pathogen isolated from opacified maxillary sinuses in children?**

Streptococcus pneumoniae.

O   **What is the most common organism cultured from the blood of patients with preseptal orbital cellulitis?**

Streptococcus pneumoniae (*Haemophilus influenzae* type b if not vaccinated).

O   **What is the significance of age in the etiology and pathogenesis of postseptal orbital cellulitis?**

In children under 9, one organism, usually a streptococcus, is responsible. Older children are more likely to be infected with multiple organisms. The likelihood of resolution with a prolonged course of intravenous antibiotics decreases with age (10% in the 9-15 year old age group to 0% in patients older than 15). At age 12, the maxillary sinus comes in contact with molar tooth roots; infection of the molars can lead to orbital cellulitis.

O   **When is lumbar puncture indicated in patients with preseptal cellulitis?**

Age less than 2 months, meningeal or focal neurologic signs, clinical toxicity.

O   **What are the 2 types of postseptal cellulitis?**

Extraconal and intraconal.

O   **What is the most common form of extraconal infection?**

Medial subperiosteal phlegmon or abscess caused by extension of bacteria from adjacent ethmoid sinusitis.

O   **What are the indications for emergent surgery?**

CT evidence of an intraconal abscess; massive proptosis with retinal or optic nerve ischemia and loss of vision; visual acuity of 20/60 or less in an immunocompromised patient with a subperiosteal abscess.

O   **T/F: The risk of intracranial complications from orbital cellulitis is higher in teenagers than infants.**

True.

O   **What is the average volume of the orbit?**

30 cc.

O   **What is the differential diagnosis of proptosis?**

Dysthyroid ophthalmopathy (Graves' ophthalmopathy), pseudotumor cerebri, lymphoma, other space occupying lesions, congenital shallowness of the orbits.

O   **What is the pathophysiology behind dysthyroid ophthalmopathy?**

Infiltration of fluid and cells into the extraocular muscles and retrobulbar structures secondary to deposition of abnormal antibody-receptor complexes and glycosaminoglycans.

O   **What is the ATA classification system for eye involvement in Graves' disease?**

Class I – lid lag and the appearance of a stare.
Class II – conjunctival chemosis, epiphora, periorbital edema, photophobia.
Class III – proptosis.
Class IV – decreased ocular mobility and diplopia.
Class V – corneal ulceration.
Class VI – optic nerve involvement.

O   **What finding on physical exam is pathognomonic for thyroidal eye disease?**

Hyperemia over the lateral rectus muscle.

O   **T/F: Treatment of Graves' disease prevents later development of exophthalmos and ameliorates eye symptoms already present.**

False.

O   **What % of these patients suffer from visual disturbances severe enough to warrant intervention?**

5%.

O   **What manifestation of dysthyroid ophthalmopathy is most likely to regress without treatment?**

Lid retraction.

O   **What is the most common cause of unilateral proptosis in adults?**

Graves' disease.

O   **What is the test of choice for the diagnosis of dysthyroid ophthalmopathy?**

Axial CT scan.

O   **Which muscles are most commonly involved in dysthyroid ophthalmopathy?**

Medial and inferior rectus muscles.

O   **What are the indications for orbital decompression?**

Optic neuropathy, severe proptosis (in excess of 24 mm), exposure keratopathy, acute deterioration in orbital status not responsive to short term corticosteroids.

O   **Which area of the orbital floor should be preserved during endoscopic orbital decompression?**

Portion lateral to the infraorbital nerve canal to prevent vertical subluxation.

O   **What is the primary advantage of the inferior orbital decompression technique?**

Large volume for decompression.

O   **What is the reduction in proptosis after endoscopic medial orbital decompression?**

3.5 mm.

O   **What is the reduction in proptosis after endoscopic medial decompression and external lateral decompression?**

5.4 mm.

O   **What is the landmark for the posterior extent of bone resection during medial orbital decompression?**

Posterior ethmoid artery.

O   **What are the complications from excessive orbital decompression?**

Intractable strabismus and hypoglobus.

O   **What complication after orbital decompression is most threatening to the vision?**

Retinal artery occlusion.

OBSTRUCTIVE SLEEP APNEA

○ **Where in the brain is the "biological clock"?**

Suprachiasmatic nuclei.

○ **What is "clock-dependent alerting"?**

Internal signal from the biological clock that opposes the tendency to fall asleep.

○ **When is clock-dependent alerting most active?**

In the afternoon.

○ **What is the prevalence of obstructive sleep apnea syndrome (OSAS)?**

24% of adult men and 9% of adult women; about 30 million people in the US.

○ **What is the definition of sleep apnea?**

Cessation of airflow due to obstruction or cessation of respiratory effort during sleep.

○ **What are the most common symptoms associated with OSAS?**

Restless sleep, loud snoring, excess daytime sleepiness, decreased intellectual capacity and memory loss, personality changes or depression, decreased libido, morning headaches (in decreasing order of frequency).

○ **What are the most common physical signs associated with OSAS?**

Obesity, systemic and pulmonary hypertension, erythrocytosis, congestive heart failure, sleep-related arrhythmias, unexplained cognitive/psychiatric disturbances.

○ **What is upper airway resistance syndrome (UARS)?**

Snoring with pathologic daytime sleepiness, poor sleep efficiency, and fragmented sleep; near-normal RDIs and oxygen saturations but abnormal negative esophageal pressures.

○ **What is considered abnormal negative esophageal pressure (-Pes)?**

More negative than –12 mm Hg.

○ **What are the 4 basic types of polysomnographies?**

Level I – standard.
Level II – comprehensive portable.
Level III – modified portable.
Level IV – continuous single or dual bioparameter.

○ **What does a standard polysomnography (PSG) record?**

EEG, EOG, EMG (submentalis and mentalis, anterior tibialis), EKG, oxygen saturation, nasal airflow, rib cage and abdominal respiratory effort.

O   What are the primary disadvantages of an outpatient study?

No EEG to assess total sleep time and no EMG to study periodic limb movements.

O   What is a split-night study?

Patient is studied for the first half of the night then placed on a CPAP machine for the latter half.

O   What is the primary disadvantage of a split-night study?

REM sleep is most concentrated in the final 1/3 of the night; OSAS is worse during REM sleep.

O   Why is OSAS worse during REM sleep?

Muscle relaxation is maximal during REM sleep.

O   What is the definition of an apneic episode?

Cessation of airflow for 10 seconds, usually associated with an arousal and/or desaturation.

O   What is the definition of a hypopneic episode?

A 50% or more decrease in flow with a drop in oxygen saturation of 4% or more.

O   What are the categories of apneic or hypopneic episodes?

Central, obstructive, or mixed.

O   What is the AHI?

Apnea-hypopnea index or # apneic and hypopneic events per hour.

O   How is an arousal defined during PSG?

Abrupt shift in EEG frequency consisting of an alpha wave, theta wave or wave with frequency >16 Hz, excluding spindle waves; must be preceded by at least 10 seconds of sleep, must last at least 3 seconds, and must be accompanied by increase in chin EMG.

O   What is an RERA (respiratory effort related arousal)?

An arousal related to an obstructive respiratory event other than apnea or hypopnea (ie, esophageal pressure crescendo, snoring, increased diaphragm EMG, or increased nasal resistance).

O   What is the respiratory arousal index?

apneas + hypopneas + RERAs per hour.

O   Neurocognitive dysfunction is most related to which two measurements on PSG?

Arousal index and hypoxemia.

○   **What level of oxygen desaturation is associated with a significantly higher incidence of PVCs?**

<60%.

○   **What proportion of patients with OSAS are obese?**

2/3.

○   **What is the Bernoulli principle?**

A column of air flowing through a conduit produces a partial vacuum or negative pressure at the margins of the column that increases as the rate of flow increases.

○   **What is the Venturi effect?**

The acceleration of flow as a current of air or liquid enters a narrowed passage.

○   **Increased electrical activity of which muscles has been demonstrated in patients with OSAS while awake?**

Genioglossus and tensor palatini muscles.

○   **What % of patients with OSAS have systemic hypertension?**

50%.

○   **What is the RDI in patients with severe OSAS?**

>30 events per hour.

○   **What disease is characterized by a decreased sleep latency time with quick onset of REM sleep on polysomnogram?**

Narcolepsy.

○   **What is the preferred treatment for OSAS in children?**

Tonsillectomy and adenoidectomy.

○   **What is the prevalence of behavioral and emotional problems in children undergoing tonsillectomy and adenoidectomy for treatment of sleep-disordered breathing?**

25%.

○   **What is Fujita's classification of airway obstruction in patients with OSAS?**

Type I – palate only (normal base of tongue).
Type II/IIA – palate and base of tongue.
Type III/IIB – base of tongue only (normal palate).

○   **What factors are associated with an increased risk of base of tongue obstruction?**

BMI >31, mandibular skeletal deficiency, and RDI >40.

O   **What is the normal thickness of the soft palate in adults?**

About 12 mm; gets thinner laterally.

O   **What is the success of UPPP for the treatment of OSAS in adults?**

Overall, 50% experience a 50% reduction in AHI or in the amount of oxyhemoglobin desaturation.

O   **What preoperative symptom best correlates with improvement in AHI after UPPP?**

Excess daytime sleepiness.

O   **What preoperative factor is associated with a positive long-term response to UPPP?**

AHI <40.

O   **Where is dehiscence most likely to occur after UPPP?**

At the inferior tonsillar poles.

O   **What is the incidence of dehiscence after UPPP?**

8%.

O   **What are the advantages of the uvulopalatal flap?**

Reversible; less pain and less incidence of dehiscence than UPPP.

O   **Why should adenoidectomy be avoided when performing UPPP?**

Increases the risk of nasopharyngeal stenosis.

O   **What is the only patient characteristic shown to increase the likelihood of OSAS?**

High body mass index.

O   **What is the relative risk for sleep-disordered breathing in a patient with allergic rhinitis?**

1.8.

O   **What are some adjunctive procedures for patients who do not improve after UPPP?**

BOT reduction, mandibular advancement with LeFort I osteotomy and maxillary advancement, genioglossus advancement, tracheostomy.

O   **How far is the genioglossus normally moved with the genioglossus advancement (GA)?**

10 – 14 mm.

O   **What is the cure rate for OSAS in patients with RDI<40 who undergo UPPP and GA with or without hyoid suspension?**

77% (Riley and Powell).

O   **What is the minimal mandibular height necessary for performing GA?**

25 mm.

O   **What are the normal dimensions of the osteotomy in GA?**

10 x 20 mm.

O   **How far from the inferior border of the mandible should the osteotomy be placed?**

8 – 10 mm.

O   **What are the possible complications of GA?**

Mandible fracture, dental injury, failure to advance, infection, anesthesia of lower lip, gums, and chin, bleeding/hematoma.

O   **What % of cases of anesthesia of the chin/lip after GA will resolve by 6 months?**

95%.

O   **When should PSG be performed after surgery for OSAS?**

6 months after surgery.

O   **What are the general indications for performing tracheostomy on patients with OSAS?**

Oxygen saturation <50%, severe arrhythmias, morbid obesity, and unable to tolerate CPAP.

O   **What is the incidence of postoperative hypertension in patients with OSAS without history of hypertension?**

63%.

O   **What is the ideal MAP after surgery for OSAS?**

Below 100 mm Hg.

O   **What % of patients with OSAS will be considered difficult to intubate?**

19%.

O   **What physical features are predictors of difficult intubation in patients with OSAS?**

Low hyoid (mental protuberance to hyoid distance >30cm), mandibular deficiency, and large neck circumference (>45.6 cm).

AUDIOLOGY

O   **What is the definition of auditory threshold?**

The lowest level at which the patient can detect a sound 50% of the time.

O   **Where is bone-conducted sound transmitted?**

Directly to the cochlea.

O   **Which part of the auditory system is assessed by air conduction tests?**

The entire auditory system.

O   **Which part of the cochlea represents high frequency sounds?**

The basal end.

O   **What range of frequencies can the human ear detect?**

20 – 20,000 Hz (greatest sensitivity is from 500 to 3000 Hz).

O   **What noise level begins to cause pain?**

140 dB.

O   **How many times louder is 60 dB than 0 dB?**

1,000,000 times.

O   **What is the significance of a negative Rinne at 256 Hz? 512 Hz? 1024 Hz?**

At least a 15 dB conductive hearing loss (CHL), 25-30 dB CHL, and 35 dB CHL, respectively.

O   **What % of the time will the Rinne test miss an air-bone gap <30dB?**

50%.

O   **A patient has a negative Rinne at 256 Hz AS. At 512 Hz and 1024 Hz it is positive as it is at all three frequencies AD. The Weber test lateralizes to the left at all three frequencies. He hears a soft whisper AD and a soft to medium whisper AS. What is his hearing loss?**

15 dB conductive HL AS.

O   **What is the glycerol test?**

An audiogram is given just prior to and 3 hours after ingesting 6 oz of D50. An improvement of 15 dB for at least one frequency, 12% SDS, or 10 dB SRT is significant for Menière's disease (the glycerol acts as a diuretic).

○   **Which frequencies are air conduction thresholds obtained from?**

250 – 8000 Hz at octave intervals.

○   **When are interoctave frequencies tested (750, 1500, and 6000 Hz)?**

When successive octave thresholds differ by more than 20 dB.

○   **How are air and bone conduction thresholds measured?**

By first obtaining a positive response, then lowering the intensity by 10 dB increments until no response is obtained.

○   **What are the stimuli used to obtain a speech reception threshold (SRT)?**

Spondees.

○   **What is a spondee?**

A two-syllable word spoken with equal stress on both syllables.

○   **What effect does pre-test familiarization with spondee words have on SRT?**

Improves speech reception threshold by 4-5 dB.

○   **How is SRT measured?**

By starting at minimal intensity and ascending in 10 dB increments until the correct response is identified.

○   **What is the spondee/speech reception threshold?**

The lowest hearing level at which half of the words are heard and repeated correctly, followed by at least 2 correct ascending steps.

○   **SRT should be within ____ dB of pure tone average (PTA).**

10 dB.

○   **What is the speech detection threshold (SDT)?**

Hearing level at which 50% of the spondaic words are detected; usually 6 – 7 dB lower than the SRT.

○   **How is speech discrimination testing performed?**

Phonetically balanced monosyllabic word lists (50) are administered at 30-50 dB above threshold and the % correct is identified.

○   **What is a normal word recognition score?**

90 – 100%.

○   **What is the significance of speech discrimination scores?**

Patients with cochlear and retrocochlear pathology will have poor to very poor scores, respectively; those with only conductive hearing loss will have normal scores when the intensity level is sufficiently loud.

O **What is rollover?**

A decrease in speech discrimination scores when presented at higher intensities; suggestive of a retrocochlear lesion.

O **A patient with a SRT of 55 dB HL and a speech discrimination score of 64% at 75 dB HL has what kind of hearing loss?**

Sensorineural.

O **What is the speech awareness threshold (SAT)?**

Lowest level at which the patient can detect the presence of speech.

O **What is interaural attenuation?**

The reduction of sound when it crosses from one ear to another.

O **What is normal interaural attenuation of air conducted tones?**

40 – 80 dB depending on whether ear inserts or headphones are used and also on the frequency being tested.

O **What is the normal interaural attenuation value for bone conduction?**

0 dB.

O **T/F: Interaural attenuation values tend to be smaller for lower frequencies than higher frequencies.**

True.

O **When should masking be used?**

When the air conduction threshold of the test ear exceeds the bone conduction threshold of the non-test ear by a value greater than interaural attenuation.

O **What is crossover?**

The attained responses represent the performance of the non-test ear rather than the test ear due to a large sensitivity difference between the ears.

O **When does masking dilemma occur?**

Bilateral 50 dB or greater air-bone gaps.

O **What is the plateau method in clinical masking?**

The non-test ear is masked by progressively greater amounts of sound until the threshold of the test ear does not continue to increase.

O **What is fatigue?**

Tone decay or adaptation where continued acoustic stimulation changes the auditory threshold… suggestive of a lesion of the VIIIth nerve or brainstem.

○   **What is the most common cause of conductive hearing loss in people 15-50 years of age?**

Otosclerosis.

○   **Where is the earliest lesion of otosclerosis most commonly found?**

Anterior edge of the oval window (fissula ante fenestrum).

○   **What is the most common cause of an air-bone gap >50dB?**

Ossicular discontinuity.

○   **Where is the peak pressure point in a normal tympanogram in an adult?**

Between –100 and +40 daPa.

○   **What would the tympanogram look like in an ear with an interrupted ossicular chain?**

Very steep amplitude, high peak (type A_d).

○   **What are normal ear canal volumes in children and adults?**

0.5 – 1.0 cc in children, 0.6 – 2.0 cc in adults.

○   **What is the acoustic reflex threshold?**

The lowest stimulus level that elicits the stapedial reflex.

○   **In the normal ear, contraction of middle ear muscles occurs at which pure tones?**

65 – 95dB HL.

○   **What are the neural pathways of the acoustic reflex?**

VIII to the ipsilateral ventral cochlear nucleus to the trapezoid body to the motor nucleus of VII to VII to the ipsilateral stapedius.

VIII to the ipsilateral ventral cochlear nucleus to the trapezoid body to the ipsilateral medial superior olive to the motor nucleus of VII to VII to the ipsilateral stapedius.

VIII to the ipsilateral ventral cochlear nucleus to the medial superior olive to the contralateral motor nucleus of VII to the contralateral VII to the contralateral stapedius.

○   **What is adaptation?**

Continuous stimulation leads to decrease in the intensity of stapedial contraction.

○   **T/F: The acoustic reflex threshold is absent in patients with middle ear disease.**

True.

○   **What does the finding of elevated acoustic reflex in the presence of normal hearing or mild SNHL and a normal tympanogram suggest?**

Retrocochlear pathology.

O   **T/F: Brainstem lesions may abolish the acoustic reflex without affecting the pure tone thresholds.**

True.

O   **What does acoustic reflex delay measure?**

The ability of the stapedius muscle to maintain sustained contraction.

O   **How is this measured?**

A signal is presented 10 dB above the acoustic reflex threshold for 10 seconds; if the response decreases to one half or less of the original amplitude within 5 seconds, the response is considered abnormal and suggestive of retrocochlear pathology.

O   **What is measured in electrocochleography?**

Cochlear microphonic action potential, action potential of VIII, the summating and compound action potentials.

O   **Where are the recording electrodes placed?**

As close as possible to the cochlea and auditory nerve (promontory, tympanic membrane, external auditory canal).

O   **When comparing the summating to the compound action potential, what value is considered abnormal?**

A ratio greater than or equal to 0.45.

O   **What does an abnormal ratio suggest?**

Menière's disease.

O   **What technique can be used to differentiate the summating potential (SP) from the nerve potential of VIII (AP)?**

AP is a neural response that will respond to higher rates of stimulation. SP is a preneural response that is not affected by higher rates of stimulation. Therefore, increasing the click rate of the stimulus will affect the AP but not the SP.

O   **What 3 audiometric test techniques are used to obtain behavioral response levels from a child?**

Behavioral observation audiometry (BOA), visual reinforcement audiometry (VRA), and conditioned play audiometry (CPA).

O   **What is behavioral observation audiometry (BOA)?**

Method of assessing hearing levels in children less than 2 by observing reflexive/behavioral responses to sound stimuli at different frequencies.

O   **What is visual reinforcement audiometry (VRA)?**

Method of assessing hearing levels in children aged 6-24 months by employing lighted transparent toys to reinforced responses (head turn) to auditory stimuli.

○   **What is conditioned play audiometry (CPA)?**

Method of assessing hearing levels in children aged 2-5 years where the child is trained to respond to auditory stimuli with a motor response (e.g., pointing to pictures)

○   **What stimulus is used to evoke the auditory brainstem response?**

A simple acoustic click, between 2000-4000 Hz.

○   **What do the peaks of the ABR represent?**

Synchronous neural discharge at various locations along the auditory pathway.

○   **What does each wave represent?**

I - *e*ighth nerve
II - *c*ochlear nucleus
III - superior *o*livary complex
IV - *l*ateral lemniscus
V- *i*nferior colliculus
[note: e.coli]

○   **Which of the waves is the largest and most consistent?**

V.

○   **T/F: The ABR is unaffected by state of sleep or medications.**

True.

○   **How is ABR most commonly used?**

To test newborns, difficult to test children, and malingerers.

○   **How is hearing threshold estimation performed using ABR?**

Wave V is tracked with decreasing sound intensity until it can no longer be observed.

○   **What does the interwave latency reflect?**

The time necessary for neural information to travel between places in the auditory pathway; any pathology which interferes with this transmission will prolong the latency.

○   **When is the interaural latency difference of wave V important?**

Used to document retrocochlear pathology when wave I is absent.

○   **When is wave I absent?**

When hearing loss exceeds 40 – 45 dB at higher frequencies.

O **When determining interpeak latencies, which waves are compared?**

I-III, I-V.

O **What is the difference in these interpeak latencies?**

Increased I-III intervals are almost always indicative of retrocochlear pathology, whereas increased I-V intervals is more likely associated with noise-induced SNHL.

O **How will a retrocochlear lesion affect the ABR?**

Prolongation of absolute wave V latency, I-V latency, and interaural wave V latency.

O **Which cells emit otoacoustic emissions (OAEs)?**

Outer hair cells.

O **What % of normal ears emit spontaneous OAEs?**

35 – 60%.

O **T/F: Females are twice as likely as males to demonstrate spontaneous OAEs.**

True.

O **What % of normal ears demonstrate evoked OAEs?**

96 – 100%.

O **What are the 3 types of evoked OAEs?**

SFOAE (stimulus frequency).
TEAOE (transient evoked).
DPOAE (distortion product).

O **Which of these has no useful clinical application?**

SFOAE.

O **Which of these is evoked by 2 pure tones?**

DPOAE.

O **What are the typical objective auditory findings in patients with auditory neuropathy?**

Decreased or absent ABR, normal OAEs, absent auditory reflexes, very poor speech discrimination, mild to profound pure tone hearing loss.

O **Why are OAEs useful as a screening tool in infants?**

Nearly 100% of people demonstrate evoked OAEs; testing is non-invasive and inexpensive; test time is short; cochlear hearing loss exceeding 30 dB can be detected.

O **What is the Stenger's test?**

Test to see if the patient is malingering; appropriate to administer if there is >20dB difference between ears in voluntary thresholds.

O   **If otoacoustic emissions are present, can retrocochlear pathology be ruled-out?**

No.

O   **T/F: The absence of the click-evoked ABR at maxiumum levels (100 dB) excludes the presence of aidable hearing.**

False.

O   **What test can be use to exclude the absence of aidable hearing when the ABR is absent at maximum levels?**

ASSEP (Auditory steady-state evoked potentials).

O   **T/F: ASSEP has little predictive value in for hearing levels in children with auditory neuropathy.**

True.

O   **T/F: ASSEP cannot distinguish between cochlear and retrocochlear hearing loss.**

True.

O   **What are the 3 general types of hearing aids?**

Analogue devices, digitally programmable systems, and digital signal processors.

O   **What is the *gain* of a hearing aid?**

Difference in the output of the instrument relative to its input.

O   **What is the *frequency response* of a hearing aid?**

The gain of the hearing aid across a range of frequencies.

O   **What is a linear amplification system?**

One in which the amplitude output is directly proportional to the signal input until saturation is reached.

O   **How do linear amplification systems limit output?**

Peak clipping.

O   **What is a nonlinear amplification system?**

The ratio of input to output is <1 (compression).

O   **Which patients benefit most from nonlinear amplification systems?**

Those with a small range between their threshold for hearing and their loudness discomfort level (LDL).

O   **What are the 3 categories of compression?**

Compression limiting, wide dynamic range compression, and automatic volume control.

O   **Which of these is most appropriate for patients with substantially reduced dynamic ranges?**

Wide dynamic range compression.

O   **What is the "half-gain rule?"**

When programming a hearing aid, the gain for each frequency is determined by multiplying the patient's hearing threshold at each frequency by 0.5.

O   **What is the basic function of assisted listening devices?**

To improve the signal-to-noise ratio at ear level by 15 – 20 dB in moderate noise and reverberation.

O   **What are the different types of assisted listening devices?**

FM systems, soundfield systems, infrared systems.

O   **What are the components of a cochlear implant?**

Implantable stimulator, headpiece and transmitter, and speech processor.

O   **What are the basic steps of sound processing performed by cochlear implants?**

Amplification, compression, filtering, and encoding.

O   **What are the criteria for cochlear implantation in adults?**

Postlingual, profound bilateral SNHL in excess of 95 dB PTA, no benefit from hearing aids (word discrimination <30% and speech detection threshold of 70 dB), psychological and motivational suitability, and no medical contraindications to surgery.

O   **What are the criteria for pediatric cochlear implantation?**

Bilateral SNHL of 90 dB HL or poorer in the better ear across the speech frequencies and no better than chance performance on open-set word and sentence materials (30%); no appreciable benefit from hearing aids, and no medical contraindication to surgery.

O   **What factor is most predictive of enhanced ability to understand speech with a cochlear implant?**

Age at onset of deafness.

O   **What is the critical period for stimulating the auditory system?**

0 – 3 years of age.

O   **How do prelingually deafened children with cochlear implants compare to those with multichannel tactile aids in open-set word recognition skills?**

Those with cochlear implants do better.

○   T/F: Speech perception of prelingually deafened children who have had cochlear implants for 5 years is likely to be equal to or better than postlingually deafened patients.

True.

○   What 2 inner ear malformations are contraindications to cochlear implantation?

Michel deformity and small internal auditory canal syndrome (<3mm).

○   What psychological problems are contraindications to cochlear implantation?

Organic brain dysfunction, mental retardation, psychosis, unrealistic expectations.

○   Into which ear is the implant placed if there is no difference acoustically between ears?

Into the better surgical ear as determined by CT scan (side with the least amount of ossification or fibrosis within the scala tympani).

○   Into which ear is the implant placed if the patient has had different durations of hearing impairment in each ear?

Into the ear that has had the shortest duration of deafness.

○   What % of patients will have new bone growth covering the round window niche and membrane during cochlear implantation?

50%.

○   What condition increases the likelihood of this happening?

History of meningitis.

○   What is the incidence of ossification after pneumococcal meningitis?

20 – 30%.

○   T/F: The electrode of the cochlear implant is normally placed into the scala tympani.

True.

○   T/F: Results of cochlear implantation in children with congenital inner ear malformations are comparable to those without malformations.

True.

○   When is monopolar electrocautery contraindicated in cochlear implant patients?

During revision and other head and neck surgery in a patient with a cochlear implant and during primary cochlear implantation in a patient with another electronic medical device.

○   What are the most common complications of cochlear implantation?

Flap complications, electrode dislocation or malinsertion, facial nerve injury, stimulation of facial nerve postoperatively.

O   **What activities are contraindicated in patients with a cochlear implant?**

Scuba and skydiving.

O   **A patient who recently had a cochlear implant placed complains of throat pain every time someone talks to him. What has happened?**

One of the electrodes of the cochlear implant is stimulating Jacobson's nerve on the promontory.

O   **How can this be treated?**

Removal of the electrode(s) stimulating the nerve (probably 17 or 18).

O   **What factors influence outcome after cochlear implantation?**

Length of auditory deprivation, pre-versus post-lingual onset of deafness, etiology of deafness, electrode insertion length, patient motivation, family support, age at the time of implantation.

INNER EAR

○ **What is the incidence of congenital hearing loss?**

1:1000.

○ **What % of these are hereditary?**

>60%.

○ **What % the hereditary cases are syndromic?**

30%.

○ **What is the typical inheritance pattern of syndromic hearing loss?**

Autosomal dominant (AD).

○ **What are the typical inheritance patterns of nonsyndromic hearing loss?**

10 – 20% AD, 75% autosomal recessive (AR), 2 – 3% X-linked, <1% mitochondrial.

○ **What genetic mutation is thought to be responsible for 50 – 80% of all AR hearing loss?**

Mutation of the DFNB1 gene on chromosome 13q encoding for connexin 26.

○ **What % of sporadic cases of congenital HL are caused by this mutation?**

27%.

○ **T/F: 1 in 31 people are carriers for the connexin 26 mutation.**

True.

○ **What is the function of connexin 26?**

Formation of gap junctions in the stria vascularis, basement membrane, limbus, and spiral prominence of the cochlea.

○ **What is the typical severity and pattern of AD hearing loss?**

Less severe, delayed-onset, high frequency hearing loss.

○ **What is the typical severity and pattern of X-linked hearing loss?**

Prelingual and more clinically diverse hearing loss.

○ **What is the term for complete agenesis of the petrous portion of the temporal bone?**

Michel aplasia.

O   **What is the term for a developmentally deformed cochlea where only the basal coil can be identified?**

Mondini aplasia.

O   **What is the most common form of inner ear aplasia?**

Scheibe aplasia (cochleosaccular dysplasia or pars inferior dysplasia).

O   **Which inner ear aplasia is characterized by high frequency hearing loss with normal low frequency hearing?**

Alexander.

O   **Which inner ear aplasia will not allow cochlear implant or amplification aids?**

Michel aplasia.

O   **Mutation of what gene is associated with enlarged vestibular aqueduct?**

Pendrin on chromosome 7q31.

O   **What inner ear malformation is associated with early onset SNHL, usually bilateral and progressive, and vertigo?**

Enlarged vestibular aqueduct.

O   **Which semicircular canal forms first? Last?**

Superior canal forms first; lateral canal forms last.

O   **What is the most commonly identified inner ear malformation on temporal bone imaging studies?**

Isolated lateral semicircular canal defects.

O   **T/F: Superior SCC deformities are always accompanied by lateral SCC deformities.**

True.

O   **What syndrome accounts for the most common form of hereditary congenital deafness?**

Waardenburg's syndrome.

O   **What is the incidence of Waardenburg's syndrome?**

1 in 4,000 births.

O   **What are the 4 clinical subtypes of Waardenburg's syndrome?**

1. SNHL (20%), heterochromia irides, pigment anomalies, dystopia canthorum.
2. As above, without dystopia canthorum (SNHL in >50%)
3. Klein-Waardenburg's syndrome: microcephaly, mental retardation, limb and skeletal abnormalities, in addition to signs of #1.
4. Shah-Waardenburg's syndrome: #2 + Hirschsprung's disease

○   **What genetic mutation is responsible for most cases of types 1 and 3 of Waardenburg's syndrome?**

Mutation of the PAX3 gene on chromosome 2q37.

○   **What is dystopia canthorum?**

Shortened and fused medial eyelids resulting in small medial sclera, lateral displacement of the inferior puncta, and hypertelorism.

○   **What syndrome is characterized by cleft palate, micrognathia, severe myopia, retinal detachments, cataracts, marfanoid habitus, and hearing loss?**

Stickler.

○   **What genetic mutations are responsible for most cases of Stickler syndrome?**

Mutations in the COL2A1 gene on chromosome 12 or the COLIIA2 gene on chromosome 6.

○   **What syndrome is characterized by SNHL and retinitis pigmentosa?**

Usher's syndrome.

○   **What are the 3 clinical subtypes of Usher's syndrome?**

I – severe-profound HL, absent vestibular function, pre-pubertal retinitis pigmentosa.
II – moderate-severe HL, normal vestibular function, post-pubertal retinitis pigmentosa.
III – progressive hearing loss.

○   **Which of these subtypes is primarily found in Norwegians?**

Type III.

○   **What test assists in the diagnosis of Pendred syndrome?**

Perchlorate challenge test… perchlorate will displace more iodine than normal from the thyroid gland in these patients.

○   **What inner ear malformations are more common in patients with Pendred syndrome?**

Mondini aplasia and enlarged vestibular aqueduct.

○   **What gene is associated with both Pendred syndrome and enlarged vestibular aqueduct?**

PDS gene, encoding for pendrin protein, on chromosome 7q31.

○   **What are the clinical features of Alport syndrome?**

Sensorineural hearing loss (SNHL) and renal failure (presenting as hematuria).

○   **What feature seen on electron microscopy is pathognomonic for Alport syndrome?**

Basket-weave configuration of the glomerular basement membrane.

○   **What is the basic defect causing Alport syndrome?**

Mutation of the COL4A5 gene producing the alpha chain of type IV collagen in basement membranes.

○   **What other test can be useful in diagnosing Alport syndrome?**

Skin biopsy.

○   **What syndrome is characterized by hearing loss, renal defects, and cervical fistula?**

Branchio-oto-renal.

○   **What is the inheritance pattern of branchio-oto-renal syndrome?**

Autosomal dominant.

○   **What % of these patients have hearing loss?**

80% (50% mixed, 30% conductive, 20% sensorineural).

○   **What gene is responsible for this syndrome?**

EYA1 on chromosome 8q13.3.

○   **What are the clinical features of Jervell and Lange-Nielsen's syndrome?**

Prolonged QT interval, syncope, sudden death, and hearing loss.

○   **What is the basic defect causing this syndrome?**

Abnormal potassium channels.

○   **What % of patients with neurofibromatosis type 1 have acoustic neuromas?**

5% and usually unilateral.

○   **What % of patients with neurofibromatosis type 2 have acoustic neuromas?**

95% and usually bilateral.

○   **Which type of neurofibromatosis is characterized by cutaneous neurofibromas?**

Type 1.

○   **What genetic mutation is responsible for neurofibromatosis type 1?**

Mutation of the NF1 gene (nerve growth factor gene) on chromosome 17q11.2.

○   **What genetic mutation is responsible for neurofibromatosis type 2?**

Mutation of the NF2 gene (tumor suppressor gene) on chromosome 22q12.2.

○   **What is the name for the subtype of osteogenesis imperfecta in which progressive hearing loss begins in early childhood?**

Van der Hoeve's syndrome.

O   **What genetic mutations are thought to be responsible for osteogenesis imperfecta?**

Mutations of the COLIA1 gene on chromosome 17q and the COLIA2 gene on chromosome 7q.

O   **What disease is characterized by cranial synostosis, exophthalmos, parrot-beaked nose, and hypoplastic mandible?**

Crouzon's disease.

O   **What is the basic defect of this disease?**

Abnormal fibroblast growth factor (FGF) receptors.

O   **What is Norrie syndrome?**

X-linked disease characterized by blindness, progressive mental retardation, and hearing loss.

O   **What syndrome is characterized by hypertelorism, short stature, broad fingers and toes, cleft palate, and conductive hearing loss?**

Otopalatodigital syndrome.

O   **What X-linked syndrome is associated with the Klippel-Feil syndrome, SNHL, and cranial nerve VI paralysis?**

Wildervanck syndrome.

O   **What disease is characterized by lower lid colobomas, downward slanting palpebral fissures, hypoplastic mandible, malformations of the external ear, cleft palate, and hearing loss?**

Treacher Collins.

O   **What is the inheritance pattern of this disease?**

Autosomal dominant.

O   **What genetic mutation is responsible for Treacher Collins syndrome?**

Mutation of TCOF1 on chromosome 5q.

O   **What protein does this gene produce?**

Treacle.

O   **What do Kearns-Sayre, MELAS, MERRF, and Leber's hereditary optic neuropathy all have in common?**

They are all mitochondrial disorders with varying degrees of hearing loss.

O   **Mitochondrial mutations have been found to produce enhanced sensitivity to the ototoxic effects of which medications?**

Aminoglycosides.

O   What are the indications for performing hearing screening in neonates if universal screening is not available?

Family history of hereditary childhood SNHL.
Congenital perinatal infection (TORCH).
Head or neck malformation.
Birth weight <1500g.
Hyperbilirubinemia requiring an exchange transfusion (>20).
Bacterial meningitis.
Apgar 0 – 4 at 1 minute or 0 – 6 at 5 minutes.
Prolonged ventilation (>5 days).
Ototoxic medications.

O   What are the indications for performing hearing screening in infants 29 days to 2 years?

Parent concern.
Developmental delay.
Bacterial meningitis.
Head trauma associated with loss of consciousness or skull fracture.
Ototoxic medications.
Recurrent or persistent otitis media with effusion for at least 3 months.

O   What are the indications for hearing evaluation every 6 months until age 3?

Family history of hereditary childhood hearing loss.
In utero infection (TORCH).
Neurodegenerative disorders.

O   What organism is most commonly associated with virus-induced congenital deafness?

CMV.

O   What % of children with congenital CMV have hearing loss?

10% are born with hearing loss, 10 – 15% eventually develop hearing loss.

O   How is congenital CMV diagnosed in the newborn?

Identification of serum anti-CMV IgM, "owl eye" bodies in the urinary sediment, and intracerebral calcifications on radiographs.

O   What are the most common organisms causing nonfatal bacterial meningitis in children >2.5 years?

Haemophilus influenzae, Neisseria meningitides, Streptococcus pneumoniae.

O   What is the incidence of post-meningitic hearing loss?

10 – 20%.

O   Which organism most commonly causes post-meningitic hearing loss?

Streptococcus pneumoniae.

O   **What sort of hearing loss is typical after meningitis?**

Bilateral, severe to profound, and permanent.

O   **At what age should children be able to say multi-word sentences?**

36 months.

O   **At what age should children be able to respond to their name and understand simple words?**

6 to 10 months.

O   **What are the only antigen-specific tests for syphilis?**

FTA-ABS and MHA-TP.

O   **What manifestation of congenital syphilis is most commonly related to SNHL?**

Interstitial keratitis.

O   **What are the 3 classic findings of congenital rubella syndrome?**

SNHL, cataracts, heart malformations.

O   **What does the audiogram typically look like in a child with SNHL secondary to rubella?**

Cookie-bite pattern.

O   **What temporal bone malformation is classic for rubella?**

Scheibe malformation.

O   **What is the incidence of hearing loss after infection with mumps?**

0.5%.

O   **How does hearing loss caused by mumps usually present?**

Hearing loss develops as the parotitis is resolving.

O   **Of all the viruses associated with hearing loss, which one is most likely to be associated with unilateral hearing loss?**

Mumps.

O   **T/F: SNHL associated with mumps usually causes vestibular dysfunction.**

False.

O   **What physical exam findings are classic for measles?**

Rash, conjunctivitis, and Koplik's spots.

O   **What is the likely diagnosis for someone who presents with vesicles on the pinna and EAC, facial nerve weakness, and SNHL?**

Ramsey-Hunt syndrome.

O   **How many words should a child age 24 – 36 months be able to say?**

50.

O   **If one parent and one sibling are deaf, what is the risk of hearing loss for subsequent offspring?**

40% risk.

O   **What % of infants with significant congenital hearing loss will not have risk factors?**

50%.

O   **Diligent workup of congenital hearing loss with state-of-the-art techniques is inconclusive what % of the time?**

30 – 40%.

O   **In the workup of congenital hearing loss, what test has the highest diagnostic yield?**

CT scan.

O   **What % of patients with unilateral tinnitus have retrocochlear pathology?**

11%.

O   **What % of patients with unilateral SNHL have an acoustic neuroma?**

1-2%.

O   **How small of a lesion can MRI with gadolinium detect?**

2 mm.

O   **How small of a lesion can fast-spin echo MRI detect?**

4-5 mm.

O   **Which is less expensive – MRI with gadolinium or fast-spin echo MRI?**

Fast-spin echo MRI.

O   **What is the primary disadvantage of fast-spin echo MRI?**

Unlikely to detect other retrocochlear etiologies of SNHL.

O   **What is the sensitivity of stacked derived-band ABR in detecting an acoustic neuroma?**

100%.

O   **What is the most common type of hearing loss from acoustic neuroma?**

High-frequency unilateral SNHL.

O   **What is a typical word discrimination score in a patient with acoustic neuroma?**

0-30% in >50% of patients with an acoustic neuroma.

O   **What is the definition of sudden SNHL?**

>20dB hearing loss over at least three contiguous frequencies occurring within 3 days.

O   **In what % of these cases can a definite cause be determined?**

10%.

O   **What % of these cases will turn out to have a vestibular schwannoma?**

Up to 4%.

O   **What are two common theories on the etiology of idiopathic sudden sensorineural hearing loss (ISSNHL)?**

Circulatory disturbance and inflammatory reaction (usually viral).

O   **What findings support the circulatory theory?**

Fisch et al (1976) showed that the perilymphatic oxygen tension was 30% lower in patients with ISSNHL versus normal subjects. Ciuffetti et al (1991) found disturbances in microcirculatory blood flow in 16 patients with ISSNHL.

O   **What evidence refutes the circulatory theory?**

Schuknecht et al (1973) reports no histologic evidence of vascular compromise to the organ of Corti in these patients.

O   **What findings support the inflammatory theory?**

Up to 1/3 of patients report URI symptoms preceding SNHL (Mattox 1977, Jaffe 1973); patients have been shown to seroconvert to a variety of viruses (Wilson et al 1983); histologic evidence consistent with viral infection (Schuknecht et al 1973).

O   **What is the current standard of care for the workup and treatment of ISSNHL?**

Otologic exam, audiogram and rule-out retrocochlear pathology… treatment with steroids, +/- antivirals, +/- diuretics.

O   **What laboratory studies are useful in the workup?**

Coagulation profile (CBC, PT, PTT), viral studies, ESR.

O   **What is the prognosis of ISSNHL?**

Overall recovery to functional hearing levels in 65-69%; no conclusive evidence that outcome is improved by medical treatment.

O   **When is spontaneous recovery of hearing more likely?**

If patient is without vestibular symptoms and suffers only partial hearing loss, particularly low-frequency (better prognosis if apex of the cochlea is involved).

O   **What treatments are used to try to optimize cochlear blood flow?**

Vasodilators (histamine, papaverine, verapamil, carbon dioxide) and blood thinners (defibrinogenation therapy, dextran, papaverine).

O   **Which of these vasodilators can override the intracranial autoregulatory mechanism of blood flow?**

Carbon dioxide.

O   **What evidence supports the use of carbon dioxide for ISSNHL?**

Fisch et al (1983) compared carbogen (95% oxygen and 5% carbon dioxide) inhalation therapy daily for 5 days to papverine and low-molecular-weight dextran for 5 days and found a statistically significant improvement in hearing levels with carbogen therapy. These findings have not been replicated.

O   **What evidence supports the use of corticosteroids for ISSNHL?**

Steroid therapy is among the few treatment methods in ISSNHL to have single modality, randomized, prospective studies demonstrating effectiveness (Wilson et al 1980, Moschowitz et al 1984).

O   **What evidence supports the use of antivirals for ISSNHL?**

No randomized, prospective studies have demonstrated this therapy to be effective.

O   **What factors lead to the best rate of recovery after ISSNHL?**

Patients treated with steroids and vasodilators, with worse initial PTA and SDS, younger age, and greater number of treatments are most likely to improve (Fetterman et al 1996).

O   **When is a middle ear exploration indicated?**

If the loss occurs in an only-hearing ear... to rule out fistula.

O   **In which area of the inner ear are immunologically active structures most commonly found?**

Endolymphatic sac.

O   **What is the predominant immunoglobulin in the endolymphatic sac?**

IgA.

O   **What is the concentration of immunoglobulins in the perilymph compared to the serum?**

1/1000[th.]

O   **What is the predominant immunoglobulin in the perilymph?**

IgG.

O   **How do lymphocytes responding to antigenic stimulation in the inner ear enter from the systemic circulation?**

Via the spiral modiolar vein.

O   **Inhalant allergy and anaphylaxis are what type of immune reactions?**

Type I, mediated by IgE.

O   **What is the mechanism of type II immune reactions?**

Antibodies directed against a specific antigen within tissues activate complement.

O   **What is the mechanism of type III immune reactions?**

Deposition of immune complexes in the microcirculation.

O   **What is the mechanism of type IV immune reactions?**

T-cell mediated delayed hypersensitivity.

O   **What is the usual presentation of autoimmune inner ear disease (AIED)?**

Progressive SNHL over weeks to months in middle-aged women, occasionally with a serous middle ear effusion.

O   **What % of patients with AIED have bilateral hearing loss?**

79%.

O   **What proportion of patients with AIED will not have any vestibular symptoms?**

1/3.

O   **What % of patients with AIED will also have a systemic autoimmune disease?**

29%.

O   **What is the most definitive test for AIED?**

Western blot immunoassay to 68 kDa antigen.

O   **The 68 kDa antigen is thought to represent what protein?**

Heat shock protein 70 (hsp 70).

O   **What % of patients with immune-mediated Menière's disease will have a positive anti-68-kD Western blot test?**

30 – 50%.

O   **What is the recommended treatment for AIED?**

First line treatment is high-dose prednisone, then methotrexate, then cyclophosphamide.

○   **What are the potential side effects of cyclophosphamide?**

Hemorrhagic cystitis, leukopenia, sterility, and malignancies of the urinary tract.

○   **What is the mechanism of action of methotrexate?**

Inhibits dihydrofolate reductase, interfering with DNA synthesis, repair, and replication.

○   **What is the most common toxicity of methotrexate?**

Abnormal liver function.

○   **What is an early sign of relapse following treatment?**

Loud tinnitus.

○   **What disease is a necrotizing vasculitis of small and medium-sized muscular arteries, most commonly involving the renal and visceral vessels, and is a potential cause of hearing loss?**

Polyarteritis nodosa.

○   **What syndrome is characterized by vestibuloauditory symptoms in association with non-syphilitic interstitial keratitis, mostly in young adults?**

Cogan's syndrome.

○   **What sort of hearing loss is most common in patients with Cogan's syndrome?**

Progressive to total deafness.

○   **What are the typical symptoms of interstitial keratitis?**

Photophobia, lacrimation, pain.

○   **What syndrome is characterized by vestibuloauditory symptoms in association with uveitis, depigmentation of periorbital hair and skin, loss of eyelashes, and aseptic meningitis?**

Vogt-Koyanagi-Harada syndrome.

○   **What disease is characterized by necrotizing granulomas with vasculitis in one or more organs and focal necrotizing glomerulonephritis?**

Wegener's granulomatosis.

○   **What is the most common otologic manifestation of Wegener's?**

Serous otitis media.

○   **What test has greater than 90% specificity for the diagnosis of Wegener's?**

c-ANCA.

○   **What disease is characterized by recurrent aphthous ulcers, ocular inflammation, cutaneous vasculitis, and SNHL?**

Behçet's disease.

O   **What is the treatment for relapsing polychondritis?**

NSAIDs, steroids, dapsone.

O   **What autoantibody is present in 75% of patients with rheumatoid arthritis (RA)?**

Rheumatoid factor.

O   **What % of patients with RA have SNHL?**

44%.

O   **Why is aspergillus infection a risk factor for ear and temporal bone tumors?**

It produces aflatoxin B, a known carcinogen.

O   **What are other risk factors for development of ear and temporal bone tumors?**

History of radiation to the head and neck, chronic chromate burns secondary to using matchsticks to clean the ear canal.

O   **What is the most common site of ear and temporal bone tumors?**

External auditory canal (EAC).

O   **What is the most common route of spread of tumors in the cartilaginous portion of the EAC?**

Through the fissures of Santorini.

O   **What is the most common histologic type of tumor involving the EAC or middle ear?**

Squamous cell carcinoma (SCCA).

O   **Where do most basal cell carcinomas of the EAC arise?**

Concha.

O   **What is the most common tumor of glandular origin to involve the EAC or middle ear?**

Adenoid cystic carcinoma.

O   **Which histologic pattern of adenoid cystic carcinoma has the best prognosis?**

Tubular pattern.

O   **Which pattern has the worst prognosis?**

Solid pattern.

O   **What are the most common types of sarcoma of the temporal bone?**

Rhabdomyosarcoma, chondrosarcoma, and osteosarcoma.

○   **What are the most common sites of origin of metastatic tumors of the temporal bone?**

Breast, lung, and kidney.

○   **Tumors that metastasize to the temporal bone hematogenously most often involve which area of the temporal bone?**

Petrous apex.

○   **Tumors that metastasize to the temporal bone via the meninges most often traverse what structure?**

Internal auditory canal.

○   **What are the most important questions to answer in the preoperative evaluation of a temporal bone tumor?**

Is the carotid artery or brain involved?

○   **What is the most common presentation of tumors of the EAC?**

Unremitting pain and serosanguinous otorrhea.

○   **What % of patients with a tumor in the EAC will present with cervical metastases?**

10%.

○   **What % of patients with a tumor in the middle ear will present with facial nerve palsy?**

20 – 40%.

○   **What histologic finding distinguishes cholesteatoma from cholesterol granuloma?**

Squamous epithelium is only present in cholesteatomas.

○   **What surgical approach is used for small, localized tumors of the cartilaginous ear canal that have not invaded deep structures?**

Sleeve resection.

○   **What surgical approach is used for tumors that involve both the cartilaginous and bony ear canal without extension into the middle ear?**

Lateral temporal bone resection.

○   **What procedures are often performed in conjunction with a lateral temporal bone resection?**

Neck dissection, parotidectomy, and occasionally, partial mandibulectomy.

○   **Is the facial nerve sacrificed during lateral temporal bone resection?**

Only if it is involved with tumor.

O   **What surgical approach is used for tumors involving the middle ear that appear confined to the temporal bone?**

Subtotal temporal bone resection.

O   **What structures are resected in a subtotal temporal bone resection?**

EAC, middle ear, petrous bone, TMJ, parotid gland with facial nerve.

O   **What other procedures are routinely performed with a subtotal temporal bone resection?**

Neck dissection, temporal craniotomy to rule-out transdural extension.

O   **T/F: After subtotal temporal bone resection, all patients will have facial nerve paralysis and a dead ear.**

True.

O   **What operation is performed for tumors that involve the medial aspect of the temporal bone in the region of the petrous apex?**

Total temporal bone resection.

O   **What is the 5-year survival for SCCA confined to the lateral EAC?**

65%.

O   **What is the 5-year survival for SCCA extending beyond the lateral EAC?**

15 – 20%.

O   **What cell patterns are characteristic of acoustic neuromas?**

Antoni A (tightly arranged) and Antoni B (loosely arranged).

O   **In which pattern are Verocay's bodies found?**

Antoni A.

O   **T/F: Tumors with a high % of Antoni A cells relative to Antoni B cells have a better prognostic outcome.**

False; outcome is independent of cell proportions.

O   **What % of cerebellopontine angle (CPA) tumors are acoustic neuromas?**

78%.

O   **What is the differential diagnosis of a CPA tumor?**

Schwannoma, meningioma, epidermoid, lipoma, arachnoid cyst, cholesterol granuloma.

O   **What % of patients with acoustic neuroma are asymptomatic at presentation?**

2.4%.

O   **An 18-year-old man with unilateral hearing loss has an enhancing lesion in the CPA and a meningioma in the occipital region. He has no skin lesions or subcutaneous nodules. What disease does he most likely have?**

Neurofibromatosis type 2.

O   **What are the three surgical approaches to resection of an acoustic neuroma?**

Translabyrinthine, middle fossa, and retrosigmoid.

O   **Which approach is best in patients with tumors > 2.5 cm with good hearing?**

Retrosigmoid.

O   **Which approach is best in patients with tumors <2.5 cm with good hearing?**

Middle fossa.

O   **Which approach offers the best exposure?**

Translabyrinthine.

O   **Which approach results in the best facial nerve outcome?**

Translabyrinthine.

O   **What is the primary disadvantage of the translabyrinthine approach?**

Destroys hearing permanently.

O   **Which approach is best in the high-risk surgical patient, regardless of tumor size?**

Translabyrinthine.

O   **Why is skull-based surgery more difficult in elderly patients?**

The dura is more fragile and prone to tearing.

O   **What are the most common complications of acoustic neuroma resection?**

SNHL, paralysis of VII, CSF leak (10-35%), meningitis (1-10%), intracranial hemorrhage (0.5-2%).

O   **What factor is most related to hearing outcome after surgery?**

Size of tumor; significantly more likely to have preservation of hearing if <1.5 cm.

O   **Following acoustic neuroma resection, what problem do patients perceive as most troublesome?**

Hearing loss.

O   **What nerve is involved in paroxysmal lacrimation?**

Nervus intermedius.

O   **Of the disorders of lacrimation, taste, and salivation, which is the first to return after injury to the nervus intermedius?**

Taste.

O   **What % of skull fractures involve the temporal bone?**

18%.

O   **What are the 3 types of temporal bone fractures?**

Longitudinal, transverse, and mixed.

O   **Which of these is most common?**

Longitudinal (80 - 90%).

O   **Which of these is associated with conductive hearing loss (CHL)?**

Longitudinal.

O   **What is the most common mechanism of CHL in longitudinal fractures?**

Incudostapedial joint dislocation.

O   **Which of these fractures is most likely to result in facial nerve paralysis?**

Transverse.

O   **Which of these accounts for the majority of facial nerve injuries?**

Longitudinal.

O   **Which of these is most likely to occur from a blow to the occiput?**

Transverse.

O   **Where are the laceration and bony disruption in the EAC most often found after longitudinal temporal bone fracture?**

Along the tympanosquamous suture line (posterior and superior).

O   **Where does the fracture line typically course in relation to the otic capsule?**

Anterior to the otic capsule.

O   **What % of patients with longitudinal temporal bone fractures have facial nerve paralysis?**

20 - 25%.

O   **Which part of the facial nerve is most often involved?**

Perigeniculate area.

O   **What are the most common etiologies of nerve dysfunction after longitudinal temporal bone fracture?**

Edema and intraneural hemorrhage.

O   **What is the most common etiology of dizziness after longitudinal temporal bone fracture?**

BPPV.

O   **What % of patients have facial nerve injury after transverse fracture of the temporal bone?**

40 - 50%.

O   **What is the typical course of the fracture line in transverse temporal bone fractures?**

Foramen magnum across the petrous apex, across the IAC and otic capsule, to the foramen spinosum or lacerum.

O   **When should middle ear exploration and ossicular reconstruction be performed after temporal bone fracture?**

At least 3 months after injury.

O   **What is temporal bone myospherulosis?**

An unusual foreign-body reaction occurring in tissues exposed to petrolatum-based products.

O   **What is the strongest predictor of poor recovery of facial nerve function following temporal bone trauma?**

Immediate onset of facial paralysis in a patient with a closed head injury.

O   **When is surgical exploration indicated after temporal bone fracture?**

For massively displaced fractures with compromise of the carotid artery or VII; or for VIIth nerve paralysis with >90% degeneration documented on ENoG within 14 days of the injury.

O   **What approach is most often used for longitudinal fractures?**

Combined transmastoid/middle fossa.

O   **What are the most common injuries encountered on surgical exploration?**

Hematoma and contusion with bony spicules impinging on the nerve sheath.

O   **What is the most accurate method of determining if otorrhea is CSF?**

Beta-2-transferrin assay.

O   **What is the most common type of temporal bone fracture in children?**

Obliquely oriented fractures.

O   **When is surgical exploration indicated for facial nerve paralysis after gunshot injuries?**

When >90% degeneration is documented on ENoG within 14 days of the injury.

O   **What is the best surgical approach for facial nerve exploration in a patient with a temporal bone fracture distal to the geniculate ganglion with intact hearing?**

Combined transmastoid/middle fossa approach.

O   **What is associated with a decreased risk of intracranial and vascular injuries after gunshot wounds to the temporal bone?**

Bullet trajectory lateral to the middle ear cavity.

O   **What are the most common associated injuries following gunshot wounds of the temporal bone?**

Intracranial injuries (53%).

O   **What substance is unique to CSF, perilymph, and vitreous humor?**

Beta-2-transferrin.

O   **What are the 2 types of non-traumatic CSF leaks?**

High pressure and normal pressure.

O   **What is the most common cause of CSF leak?**

Non-surgical trauma.

O   **What % of CSF leaks are from non-traumatic causes?**

3 – 4%.

O   **What % of basilar skull fractures result in CSF leak?**

10 – 30%.

O   **What % of patients with CSF leak secondary to non-surgical trauma will develop meningitis?**

10 – 25%.

O   **What is the most common site of CSF leakage from the inner ear into the middle ear in children?**

Oval window (especially in patients with Mondini dysplasia).

O   **What are the characteristics of CSF in the presence of meningitis?**

Elevated protein, WBC, and pressure; decreased glucose.

O   **What is the mortality rate of patients who develop meningitis with a traumatic CSF leak?**

10%.

O   **What % of CSF leaks are cranio-nasal?**

80%.

O   **T/F: Cranio-aural CSF leaks are more likely to spontaneously close than cranio-nasal CSF leaks.**

True.

O   **What signs on physical exam are suggestive of CSF leak?**

Halo sign and reservoir sign.

O   **What is the reservoir sign?**

A rush of clear rhinorrhea occurs with sudden upright position.

O   **What laboratory tests can be used to diagnose CSF leak?**

Measurement of glucose (nasal secretions are devoid of glucose), beta-2-transferrin.

O   **What other tests can be used to diagnose CSF leak?**

Radionuclide cisternography, CT cisternography, intrathecal fluorescein.

O   **What is the medical management of CSF leak?**

Elevation of the head of bed, antitussives, laxatives, anti-hypertensives, analgesics, bedrest, lumbar drain.

O   **What is a serious complication of lumbar drainage?**

Tension pneumocephalus.

O   **What are the two types of congenital defects that lead to spontaneous CSF otorrhea?**

Preformed bony pathway around the bony labyrinth, often associated with a meningocele and aberrant arachnoid granulations located over a pneumatized area of the skull.

O   **Which of these is associated with meningitis?**

Preformed bony pathway around the bony labyrinth.

O   **How does the defect caused by arachnoid granulations usually present?**

Presents after age 50 as unilateral serous otitis which is at first recurrent and then persistent.

O   **Why does spontaneous CSF otorrhea present late when caused by arachnoid granulations?**

Arachnoid granulations become larger with time; the normal pulsation of CSF pressure can cause bony erosion.

O   **What are the 2 main categories of tinnitus?**

Non-pulsatile and pulsatile.

O   **Which is more common?**

Non-pulsatile.

O   **T/F: The pitch of the tinnitus usually corresponds to the frequency of hearing loss.**

True.

O   **What is the most common cause of hearing loss and associated tinnitus?**

Noise exposure.

O   **What are the indications for MRI in a patient with tinnitus?**

Unilateral unexplained tinnitus with or without hearing loss; bilateral symmetrical or asymmetrical hearing loss suspicious for retrocochlear etiology (poor discrimination, absent acoustic reflexes, acoustic reflex decay, abnormal ABR).

O   **What auditory tests are performed in tinnitus analysis?**

Pitch matching, loudness matching, minimum masking level (MML), and residual inhibition.

O   **How can one determine if maskers will be effective in the treatment of tinnitus?**

Measure the MML and loudness matching; if the MML is lower or equal to the loudness matching, maskers will likely be effective.

O   **What is residual inhibition?**

Decreased or absent tinnitus following exposure to MML plus 10 dB for 1 minute.

O   **What % of patients with severe tinnitus are successfully treated with masking devices?**

58-64%.

O   **What type of masking device is recommended for patients with hearing loss?**

Behind-the-ear hearing aid.

O   **Why are in-the-ear hearing aids not recommended in patients with tinnitus?**

They can produce too much occlusion effect and amplification of the lower frequencies, resulting in exacerbation of tinnitus.

O   **What devices are used in the habituation technique for the treatment of tinnitus?**

Viennatone maskers.

O   **What is the habituation technique for the treatment of tinnitus?**

Binaural broad-band noise generators are worn for at least 6 hours everyday for at least 12 months; in a study by Mattox et al., tinnitus was significantly improved in 84%.

O   **T/F: Cochlear implantation has been shown to relieve tinnitus in a large % of profoundly deaf individuals.**

True.

O   **Tricyclic antidepressants are most likely to benefit patients with tinnitus who have what other problem?**

Insomnia.

O   **T/F: The majority of patients with pulsatile tinnitus do not have a treatable underlying cause.**

False.

O   **What is the most common cause of pulsatile tinnitus in patients older than 50?**

Atherosclerotic carotid artery disease.

O   **What is the most common cause of venous pulsatile tinnitus?**

Idiopathic intracranial hypertension syndrome (pseudotumor cerebri, benign intracranial hypertension).

O   **What is the most common cause of pulsatile tinnitus in young female patients?**

Idiopathic intracranial hypertension (IIH) syndrome.

O   **T/F: Absence of papilledema excludes IIH syndrome.**

False.

O   **How is the diagnosis of IIH syndrome made?**

Exclusion of lesions producing intracranial hypertension, lumbar puncture with CSF pressure of more than 200 mmH$_2$O and normal CSF constituents.

O   **What proportion of these patients will have an abnormal ABR?**

1/3.

O   **In patients with IIH, what is the usual pitch of the tinnitus?**

Low frequency.

O   **What are 5 other venous etiologies of pulsatile tinnitus?**

Jugular bulb abnormalities; hydrocephalus associated with stenosis of the sylvian aqueduct; increased intracranial pressure associated with Arnold-Chiari syndrome; abnormal condylar and mastoid emissary veins; idiopathic or essential tinnitus.

O   **What maneuvers on physical exam will decrease or completely eliminate pulsatile tinnitus of venous origin?**

Light digital pressure over the ipsilateral internal jugular vein and head turning towards the ipsilateral side.

○   **What is the initial test of choice in patients with pulsatile tinnitus and normal otoscopy?**

Duplex carotid ultrasound and echocardiogram in patients suspected of ACAD; otherwise, MRI/MRA/MRV.

○   **What is the initial test of choice in patients with pulsatile tinnitus and a retrotympanic mass?**

CT scan of the temporal bones.

○   **What is the treatment for IIH?**

Weight reduction and acetazolamide (250 mg TID) or furosemide (20 mg BID); lumbar-peritoneal shunt for patients with visual deterioration, persistent headaches or disabling tinnitus.

VERTIGO AND DIZZINESS

O   **Name the most likely etiology of vertigo--**

Positional vertigo, lasting seconds, associated with rotatory nystagmus:

BPPV.

Acute, non-progressive, episodic vertigo lasting for hours to days; no hearing loss:

Vestibular neuritis.

Acute, episodic vertigo lasting at least 20 minutes, low frequency SNHL:

Menière's disease.

Constant, progressive dizziness, Brun's nystagmus, SNHL:

CPA tumor.

Transient, orthostatic dizziness with vertical nystagmus:

Vertebrobasilar insufficiency (VBI).

Constant dizziness, high frequency SNHL, oscillopsia, head-shake nystagmus:

Ototoxicity.

O   **Which part of the vestibular labyrinth detects angular acceleration?**

Semicircular canals.

O   **What do the utricle and saccule detect?**

Linear acceleration.

O   **Where are cupula found?**

Semicircular canals.

O   **Balance is determined by what 3 systems?**

Vestibular, vestibulo-ocular (visual), and vestibulospinal (proprioceptive) systems.

O   **What disorders are associated with down-beating nystagmus?**

Arnold-Chiari, cerebellar degeneration, multiple sclerosis, brainstem infarction, lithium intoxication, magnesium and thiamine deficiency.

O   **What disorders are associated with up-beating nystagmus?**

Brainstem tumors, congenital abnormalities, multiple sclerosis, hemangiomas, vascular lesions, encephalitis, and brainstem abscess.

○   **What disorders are associated with bidirectional gaze-fixation nystagmus?**

Barbiturate, phenytoin, and alcohol intoxication.

○   **What clinical findings are diagnostic of central vestibular disorders?**

Disconjugate eye movements, skew deviation, vertical gaze palsy, inverted Bell's phenomenon, seesaw nystagmus, bidirectional nystagmus, periodic alternating nystagmus, and nystagmus that is greater with eyes open and fixed on a visual target than in darkness.

○   **What clinical finding is pathognomonic for a lesion at the craniocervical junction?**

Spontaneous downbeat nystagmus with the eyes open, in the primary position that increases with lateral gaze or head extension.

○   **What is the treatment for otosyphilis?**

2.4 million U of benzathine penicillin IM q week for at least 3 weeks (up to 1 year) or 10 million U of penicillin G IV qd for 10 days followed by 2.4 million U of IM benzathine penicillin q week for 2 weeks plus prednisone 40 – 60 mg qd for 2 – 4 weeks followed by a taper.

○   **What is the primary problem of IM penicillin therapy for otosyphilis?**

Fails to achieve treponemicidal levels in the CSF.

○   **What medication extends the half-life and facilitates CSF penetration of penicillin?**

Probenecid.

○   **What is the Jarisch-Herxheimer reaction?**

Fever and flu-like symptoms beginning within 4 hours of commencing treatment for secondary syphilis.

○   **What % of patients with vertigo secondary to otosyphilis improve with penicillin and steroid therapy?**

58 – 86%.

○   **What % of patients with hearing loss secondary to otosyphilis improve with penicillin and steroid therapy?**

31%.

○   **What are the most common manifestations of VBI?**

Abrupt, transient attacks of vertigo associated with bilaterally reduced caloric responses.

○   **What is the treatment for vertigo secondary to VBI?**

Aspirin or ticlid if aspirin-sensitive.

○   **Why is ticlid only warranted in patients unable to tolerate aspirin?**

Risk of life-threatening neutropenia.

○   **What % of patients with classic migraine experience vertigo?**

30 – 40%.

○   **What are the most widely used agents for treatment of acute migraine?**

Ergotamine tartrate and sumatriptan.

○   **What are the most widely used agents for prophylaxis of migraine?**

Beta-blockers and calcium antagonists.

○   **What syndrome is characterized by recurrent episodes of vertigo and ataxia in several members of a family?**

Familial ataxia syndrome.

○   **What is the treatment for this syndrome?**

Acetazolamide.

○   **Which patients are least likely to benefit from vestibular rehabilitation programs?**

Patients with fluctuating nonstable vestibular lesions such as with Menière's disease; patients in whom no provocative maneuvers or postural control abnormalities are found on examination.

○   **What does computerized dynamic platform posturography specifically measure?**

Postural stability and sway.

○   **What are the clinical features of BPPV?**

10-20 second attacks of rotational vertigo, precipitated by head movements, with spontaneous resolution after several weeks to months in 80-90%.

○   **What are the physical exam findings in patients with BPPV?**

With the Dix-Hallpike maneuver, rotatory nystagmus towards the undermost ear accompanied by vertigo, both with a latent period of 5-30 s and duration <30 s.

○   **What features distinguish BPPV from vertigo due to CNS disease?**

CNS disease: no latent period, direction of nystagmus varies, nystagmus and vertigo are nonfatiguable.

○   **What are the 2 main theories of the pathophysiology of BPPV?**

Cupulolithiasis theory: deposits gravitate, attach to, and stimulate the cupula.
Canalolithiasis theory: deposits float freely within the semicircular canals (SCC) under the influence of gravity.

○   **What % of cases occur in the posterior SCC? Horizontal SCC?**

Posterior 80 – 95%; horizontal 5 – 20%.

O   **Which theory is currently more favored?**

Canalolithiasis.

O   **How does this theory account for the latency of onset of nystagmus?**

Delay is due to the adherence of deposits to the membranous wall of the labyrinth.

O   **What are the deposits thought to consist of?**

Calcium carbonate crystals, possibly resulting from microfractures of the temporal bone near the round window niche (also near the ampulla of the posterior SCC).

O   **What therapeutic maneuver is based on the cupulolithiasis theory?**

Semont.

O   **What therapeutic maneuver is based on the canalolithiasis theory?**

Epley.

O   **What is the success rate of the Epley maneuver after only 1 manipulation?**

50 – 77%.

O   **What is the success rate after 2 manipulations?**

95 – 97%.

O   **What is the rate of recurrence?**

30 – 50% eventually have a recurrence; 10 – 20% within 1 – 2 weeks of the maneuver.

O   **What are the indications for surgical treatment of BPPV?**

Incapacitating symptoms >1 year, confirmation of BPPV with Dix-Hallpike on at least 3 visits, failure of conservative treatment, normal head MRI.

O   **What are the surgical options for treatment of BPPV?**

Singular neurectomy, posterior SCC ablation.

O   **What is the success rate of singular neurectomy?**

79 – 94%.

O   **What are the disadvantages of singular neurectomy?**

Technically difficult, 10% risk of SNHL, and nerve may be inaccessible under the basal turn of the cochlea in a small number of patients.

O   **Why is posterior SCC ablation most often the procedure of choice?**

Relatively easier, less risk to hearing, excellent long term results (approaches 100%).

O **According to AAO-HNS, what are the criteria for "definite" Menière's disease?**

1) 2 or more episodes of spontaneous rotational vertigo lasting 20 minutes or longer.
2) Audiometrically documented hearing loss on at least one occasion.
3) Tinnitus or aural fullness in the affected ear.
4) Exclusion of other causes.

O **What are the criteria for "certain" Menière's disease?**

The above criteria plus histopathologic confirmation.

O **What are the criteria for "probable" Menière's disease?**

Only 1 episode of vertigo plus the other criteria for "definite" disease.

O **What are the criteria for "possible" Menière's disease?**

Cochlear or vestibular variants of Menière's for which other causes have been excluded.

O **A patient with Menière's disease is able to work, drive, and travel but must exert a great deal of effort to do so and is "barely making it." What functional level is he/she?**

4 (out of 6).

O **A patient with Menière's disease has been disabled for >1 year and is on disability. What functional level is he/she?**

6.

O **What % of patients have bilateral Menière's disease?**

After 2 years, 15% of patients; after 10 years, 25 – 35%; and after 20 years, 40 – 60%.

O **What is the most consistently reliable objective test for hydrops?**

Transtympanic electrocochleography (ECochG).

O **What 3 variables does it measure?**

Action potential (AP), summating potential (SP), and cochlear microphonic (CM).

O **What happens to the SP when the basilar membrane is displaced towards the scala media?**

Decreases or reverses polarity.

O **What happens to the SP when the pressure increases inside the scala media?**

Increases (basilar membrane is displaced towards the scala tympani).

O **What is the earliest indicator of hydrops on ECochG?**

Ratio of SP to AP >30%.

○   **What happens to the SP in the presence of hydrops?**

36% of patients will have a normal SP; 32% will have a moderately enhanced negative SP; 27% will have a very enhanced negative SP; 5% will have no SP or action potential.

○   **What happens to CM in the presence of hydrops?**

Diminishes; after-ringing may occur.

○   **How is ECochG helpful prior to destructive surgery for Menière's disease?**

In patients with unilateral disease, abnormalities in the asymptomatic ear (SP:AP >35%, distorted CM with after-ringing) predict development of hydrops in that ear.

○   **What is the prognostic significance of a normal AP-SP prior to surgery?**

Outcomes are significantly better.

○   **What is the glycerol test for Menière's?**

Glycerol given orally increases the serum osmolality, causing a shift of water and electrolytes from the perilymph and CSF to the serum, and increases cochlear blood flow. In most patients with Menière's, this will result in an improvement in hearing.

○   **What is the significance of a positive test?**

Indicates hydrops, which can be caused by Menière's, late syphilis, Cogan's disease, otosclerosis, or acoustic neuroma.

○   **What is the mainstay of treatment for Menière's disease?**

Diuretics and dietary salt restriction.

○   **What are the metabolic effects of prolonged thiazide diuretic therapy?**

Metabolic alkalosis with hypokalemia and hypochloremia, hyperglycemia.

○   **What % of patients with Menière's disease do not respond adequately to salt restriction and diuretics?**

10%.

○   **In terms of functional level, which patients with Menière's disease are candidates for chemical or surgical labyrinthectomy?**

Patients with functional levels of 4, 5, or 6.

○   **What is the most common and most difficult to manage problem after any vestibular destructive surgery?**

Persistent dysequilibrium (20%).

○   **After aminoglycoside treatments, when is the usual onset of dysequilibrium?**

4 days after treatment.

O   **What is the most important factor in the ototoxic effect of aminoglycosides?**

Total cumulative dose.

O   **How do aminoglycosides exert their toxic effects on the hair cells of the inner ear?**

Bind to the plasma membrane and displace calcium and magnesium; once transported into the cell, bind with phosphatidylinositol, causing disruption of the plasma membrane and inhibition of inositol triphosphate, resulting in cell death.

O   **Which aminoglycosides are primarily vestibulotoxic?**

Gentamicin and streptomycin.

O   **Which aminoglycosides are primarily cochleotoxic?**

Amikacin, dihydrostreptomycin, kanamycin, and streptomycin at high doses.

O   **What region of the inner ear is most susceptible to permanent loss of hair cells?**

Basal turn of the cochlea.

O   **What are the surgical options for treatment of Menière's?**

Endolymphatic shunt, destructive labyrinthectomy, and vestibular nerve section.

O   **Which of these is the only surgical procedure considered in an only-hearing ear?**

Endolymphatic shunt.

O   **Which of these is most commonly performed?**

Endolymphatic shunt.

O   **Where is the endolymphatic sac?**

Anterior to Trautmann's triangle within the dura, medial and inferior to the posterior semicircular canal.

O   **What is the incidence of total SNHL after endolymphatic sac surgery?**

1 – 2%.

O   **What % of patients will have improved tinnitus and hearing after endolymphatic sac surgery?**

50% experience improvement in tinnitus and 30 – 40% experience improvement in hearing.

O   **What % of patients have improvement of vertigo after endolymphatic sac surgery?**

70% experience complete relief, 20% experience decreased vertigo.

O   **What are the 4 primary approaches to vestibular nerve section?**

Middle fossa, retrosigmoid, transcochlear, and retrolabyrinthine.

○   **Which of these is associated with the greatest risk of damage to VII?**

Middle fossa.

○   **Which of these is most likely to result in postoperative headaches?**

Retrosigmoid.

○   **What increases the likelihood of headaches after the retrosigmoid approach?**

Drilling out of the medial portion of the IAC.

○   **Which way is the sigmoid sinus retracted in the retrosigmoid approach to vestibular nerve section?**

Anteriorly.

○   **Which way is the sigmoid sinus retracted in the retrolabyrinthine approach to vestibular nerve section?**

Posteriorly.

○   **Which of these approaches is at higher risk for a CSF leak?**

Retrolabyrinthine.

○   **What portion of the VIIIth nerve is sectioned in vestibular nerve section?**

Lateral portion (superior and inferior vestibular nerves) in the IAC.

○   **What are the landmarks for identification of the IAC during middle fossa approach to vestibular nerve section?**

Greater superficial petrosal nerve, malleus head, and superior SCC.

○   **What is the success rate of vestibular nerve section?**

For the middle fossa approach, complete elimination of vertigo is achieved in >90%; for the posterior approaches, complete elimination of vertigo is achieved in >80%.

○   **What are the contraindications to vestibular nerve section?**

Only hearing ear, signs of central vestibular dysfunction, poor medical health.

○   **What are the 2 approaches to labyrinthectomy?**

Transmastoid and transcanal.

○   **Which of these is superior in complete elimination of vertigo?**

Both are equally effective.

EXTERNAL EAR DISEASES

O   **What is the typical presentation of an auricular endochondral pseudocyst?**

Painless, fluctuant outpouching on the upper anterior surface of the auricle, often preceded by low-grade chronic trauma.

O   **What are the two types of bony growths in the EAC?**

Diffuse exostoses and osteomata.

O   **Which is more common?**

Exostoses.

O   **Which is usually attached to the tympanosquamous suture line?**

Osteomata.

O   **Which has a male predilection?**

Both.

O   **Which is more likely to be bilateral?**

Exostoses.

O   **Which is more likely to be seen in surfers?**

Exostoses.

O   **What are the indications for removal of exostoses?**

Less than 1mm aperature, recurrent otitis externa, water trapping.

O   **What is the term for a keratin plug occluding the EAC?**

Keratosis obturans.

O   **How do patients with keratosis obturans usually present?**

Conductive hearing loss, acute severe otalgia, usually bilaterally; otorrhea is rare.

O   **What are the physical findings in a patient with keratosis obturans?**

Thickened TM, widened EAC medially, hyperemic canal skin with granulation tissue.

O   **How do patients with EAC cholesteatoma present?**

Chronic dull pain, usually unilaterally, with otorrhea and normal hearing.

O   **What are the physical findings in a patient with EAC cholesteatoma?**

Localized erosion and periostitis of the posterior-inferior EAC associated with otorrhea.

O   **What are the symptoms of patulous eustachian tube?**

Aural fullness, autophony, tympanophonia that improve when the head is placed down between the legs; onset often occurs with weight loss or after irradiation to the nasopharynx.

O   **What is tympanophonia?**

Audition of one's own breath sounds.

O   **What are some treatments for patulous eustachian tube?**

Reassurance, weight gain, SSKI (10 gtt in juice po TID), Premarin nasal spray (25 mg in 30 cc NS, 3 gtt per nose TID), occlusion of the ET, and myringotomy and tympanostomy tube placement.

O   **What signs and symptoms are specific for necrotizing otitis externa (NOE)?**

Persistent otalgia for longer than 1 month.
Persistent, purulent otorrhea with granulation tissue for several weeks.
Diabetes mellitus, another immunocompromised state, or advanced age.
Cranial nerve involvement.

O   **Why are diabetics more prone to NOE?**

The pH of their cerumen is higher and more conducive to bacterial growth.

O   **How does the infection spread from the external canal to the skull base?**

Through the fissures of Santorini.

O   **What is the most causative organism of NOE?**

Pseudomonas aeruginosa.

O   **Which cranial nerves are most commonly involved in NOE?**

VII (75%), X (70%), XI (56%).

O   **What imaging studies are used to diagnose NOE?**

CT scan with contrast, technetium-99m bone scan.

O   **What study is used to monitor the response to therapy?**

Gallium-67 scan.

O   **How is NOE treated?**

6 weeks of 2 different IV antibiotics directed against the organism cultured; alternatively, ciprofloxacin and rifampin for several months; hyperbaric oxygen is recommended for advanced NOE.

O   **Why is ciprofloxacin contraindicated in children?**

It has been shown to cause arthropathy of the weight-bearing joints in immature animals.

O   **What medication reduces the absorption of ciprofloxacin?**

Antacids containing calcium or magnesium salts.

O   **When is surgery indicated in the treatment of NOE?**

Progression of pain despite aggressive medical therapy, persistence of granulations, and development of cranial nerve involvement.

O   **Why is it difficult to treat infections involving the perichondrium or cartilage?**

The metabolic demands of cartilage are low, and its blood supply is hence diminished.

O   **How can one differentiate between relapsing polychondritis involving the ear and other causes of external otitis?**

Relapsing polychondritis spares the lobule.

O   **What is the incidence of congenital aural atresia?**

1:10,000 – 20,000.

O   **What % of these are bilateral?**

33%.

O   **What does stenosis of the external auditory canal predispose to?**

Canal cholesteatoma.

O   **Which portion of the ossicular chain is least likely to be malformed in patients with congenital aural atresia?**

Stapes footplate.

O   **What is the incidence of facial nerve displacement in congenital aural atresia?**

25 – 30%.

O   **Using the rating system developed by Jahrsdoefer, what score is associated with the best outcome after surgical treatment of aural atresia?**

8 or greater (80% chance of obtaining an SRT 15 – 25 dB).

O   **T/F: A patient with a score of 5 or less is considered a very poor operative candidate.**

True.

O   **What is the most important factor in assessing the possibility of surgery in a patient with congenital aural atresia?**

Presence of the stapes.

O   **Why is it particularly difficult to assess the auditory function in patients with bilateral atresia?**

Masking dilemma.

O   **What test should be used to assess auditory function in these patients?**

ABR.

O   **Which wave of the ABR is ear-specific?**

Wave I.

O   **In a patient with aural atresia and no evidence of SNHL, when should a CT scan of the temporal bones be obtained?**

Age 4 or 5.

O   **On CT imaging, which ear structures are best seen on *axial* views?**

Body of the malleus and incus, incudostapedial joint, and the round window.

O   **On CT imaging, which ear structures are best seen on *coronal* views?**

Stapes, oval window and the vestibule.

O   **Why should surgery be delayed until age 5?**

To allow for completion of pneumatization of the temporal bone.

O   **T/F: Surgery is contraindicated in children with unilateral atresia.**

False; many will operate if the patient is likely to achieve a residual conductive deficit of 30 dB or less.

O   **What factors are considered contraindications to correction of unilateral atresia?**

Poor mastoid pneumatization, anterior displacement of the middle ear, and facial nerve anomalies.

O   **What are the 2 basic approaches for repair of aural atresia?**

Transmastoid and anterior approaches.

O   **What are the 2 most important landmarks of the anterior approach?**

The middle cranial fossa dura superiorly and the TMJ anteriorly.

O   **What advantage does hugging the middle fossa dura have on protecting the facial nerve?**

One will enter the middle ear first in the epitympanum; the facial nerve will always lie medial to the ossicular heads in the epitympanum.

O   **What are the reasons for persistent conductive hearing loss after aural atresia repair?**

Inadequate mobilization of the ossicular mass from the atretic bone, an unrecognized incudostapedial joint discontinuity, or a fixed stapes.

О   **What are the reasons for recurrent conductive hearing loss after aural atresia repair?**

Refixation of the ossicular chain or tympanic membrane lateralization.

О   **What structure is most at risk during removal of a 1st branchial arch sinus?**

Facial nerve.

О   **What is the most likely diagnosis of a fistula 1 cm anterior to the tragus associated with a cystic bulge in the anterior ear canal in an 8-month-old infant?**

1st branchial arch sinus, type 2.

FACIAL NERVE

○ **What are the limits of the tympanic segment of VII?**

Geniculate ganglion to the 2nd genu (adjacent to the pyramidal process).

○ **What are the limits of the mastoid segment of VII?**

Pyramidal process to the stylomastoid foramen.

○ **What are the surgical landmarks for the tympanic segment of VII?**

Cochleariform process, oval window, pyramidal process, semicanal for the tensor tympani, vertical groove on promontory for the tympanic nerve.

○ **Where does the facial nerve lie in relation to the cochleariform process?**

Posterosuperior.

○ **How is the facial nerve identified using the semicanal for the tensor tympani?**

When followed posteriorly, its inferior border is continuous with the upper margin of the oval window and the inferior border of VII.

○ **How is the facial nerve identified using the tympanic nerve?**

Groove for the tympanic nerve is followed superiorly to the cochleariform process.

○ **What are the surgical landmarks for VII in its mastoid segment?**

Lateral SCC, fossa incudis, and the digastric ridge.

○ **What is the relation of the lateral SCC to the fossa incudis?**

Short crus of the incus is inferolateral to the lateral SCC; the fossa incudis is at the tip of the short crus.

○ **What is the relationship of VII to the lateral SCC and the fossa incudis?**

Medial to the fossa incudis and inferior to the lateral canal.

○ **What are the landmarks of the tympanic segment of VII from the mastoid approach?**

Lateral SCC and the cog.

○ **What is the cog?**

A ridge of bone that extends inferiorly from the tegmen epitympanum and partially separates the anterior epitympanic compartment from the mesoepitympanum.

○ **What is the relationship of the tympanic portion of VII to the cog?**

VII lies anterior to the cog in the floor of the anterior epitympanum.

O   **Where is the facial nerve most commonly injured during mastoid surgery?**

Near the 2nd genu as it enters the mastoid cavity.

O   **What is the relationship of the 2nd genu of the facial nerve to the lateral semicircular canal and short process of the incus?**

Inferior to the lateral semicircular canal and medial to the short process of the incus.

O   **What is the management of intraoperative facial nerve transection?**

Immediate repair with primary anastomosis if possible.

O   **What if primary anastomosis is not possible?**

Use a cable graft with great auricular nerve as the donor.

O   **What if the nerve is only partially transected?**

If greater than 1/2 remains, reapproximate the remaining nerve and perform regional decompression. If less than 1/2 remains, remove the injured segment and repair as with complete transection.

O   **What prognostic information does ENoG provide?**

Patients with 95% degeneration or greater have a 50% chance of unfavorable recovery; if at least 10% function is retained in the 1st 21 days of paralysis, 80 – 100% functional recovery is highly likely.

O   **What is the next most accurate test when ENoG is unavailable?**

Maximal stimulation test.

O   **How long does it take for 100% Wallerian degeneration to occur after complete nerve transection?**

3 – 5 days.

O   **How long does it take for 100% Wallerian degeneration to occur after a compressive conduction block?**

14 – 21 days.

O   **Between which days after injury is the degree of axonotmesis and neurotmesis unclear?**

6 – 14.

O   **What test should be performed when 100% neural degeneration is recorded with ENoG?**

Voluntary EMG recording; regenerating nerve fibers conducting at different rates can result in an overestimation of neural degeneration on ENoG.

O   **What should be done if motor unit potentials are detected on EMG?**

No further therapy is indicated.

O   **When is ENoG evaluation meaningful?**

Between days 3 and 21 after complete loss of voluntary function.

O   **What electrophysiologic test is more useful 3 weeks after the onset of complete facial paralysis?**

EMG.

O   **What sort of EMG pattern is associated with nerve regeneration?**

Polyphasic action potentials.

O   **What sort of EMG pattern is associated with nerve degeneration?**

Fibrillation potentials.

O   **What is the most common area of facial nerve injury following trauma?**

Perigenicular area.

O   **What are the indications for surgical exploration of the facial nerve following temporal bone trauma?**

NET >3.5 mA side-to-side threshold differences or ENoG >90% degeneration.

O   **Which approach is best in patients with normal hearing?**

Supralabyrinthine approach.

O   **What are the 3 types of nerve injury?**

Neuropraxia, axonotmesis, and neurotmesis.

O   **Which of these result in Wallerian degeneration?**

Axonotmesis and neurotmesis.

O   **Which of these has a more rapid rate of Wallerian degeneration?**

Neurotmesis.

O   **What is Sutherland's classification for nerve injury?**

1st degree: reversible conduction block.
2nd degree: Wallerian degeneration occurs but endoneurium stays intact and recovery is usually complete.
3rd degree: endoneurium is destroyed but perineurium stays intact and recovery is incomplete.
4th degree: all is destroyed except for the epineurium; recovery is poor.
5th degree: complete nerve transection; untreated recovery is not expected.

O   **What is the most accurate predictor of poor recovery of facial nerve function following injury?**

Total paralysis of immediate onset.

○   **What is the most commonly proposed theory of the etiology of Bell's palsy?**

Activation of a latent virus present within the geniculate ganglion leading to entrapment, ischemia, and degeneration of the labyrinthine segment of VII.

○   **What viruses are most commonly implicated in the etiology of Bell's palsy?**

Herpes simplex and herpes zoster viruses.

○   **T/F: Enhancement of the facial nerve is commonly seen on MRI of patients with Bell's palsy and is likely to resolve in 2 – 4 months.**

True.

○   **What is the outcome of Bell's palsy left untreated?**

Complete recovery in 71%; permanent diminished function in 16%; poorer prognosis if >60 years of age and if onset of recovery >3 months after initial onset of paralysis.

○   **What is the narrowest intratemporal portion of the fallopian canal?**

Entrance to the fallopian canal at the lateral aspect of the IAC (fundus).

○   **T/F: Addition of acyclovir to prednisone for treatment of Bell's palsy has not been shown to result in significant improvement of facial nerve function.**

False.

○   **What is the outcome of patients with Bell's palsy who have 90% or more degeneration on ENoG within the 1st 14 days of onset and undergo decompression?**

91% have a good outcome (House I or II) 7 months after paralysis.

○   **What is the outcome of these patients who are treated with steroids alone?**

42% have a good outcome.

○   **What is the outcome of these patients who undergo surgical decompression >14 days after injury?**

Similar outcome as patients treated with steroids.

○   **What is the incidence of recurrent facial palsy?**

5 – 7%.

○   **What is the mean interval to the 1st recurrence?**

9.8 years.

○   **What factors increase the risk of recurrent Bell's palsy?**

Diabetes mellitus and family history.

○ **What is the incidence of diabetes mellitus in patients with recurrent Bell's palsy?**

31%.

○ **The triad of recurrent facial palsy, orofacial edema, and lingua plicata is classic for what disease?**

Melkersson-Rosenthal syndrome (orofacial granulomatosis).

○ **What is lingua plicata?**

Scrotal tongue.

○ **What differentiates herpes zoster oticus from Ramsay Hunt syndrome?**

Ramsay Hunt syndrome is herpes zoster oticus + facial nerve paralysis.

○ **What % of patients with Ramsay Hunt syndrome have VIIIth nerve involvement?**

20%.

○ **Which etiology of facial nerve palsy has a worse prognosis: Bell's palsy or Ramsay Hunt syndrome?**

Ramsay Hunt syndrome.

○ **What are negative prognostic factors for Ramsay Hunt syndrome?**

Increased age and a simultaneous onset of paralysis with vesicular eruption.

○ **T/F: Evidence of viral etiology for Ramsay Hunt syndrome is well documented.**

True.

○ **T/F: Evidence of viral etiology for Bell's palsy is well documented.**

False.

○ **Why must the dose of acyclovir be larger for patients with varicella zoster virus (VZV)?**

The thymidine kinase of VZV is much less sensitive to acyclovir than the herpes simplex virus.

○ **What is the recommended treatment for Ramsay Hunt syndrome?**

Acyclovir 800 mg five times a day x 10 days and prednisone taper x 14 days.

○ **What is the treatment for otogenic facial palsy in association with acute suppurative otitis media?**

Wide myringotomy, cultures, and IV antibiotics.

○ **What organisms are most often associated with facial palsy due to chronic otitis media?**

Gram-negative organisms and *Staphylococcus aureus*.

O **What is the incidence of facial palsy as the presenting symptom of tuberculous mastoiditis?**

39%.

O **What % of patients with Lyme disease have facial nerve paralysis as the sole manifestation?**

20%.

O **What is the most likely cause of bilateral facial palsy in a young adult?**

Sarcoidosis.

O **Where are intracranial lesions that cause bilateral facial paralysis located?**

Pons.

O **What is Heerfordt's syndrome?**

Facial nerve palsy with anterior uveitis, parotid gland enlargement, and fever.

O **What is Tangier's disease?**

Autosomal recessive disorder of lipid metabolism characterized by low apolipoprotein A-1 and HDL levels. Clinical features include facial diplegia, neuropathy, and coronary artery disease.

O **What test should be performed on Afro-Caribbean migrants with idiopathic facial nerve palsy?**

HTLV-1 antibody screen.

O **What causes hemifacial spasm?**

A vascular loop, most commonly of the anterior or posterior inferior cerebellar artery, impinging on the root of VII.

O **What is the initial treatment for hemifacial spasm?**

Baclofen.

O **What is the procedure of choice for patients with hemifacial spasm?**

Microvascular decompression.

O **What is the most common cause of unilateral facial palsy in a newborn infant?**

Forceps delivery.

O **When the facial nerve is sacrificed, what must be done prior to reconstruction?**

Frozen section confirmation of negative nerve margins.

O **Branches of the facial nerve anterior to _____ do not require reconstruction for return of function.**

Vertical line from lateral canthus.

○ **Which methods of facial nerve reconstruction have the potential for spontaneous emotional response?**

Direct anastomosis and cable grafting.

○ **After primary anastomosis, what is the typical return of facial nerve function?**

House grade II or III.

○ **T/F: There is a consistent topographic representation of fibers from a specific section of a nerve innervating certain parts of the face.**

False.

○ **T/F: Primary anastomosis after rerouting generally leads to a better functional outcome than cable grafting.**

True.

○ **Defects greater than _____ cannot be rerouted and require cable grafting.**

15 – 17 mm.

○ **What are some possible nerves used for cable grafting?**

Sural, greater auricular, dorsal radial cutaneous, supraclavicular nerves.

○ **Which of these is used most often?**

Greater auricular nerve.

○ **Which of these can provide the most length?**

Sural nerve (35 cm).

○ **What is the advantage of the dorsal radial cutaneous nerve?**

It branches as it approaches the wrist, making distal separation into bundles for facial nerve branch anastomosis easier.

○ **What is the best functional outcome of cable grafting?**

House grade III or IV.

○ **Which anastomotic technique is preferred by most surgeons?**

Epineural anastomosis using 3 – 8 sutures of 8-0 or 10-0 synthetic monofilament suture.

○ **T/F: No improvement in functional outcome has been demonstrated with the use of tubes or conduits in facial nerve anastomosis or grafting.**

True.

○   **T/F: Postoperative radiation does not significantly affect the outcome after facial nerve grafting.**

True

○   **What is the minimal time for functional return of the facial nerve after anastomosis or grafting?**

4 – 6 months.

○   **Which reconstructive options restore facial nerve function most quickly?**

Static slings, gold weights, tarsorrhaphies.

○   **If a tumor-free proximal nerve stump is unavailable for nerve grafting, what method should be used for optimal functional outcome?**

If reconstruction is undertaken within 2 years of division, grafting of the proximal portion of another cranial nerve to the distal stump of the facial nerve is the next best choice.

○   **Which cranial nerve is most often grafted to the distal facial nerve?**

Ipsilateral hypoglossal.

○   **What is a major contraindication to this procedure?**

Paralysis of IX or X.

○   **What is the primary drawback of hypoglossal-facial nerve grafting?**

Ipsilateral tongue paralysis.

○   **What can be done to ameliorate this problem?**

Use of a mid-tongue Z-plasty; use of only part of the hypoglossal nerve (jump graft); reinnervation of the hypoglossal nerve with the ansa cervicalis.

○   **What is a jump graft?**

The greater auricular nerve is sutured end-to-side to XII and end-to-side to the distal facial nerve.

○   **How can dynamic rehabilitation be achieved in a patient with a 10-year history of facial paralysis following radical parotidectomy?**

Crossfacial nerve graft plus microneurovascular muscle transfer.

○   **What are other indications for free muscle transposition surgery for facial reanimation?**

Möbius syndrome or destruction of muscles secondary to trauma.

○   **What is the advantage of the microneurovascular muscle transfer over the temporalis muscle sling in the treatment of facial paralysis?**

Has the potential to restore spontaneous muscle expressions.

◯   **After microneurovascular muscle transfer, what is the maximum muscle power attainable compared to normal?**

55%.

◯   **What are some other options for improvement of function after facial paralysis?**

Static fascial slings, dynamic muscle slings, free muscle transfers, gold weight upper lid implants, lid-tightening procedures, brow lift.

◯   **Can a patient with a gold weight have an MRI?**

Yes.

◯   **What is the significance of the Bell's phenomenon prior to gold weight implantation?**

If the patient has a good Bell's reflex, then the surgeon can be more conservative, choosing a lighter implant to avoid ptosis.

◯   **Into which plane is a gold weight placed?**

Suborbicularis.

◯   **What happens if the implant is placed too deep?**

Can damage the levator muscle, causing ptosis.

◯   **Where on the lid is the implant placed?**

2 mm above the lash line.

◯   **What are the complications of gold weight implantation?**

Induced astigmatism, ptosis, migration, extrusion, persistent inflammation.

MIDDLE EAR

O **What are the 2 types of tympanic membrane perforations?**

Central and marginal.

O **Which of these is associated with cholesteatoma?**

Marginal.

O **What are the indications for performing a lateral tympanoplasty?**

Anterior or large perforations, revision tympanoplasty, or if the anterior canal wall is in the way.

O **What are the advantages of lateral tympanoplasty?**

Excellent exposure, high graft take rate (95%), most versatile approach.

O **What are the disadvantages of lateral tympanoplasty?**

Longer healing time, potential for anterior blunting or lateral healing, technically more difficult.

O **What are the complications of lateral tympanoplasty?**

Anterior blunting, lateralization, epithelial pearls, canal stenosis.

O **T/F: Postoperative hearing improvement and reperforation rates are similar for medial and lateral tympanoplasty.**

True.

O **What are the 3 principle theories regarding the etiology of cholesteatoma?**

Congenital theory (von Remak, 1854 and Virchow, 1855); metaplasia theory (Trolscht, 1873); migration theory (Habermann, 1888).

O **What are the 2 parts of a cholesteatoma?**

Amorphous center surrounded by keratinized squamous epithelium.

O **What are the 2 types of cholesteatomas?**

Congenital and acquired.

O **What are the 2 types of acquired cholesteatomas?**

Primary and secondary.

O **What is the difference between a primary and a secondary cholesteatoma?**

Primary usually occurs in the attic at Shrapnell's membrane and starts as a retraction pocket; secondary is associated with chronic middle ear infection and TM perforations.

○   **Which ossicle is most commonly involved in patients with cholesteatoma?**

Incus.

○   **What % patients have erosion of the scutum with cholesteatoma?**

42%.

○   **What are the most common sites of origin of primary acquired cholesteatomas?**

Posterior epitympanum, posterior mesotympanum, and anterior epitympanum (in descending order of frequency).

○   **What is the typical route of spread of cholesteatomas originating in the posterior epitympanum?**

Starting from Prussak's space, penetrate posteriorly to the superior incudal space lateral to the body of the incus and progress to the aditus and the antrum.

○   **What is the typical route of spread of cholesteatomas originating in anterior mesotympanum?**

Descend to the pouch of Von Troeltch, and may involve the stapes, sinus tympani, or facial recess.

○   **What % of cholesteatomas are complicated by a labyrinthine fistula?**

5 – 10%.

○   **Where does this most often occur?**

Lateral semicircular canal (75%).

○   **In a patient with a cholesteatoma, what factors make presence of a fistula highly unlikely?**

Disease <20 years, normal bone conduction, negative fistula test, no history of dizziness, and normal facial nerve function.

○   **What are the indications for simple mastoidectomy?**

Acute coalescent mastoiditis with complications or acute mastoiditis that does not resolve after appropriate antibiotic therapy and myringotomy.

○   **What is a modified radical mastoidectomy?**

Conversion of the mastoid, epitympanum, and external auditory canal into a common cavity by removal of the posterior and superior external bony canal walls.

○   **T/F: The modified radical mastoidectomy does not involve a tympanoplasty.**

True.

○   **What is a radical mastoidectomy?**

Conversion of the mastoid, antrum, and middle ear into a common cavity, with removal of the tympanic membrane, malleus, incus, chorda tympani, and mucoperiosteum.

O   **Should a cholesteatoma be removed over a fistula?**

Controversial, in that leaving a piece of matrix to seal the fistula increases the risk of recurrent cholesteatoma, while completely removing the matrix and exposing the fistula increases the risk of hearing loss and vertigo.

O   **What is the significance of pain in a patient with cholesteatoma or chronic otitis media?**

Expanding mass or empyema in the antrum.

O   **What is the incidence of facial nerve paralysis in patients with chronic otitis media and cholesteatoma?**

1%.

O   **How is this treated?**

Expedient elimination of infection.

O   **In patients with chronic otitis media but not cholesteatoma, what level of hearing loss is associated with ossicular chain disruption or fixation?**

30 dB or more.

O   **What is a congenital cholesteatoma?**

Embryonal inclusion of undifferentiated squamous epithelium in the middle ear behind an intact TM, usually with no history of otitis media.

O   **Other than the middle ear, where else may congenital cholesteatomas arise?**

Petrous apex, cerebellopontine angle, mastoid, external auditory canal.

O   **What % of congenital cholesteatomas are bilateral?**

3%.

O   **What is the mean age of presentation for congenital cholesteatoma?**

4.5 years.

O   **What is the significance of hearing loss in the absence of middle ear effusion in patients with congenital cholesteatoma?**

Most lesions begin anterosuperiorly and extend posteriorly with growth. Hearing loss indicates posterior extension with involvement of the stapes superstructure and/or the lenticular process of the incus.

O   **T/F: The mastoid bones of patients with congenital cholesteatoma are most often well-aerated.**

True.

O   **What are the indications for 2nd look surgery after removal of a congenital cholesteatoma?**

Obvious recurrent disease, unexplained deterioration in hearing, concern about the adequacy of the initial surgery or disease found to extend into the antrum or mastoid.

O   **How do the surgical findings differ during removal of congenital cholesteatoma from removal of cholesteatoma associated with chronic suppurative otitis media?**

Absence of inflammatory changes/adhesions and easier removal with potential for complete preservation of the middle ear mucosa.

O   **What are the boundaries of the facial recess?**

Chorda tympani laterally, upper mastoid segment of VII medially, bone of fossa incudis superiorly.

O   **What type of cholesteatoma is most frequently found in the facial recess?**

One associated with a perforation below the posterior malleolar fold.

O   **Which areas of the middle ear are most difficult to see during mastoidectomy?**

Infrapyramidal and tympanic recesses.

O   **According to Sheehy, in which situations is the canal wall down (CWD) approach most appropriate?**

Only-hearing ear, very contracted mastoid, mastoid with a labyrinthine fistula, or presence of canal wall erosion due to disease.

O   **What are the disadvantages of the CWD procedure in the management of cholesteatoma?**

Healing is slower, indefinite periodic cleaning and dry ear precautions are required, and hearing aids are more difficult to fit in the meatus.

O   **What are the 2 most important principles of CWD procedures?**

Lowering the posterior canal wall to create a round cavity and creating a large meatus.

O   **Why is it important to saucerize the cavity margins?**

The soft tissues and auricle will assume a more medial position during healing, resulting in a smaller cavity.

O   **What is the benefit of amputating the mastoid tip?**

Reduces cavity size and eliminates a dependent cavity area that is not visible.

O   **Which portions of the ossicular chain are always removed in CWD procedures?**

Incus and head of the malleus.

O   **If a CWD procedure is used to treat a posterior-superior retraction cholesteatoma, what would be the most likely site of residual cholesteatoma?**

Sinus tympani.

O   **What are the disadvantages of the canal wall up (CWU) approach?**

Limited exposure of the anterior epitympanum, sinus tympani, and facial recess.

O   **If the CWU procedure is chosen, what are the indications for a 2nd look?**

Missing middle ear mucosa or extensive cholesteatoma.

O   **What is the single most important factor affecting hearing results after CWD tympanomastoid surgery?**

Maintenance of a pneumatized space juxtaposed to the round window.

O   **What techniques can be used to accomplish this?**

Placement of the fascia graft such that it does not obliterate the space between the eustachian tube orifice and the round window; placement of silastic crescent in the hypotympanum.

O   **What other techniques can help improve hearing results?**

Shielding the round window to increase the difference in sound pressure between the oval and round windows; placing the graft directly atop the head of the stapes when the suprastructure is present; using a TORP or placing the graft directly on the stapes footplate when the suprastructure is not present (type IV tympanoplasty).

O   **What are the potential problems with a type IV tympanoplasty?**

Narrowing of the middle ear space and graft lateralization.

O   **What are the indications for using a TORP when the stapes suprastructure is present?**

Stapes tilted towards the promontory, partial arch necrosis, and unusually deep oval window niche where a PORP might contact the fallopian canal and/or promontory.

O   **What are the expected residual hearing levels after PORP and TORP?**

15 dB conductive hearing loss PORP; 25 dB conductive hearing loss TORP.

O   **What are the advantages of using porous polyethylene prostheses over fitted autograft ossicles?**

Hearing is more stable, decreased incidence of residual and recurrent cholesteatoma.

O   **What is the most common cause of failure using a fitted ossicle for middle ear reconstruction?**

Separation of the ossicle from the stapes.

O   **What is the rate of extrusion of middle ear prostheses?**

4 – 7%.

O   **What factors contribute to extrusion?**

Eustachian tube dysfunction (70%), graft failure, cartilage resorption.

O   **What is the overall success (accounting for extrusion, HL, and graft take) at 4 months using TORP or PORP?**

58% TORP; 64% PORP.

○   **How should an extruded prosthesis be managed?**

Allow spontaneous extrusion; TM may heal and make a spontaneous connection.

○   **What are the indications for using plastic sheeting in middle ear surgery?**

Absence of mucosa on the promontory, in most of the middle ear, or in the middle ear cleft (except in the eustachian tube).

○   **What is the purpose of the plastic sheeting in these conditions?**

To prevent adhesions from forming and to allow mucosa to grow over denuded areas.

○   **What are the indications for staging a tympanoplasty without mastoidectomy?**

Extensive mucous membrane destruction, stapes fixation.

○   **What can cause persistent cavity discharge after CWD procedures?**

High facial ridge, particularly large cavity, open middle ear space, inadequate meatal opening, poor postoperative care leading to infection.

○   **What are the options for surgical management of the chronically draining mastoid cavity?**

Autologous cultured epithelial graft (from buccal mucosa), large meatoplasty, revision mastoidectomy, reconstruction of canal wall with an aerated cavity, mastoid cavity obliteration, and mastoid/middle ear obliteration.

○   **When is mastoid and middle ear obliteration most appropriate?**

In a dead ear, without cholesteatoma.

○   **What is the Palva flap?**

Technique used for mastoid obliteration where the soft tissue off the back of the ear is swung into the mastoid.

○   **What are the intracranial complications of otitis media (OM)?**

Epidural abscess/granulation tissue, sigmoid sinus thrombosis, meningitis, brain abscess, subdural abscess.

○   **What are the extracranial complications of OM?**

Subperiosteal (Bezold's) abscess, petrositis, labyrinthitis, facial nerve paralysis.

○   **What factors predispose one to complications from OM?**

Chronic infection, history of mastoid surgery, cholesteatoma, diabetes, immunocompromise.

○   **What is the most common complication of acute mastoiditis?**

Subperiosteal abscess.

O   **What is the treatment for uncomplicated acute mastoiditis?**

Tympanocentesis for culture and IV antibiotics.

O   **When is a CT scan obtained?**

If signs of progression arise while on IV antibiotics or if the patient presents with possible intracranial complications.

O   **When is mastoidectomy indicated?**

If the CT scan shows coalescent mastoiditis and/or intracranial involvement.

O   **What are the early signs and symptoms of intracranial infection?**

Prolonged suppurative OM, fetid discharge and persistent pain despite adequate treatment, bony destruction of inner cortex of mastoid on CT scan.

O   **What are the three most common organisms of OM that result in intracranial infections?**

Streptococcus faecalis, Proteus, Bacteroides fragilis.

O   **What is the most common complaint of patients with an epidural abscess/granulation tissue?**

Deep, constant pain in the temporal area that is very steroid responsive.

O   **What are the most common signs and symptoms of sigmoid sinus thrombosis?**

Picket fence fever, cannon ball infiltrates on CXR, torticollis, jugular foramen syndrome, otitic hydrocephalus.

O   **What are the radiographic findings of sigmoid sinus thrombosis?**

Delta sign on CT scan with contrast and central nonenhancement of the sigmoid sinus; decreased intraluminal signal on MRI with gadolinium.

O   **What are the three most common organisms causing meningitis secondary to OM?**

Haemophilus influenzae, type B, S*treptococcus pneumoniae, Neisseria meningitides.*

O   **What factor strongly correlates with survival and long term neurologic deficits in patients with a brain abscess?**

Patient's level of consciousness at the time of diagnosis.

O   **Where is dehiscence of the bony facial canal most common?**

Over the oval window.

O   **What vessels can be injured in the middle ear during tympanoplasty?**

Persistent stapedial artery, superficial petrosal branch of the middle meningeal artery, high-riding jugular vein, and anomalous carotid artery.

O   **What is the most common postoperative complication of pressure equalizing tube insertion?**

Persistent otorrhea.

O   **What are the most common pathogens cultured from otorrhea after tympanotomy tubes in children younger than 3?**

Haemophilus influenza and *Diplococcus pneumoniae*.

O   **What are the most common pathogens cultured from otorrhea after tympanotomy tubes in children older than 3?**

Staphylococcus aureus and *Pseudomonas aeruginosa*.

O   **In a child with spontaneous CSF leak to the middle ear, where is the leak most commonly located?**

Around the stapes footplate.

O   **What is the most common etiology of spontaneous CSF leak to the middle ear in adults?**

Through a defect in the mastoid tegmen secondary to a meningoencephalocele.

O   **What is the incidence of tympanic membrane perforation 6 months after pressure equalizing tube extrusion?**

0.5 – 2%.

O   **What are the most common reasons for recurrent conductive hearing loss after tympanoplasty?**

Recurrent perforation, blunting of the angle between the tympanic membrane and the external auditory canal, graft lateralization, graft thickening and adhesions, severe graft atelectasis.

O   **What technique is employed during ossiculoplasty to decrease the risk of prosthesis extrusion?**

Placement of cartilage between the prosthesis and the tympanic membrane.

O   **What is the management of injury to the sigmoid sinus during mastoidectomy?**

Apply gentle pressure, place a Surgicel or Gelfoam patch, and continue with surgery.

O   **What is the management of injury to the dura with CSF leak during mastoidectomy?**

Repair with temporalis fascia held in place with sutures or packing and continue with surgery; small tears can be managed with a Surgicel or Gelfoam patch.

O   **Unbeknownst to the surgeon, the dura is torn during mastoidectomy, and postoperatively, the patient develops a severe headache, followed by hemiplegia and coma. What has likely happened?**

Pneumocephalus; torn dura can create a ball valve-like effect and trap air from the middle ear. Influx of air may occur during Valsalva or as a result of high intracranial negative pressure due to the rapid escape of CSF through the tear.

O   **What is the most common cause of perilymph fistula?**

Otologic surgery (stapedectomy).

O   **What congenital ear malformation is most commonly associated with perilymph fistula in children?**

Mondini deformity.

O   **What is the most common location for iatrogenic labyrinthine fistula formation during mastoidectomy?**

Lateral semicircular canal.

O   **What is the management of intraoperative violation of the labyrinth?**

Immediate application of a Gelfoam patch or other tissue seal (other than fat).

O   **What is the prognosis after such an injury?**

Good if immediately recognized and treated.

O   **What are the most common reasons for mastoid surgery failure without recurrent cholesteatoma?**

Persistent suppurative disease in unexenterated air cells (most commonly at the sinodural angle and along the tegmen) and technical factors such as high facial ridge or meatal stenosis.

O   **During stapedectomy, the entire stapes footplate falls into the vestibule. What should be done?**

It should be left in the vestibule, as attempts to retrieve it are more likely to cause damage than leaving the footplate where it is.

O   **What is a "perilymph gusher"?**

Rapid release of perilymph after stapes footplate fenestration due to pressure and fluid from the CSF compartment venting through the inner ear.

O   **What are the symptoms and signs of a poststapedectomy perilymph fistula?**

Episodic vertigo, especially with exertion, sensorineural hearing loss, loss of speech discrimination, and nystagmus with changes of air pressure on the TM.

O   **What are the 5 primary causes of conductive hearing loss after stapedectomy?**

Failure to recognize obliterative otosclerosis of the round window; displacement of the prosthesis after head trauma or large changes in middle ear pressure; necrosis of the long process of the incus; migration of the prosthesis in the oval window; and adhesions.

O   **How is the round window evaluated for normal movement?**

The membrane is not readily visible, so a drop of saline is placed in the niche and movement is seen as a change in light reflection on the meniscus when the prosthesis is palpated.

O   **Revision stapedectomy is performed. What should be done with the original prosthesis?**

If possible, it should be left in place, and a second fenestra and prosthesis should be placed.

○   **What are the three layers of the otic capsule?**

Outer periosteal layer, inner periosteal layer (endosteum) and the middle endochondral layer.

○   **Which of these layers does otosclerosis involve?**

Middle endochondral layer.

○   **What are the terms used to describe involvement of the oval window and cochlea?**

Fenestral otosclerosis and retrofenestral otosclerosis, respectively.

○   **What does the "Blue Mantles of Manasse" refer to?**

Basophilic appearance on hematoxylin and eosin staining of bone in the active stage of otosclerosis.

○   **What is "Schwartze's sign"?**

Reddish hue on the promontory associated with otosclerosis.

○   **What is the most commonly involved site of otosclerosis in the temporal bone?**

Anterior to the oval window at the fissula ante fenestrum.

○   **What % of cases of otosclerosis are bilateral?**

85%.

○   **At what age does otosclerosis peak in incidence?**

Third decade.

○   **What conditions accelerate hearing loss in patients with otosclerosis?**

Pregnancy, estrogen replacement.

○   **What genetic mutation has been implicated as a possible cause of otosclerosis?**

Mutation of the COLIA1 gene on chromosome 17q.

○   **What virus is thought to play a role in the etiology of otosclerosis?**

Measles.

○   **What is the inheritance pattern of otosclerosis?**

Autosomal dominant with incomplete penetrance (only 25 – 40% of carriers express the phenotype).

○   **In patients with bilateral otosclerosis, which ear should be operated on first?**

Poorer hearing ear.

○   **In patients where one ear has previously been operated on and hearing loss is equal bilaterally, which ear should be operated on?**

The unoperated ear.

○ **In patients with bilateral otosclerosis and equal hearing loss, which ear should be operated on?**

Right-handed surgeon should work on the left ear (or patient preference).

○ **When is stapedectomy contraindicated?**

In young children until it has been demonstrated that they are not prone to otitis media, in the presence of active middle or external ear disease or active URI, tympanic membrane perforation, Menière's disease.

○ **Why is stapedectomy dangerous in patients with Menière's disease?**

A dilated saccule may sit immediately beneath the footplate and be injured upon entry into the vestibule.

○ **What is the medical treatment for otosclerosis?**

Sodium fluoride, vitamin D.

○ **What is obliterative otosclerosis?**

Margins of the footplate cannot be seen or removed.

○ **What is the significance of a white versus a blue floating footplate?**

Hearing success is much less in the presence of a white floating footplate (52%) versus a blue floating footplate (97%).

○ **What is the advantage of using a laser for stapedectomy?**

No-touch technique with less risk of a floating footplate.

○ **What is the significance of sensorineural hearing loss after stapedectomy?**

If no tissue graft was used, 50% of SNHL will be due to fistulas and should be revised.

○ **What is Tullio's phenomenon?**

Vertigo with loud noise.

○ **What is the significance of Tullio's phenomenon after stapedectomy?**

Suggests that the prosthesis is too long and impinging on the saccule.

○ **What is the incidence of malleus ankylosis during primary surgery for otosclerosis?**

0.4 – 1.6%.

○ **What is the incidence of malleus ankylosis during revision surgery for otosclerosis?**

4.5 – 13.5%.

○ **What is the most common cause of malleus ankylosis?**

Congenital.

O   **What is thought to cause congenital malleus ankylosis?**

Poor development of the epitympanic space leaves the head of the incus and malleus in close contact with the tegmen; a bony bridge can result between the epitympanum and the head of the malleus.

O   **T/F: Histologically, the bony structures are normal, without evidence of otosclerosis, in cases of malleus ankylosis.**

True.

O   **How does the hearing impairment from malleus ankylosis differ from that of otosclerosis?**

In patients with malleus ankylosis, hearing impairment is mostly unilateral (78%); the air-bone gap is smaller (majority less than 20 dB); sensorineural hearing loss is more frequent, particularly at 4 kHz; acoustic reflex is more likely to be present on the contralateral ear and absent on the impaired ear.

O   **Is the acoustic reflex present in patients with otosclerosis?**

Usually it is absent bilaterally, even if the disease is unilateral.

O   **T/F: In cases of malleus fixation, mobilization of the malleus usually results in lasting hearing improvement.**

False.

O   **What is the optimal treatment of malleus fixation?**

Removal of the head of the malleus and interposition of the incus between the manubrium and the stapes head.

O   **How is far-advanced otosclerosis (FAO) defined?**

Otosclerosis with an air conduction threshold greater than 85 dB and a bone conduction threshold not measurable.

O   **What are the histopathologic findings of patients with FAO?**

Invasion of otosclerotic foci into the cochlear endosteum and the stapes footplate.

O   **What features on history distinguish FAO from profound SNHL?**

Family history of otosclerosis; progressive hearing loss usually of long duration; history of hearing aid use that is no longer beneficial or present use of a hearing aid with benefit beyond that which would be expected for the severity of the hearing loss; paracusis; and previous audiograms indicating an air-bone gap.

O   **What features on physical exam distinguish FAO from profound SNHL?**

Patients with FAO more likely will have a soft voice with better quality than expected for the degree of hearing loss and the ability to hear a 512 Hz tuning fork placed on the teeth, dentures, or gums.

O   **How much more bone conduction will dental conduction provide than mastoid conduction?**

11 dB.

○ **What is the significance of the ability to hear a tuning fork placed on the teeth?**

Indicates that cochlear reserve is present and surgery may be beneficial.

○ **What is the most common tumor of the middle ear?**

Glomus tympanicum.

WOUND HEALING 101

O   **The dermis primarily contains what type(s) of collagen?**

Type I (80%) and Type III (15%).

O   **What is the ratio of Type I to Type II collagen in the skin?**

8:1.

O   **Which type of collagen is a crucial component of the basement membrane?**

Type IV.

O   **What is the predominant type of collagen in scar tissue?**

Type I.

O   **T/F: Scar maturation occurs more rapidly in children than in adults.**

False.

O   **What is the single best measure of nutritional status?**

Serum albumin level.

O   **What serum albumin level is associated with malnutrition?**

Less than 3 g/dl.

O   **Which serum proteins can be used to assess short-term nutritional status?**

Transferrin (half-life of 8 to 9 days), prealbumin (half-life of 2 days) and retinal-binding globulin (half-life of 12 hours).

O   **What are the products of platelet degranulation?**

TGF-ß and platelet derived growth factor (PDGF).

O   **T/F: TGF-ß stimulates endothelial cell proliferation.**

False. It inhibits it.

O   **T/F: Large doses of vitamin E enhance wound healing.**

False.

O   **What is the main difference between a keloid and a hypertrophic scar?**

Keloids extend beyond the boundary of the original tissue injury; hypertrophic scars do not.

O   **Which hormone normally regulates protein synthesis and breakdown?**

Insulin.

O   **Which amino acid is a key fuel for rapidly dividing cells?**

Glutamine.

O   **How much time does it take for a surgical wound to fully heal?**

2 years.

O   **Under what conditions is epithelial migration and replication most facilitated?**

Moist wound surfaces under gas-permeable dressings.

O   **T/F: Epithelialization produces a watertight seal within 48 hours.**

True.

O   **T/F: Epithelialization is more rapid under moist conditions than dry conditions.**

True.

O   **Deficiency of which white blood cell is most likely to compromise wound healing?**

Macrophages.

O   **What is the maximum tensile strength of a surgical scar?**

80% of normal uninjured tissue.

O   **When does tensile strength correlate with total collagen content during wound healing?**

For about the first 3 weeks of wound healing.

O   **What are the 3 stages of normal surgical wound healing?**

Inflammation (d1-3), proliferation (d3-week 4), maturation (week 4 – 2 years).

O   **Which stage is most sensitive to the effects of chemoradiation?**

Inflammatory stage.

O   **What are the first inflammatory cells to enter the wound space?**

Neutrophils.

O   **What is the tensile strength of a wound during the inflammatory stage?**

Less than 5% of normal.

O   **What is the major event during the proliferative phase?**

Accelerated production of collagen.

O   **When does the production of collagen peak during wound healing?**

Day 7 after wound closure (continues at this pace for 2 – 3 weeks).

O   **What is the tensile strength of a wound after 4 weeks?**

30% of normal.

O   **What are the main events of the maturation stage?**

Reduction in the number of fibroblasts and macrophages, increase in collagen content, gradual increase in tensile wound strength.

O   **What is the function of epidermal growth factor (EGF)?**

It stimulates DNA synthesis and cell division in a variety of cells, including fibroblasts, keratinocytes and endothelial cells.

O   **What is the wound bursting strength?**

A direct measure of the force required to separate a healing, linear incision.

O   **What effect does radiation therapy (RT) have on the wound bursting strength?**

Significantly decreases it... after 18 Gy, it is 52% of normal.

O   **T/F: Exogenous use of TGF-ß appears to improve healing in tissues injured by RT.**

True.

O   **Poor wound healing after RT is primarily due to injury to which cell?**

Fibroblasts.

O   **When is the wound tensile strength of irradiated tissues equivalent to that of non-irradiated tissues?**

3 weeks after RT.

O   **What can the surgeon do to prevent wound complications after salvage surgery?**

Handle tissues carefully; leave fascia and underlying muscle attached to subcutaneous tissue; fill all potential dead space; drain wounds; close incision without tension; leave sutures in for a prolonged length of time but remove before RT begins.

O   **What lines are perpendicular to the line of force of the underlying muscle?**

Relaxed skin tension lines.

O   **What is the appropriate ratio of the long and short axes for elliptical incisions?**

4:1.

○   **What complication will occur if the above ratio is not met?**

A dog-ear deformity.

○   **What is the best level for undermining skin flaps?**

In the subdermal layer.

○   **What suture material loses its strength within 7 days?**

Plain catgut.

○   **Which suture materials incite the greatest inflammatory response?**

Plain catgut and chromic catgut.

○   **What is the absorption rate of chromic catgut sutures?**

20 days.

○   **When should scar revision take place?**

Not for at least 1 year after injury.

○   **What are 4 ways to correct hypertrophic or wide scars?**

Excision/undermining, Z-plasty or W-plasty, geometric broken line closure, and dermabrasion.

○   **When does irreversible ischemia of peripheral nerves occur?**

Within 8 hours of warm ischemia.

○   **When is return of sensation after skin grafting considered maximal?**

After 2 years.

○   **What are the differences between thin and thick split thickness skin grafts?**

Thin grafts take better, but thick grafts have better color match, less contraction, and are more resistant to trauma.

○   **What is the most important factor in minimizing hyperpigmentation of skin grafts?**

Protection from UV light for a full year postoperatively.

○   **How long can skin grafts be stored when banked in saline-soaked gauze sponges at 4° Celsius?**

Up to 21 days.

○   **T/F: Split-thickness skin grafts (STSG) contract more than full-thickness skin grafts (FTSG).**

True.

○   **What are the 3 phases of healing for skin grafts?**

Imbibition, inosculation and neovascularization.

○   **What process allows survival of skin grafts in the first 48 hours?**

Plasmatic imbibition.

○   **What is meant by inosculation with regard to skin grafts?**

The process by which vascular buds from the recipient bed make contact with capillaries within the graft.

RECONSTRUCTIVE FLAPS

O   **What is the maximum length to width ratio for local flaps?**

3:1.

O   **T/F: Axial flaps are more reliable than random flaps.**

True.

O   **What is the blood supply of a random flap?**

The dermal and subdermal plexuses.

O   **What is the term for a flap that is raised and pivoted into a defect, leaving a secondary defect that must be repaired?**

Transposition flap.

O   **What is the term for a flap that is raised from a nearby region and moved to a defect across intact skin?**

Interpolation flap.

O   **Considering rotation flaps, myocutaneous flaps, and random flaps, which of these has the strongest blood supply?**

Rotation flap.

O   **T/F: The surviving length of an axial pattern flap remains constant regardless of flap width.**

True.

O   **How does delaying (elevating the flap in 2 stages 2-3 weeks apart) improve flap survival?**

Conditions tissue to ischemia, closes A-V shunts, and increases blood flow by sympathectomy.

O   **What is a V-Y advancement?**

Closure of a rectangular defect by incising an adjacent triangle of tissue and advancing it into the defect.

O   **What is the major vascular pedicle for the platysma myocutaneous flap?**

Submental branch of the facial artery.

O   **Why should a rhomboid flap not be used to close a scalp defect?**

Causes improper orientation of the hair.

O   **Why do cranial bone grafts have superior resistance to resorption when compared to other donor sites (eg, rib or iliac bone)?**

Cranial bone originates from membranous bone whereas the other donor sites originate from endochondral bone; cranial bone revascularizes more quickly.

O   **What complications are specific to the iliac crest donor site?**

Injury to abdominal contents or the ilio-femoral joint, detachment of the inguinal ligament, interference with tensor fascia lata function, or damage to nearby peripheral nerves.

O   **What complications are specific to the rib donor site?**

Pneumothorax, hemothorax, and intercostal nerve injury.

O   **What complications are specific to the cranial bone harvest?**

Dural exposure, meningitis, CSF leak, sagittal sinus injury, and brain injury.

O   **What are the different types of cranial bone grafts?**

Full thickness calvarium, split thickness calvarium, bone chips, and bone dust.

O   **What is the minimum age at which the calvarium can be split?**

Age 4 or 5 (layers of the skull are not defined until then).

O   **What is the thickest part of the skull?**

Parietal bone.

O   **What is the thinnest part of the skull?**

Squamous portion of the temporal bone.

O   **T/F: Sagittally oriented scalp incisions tend to cause less scalp sensory disturbance than do coronally oriented incisions.**

True.

O   **What can be done to minimize the visibility of the bicoronal incision?**

Perform a wavy line incision.

O   **What is the maximum size of graft that can safely be obtained in-situ?**

3 – 4 cm wide.

O   **What is the preferred site for harvesting calvarial bone?**

Parietal bone (anterior for a flat graft; posterior for a curved graft).

O   **How is the diploic layer of the skull recognized during in-situ harvesting?**

Color changes from yellow-white to red and increased bleeding occurs.

○   **What is the best way to avoid injury to the superior sagittal sinus during harvesting of calvarial bone?**

Maintain at least a 2 cm distance from the sagittal suture.

○   **What factor is most essential to the success of a vascularized bone graft to the mandible?**

Good immobilization.

○   **What is the primary blood supply to the deltopectoral flap?**

Perforating branches of the internal mammary artery (4 branches, with the 2nd and 3rd branches representing the dominant blood supply).

○   **What is the primary blood supply to the pectoralis major flap?**

Perforating arteries of the thoracoacromial artery.

○   **Where should the medial incision be placed when raising the pectoralis major flap?**

Lateral to the perforating branches of the internal mammary artery to preserve the blood supply of a deltopectoral flap should it be needed in the future.

○   **What is the primary blood supply to the trapezius flap?**

Transverse cervical artery.

○   **Which musculocutaneous flap has the largest area of skin available for transfer to the head and neck?**

Latissimus dorsi.

○   **What is the primary blood supply to this flap?**

Thoracodorsal artery.

○   **How long does it take for complete regeneration of the endothelium across a microvascular anastomosis?**

2 weeks.

○   **In institutions performing high volume microsurgical reconstruction, what is the success rate? Re-exploration rate?**

98%; 2%.

○   **What flaps are ideal for reconstruction of extensive scalp defects?**

Free latissimus dorsi surfaced with non-meshed split thickness skin graft; if entire scalp is involved, latissimus dorsi with serratus anterior.

○   **What is the best material for dural reconstruction?**

Fascia lata.

○ **What if the skull is involved?**

Can use a split calvarial, split rib, or methyl methacrylate plus latissimus dorsi flap.

○ **How can extensive midface defects involving the orbit and/or maxilla be reconstructed?**

With a prosthesis or latissimus dorsi flap with multiple skin paddles.

○ **What is the major limit of microsurgical reconstruction in this area?**

Difficult to restore normal contour.

○ **What if the skull base is involved?**

Reconstruction requires microsurgery with latissimus dorsi, rectus abdominus, or free omental flap.

○ **What is the optimal flap for oral cavity soft tissue defects?**

Radial forearm free flap (RFFF).

○ **What are the best flaps for through-and-through cheek or oral cavity defects?**

Folded RFFF or double paddle scapula flap.

○ **What is the optimal flap for reconstruction of anterior mandibular defects?**

Fibular free flap (FFF).

○ **What is the primary blood supply to the FFF?**

Peroneal artery.

○ **Where does the common tibial-peroneal trunk originate in relation to the head of the fibula?**

2 – 7 cm distal.

○ **Between which muscles does the peroneal artery run?**

Tibialis posterior and soleus muscles.

○ **On average, how much skin is perfused by the peroneal artery in the FFF?**

Approximately 10 x 21 cm.

○ **What are the 3 different types of skin branches off the peroneal artery?**

Type A: musculocutaneous.
Type B: musculocutaneous and septocutaneous.
Type C: septocutaneous.

○ **Which of these supplies the most blood to the skin ?**

Septocutaneous.

O   **Which of these are most numerous?**

Musculocutaneous.

O   **Through which muscle compartment do the musculocutaneous branches course?**

The deep posterior compartment containing the soleus and flexor hallicus longus muscles.

O   **Why is the FFF optimal for reconstruction of mandibular defects?**

It provides enough length to reconstruct any size defect, can be harvested in the supine position and in tandem with tumor resection, has low donor site morbidity, and provides soft tissue for intraoral defects.

O   **What is the average length of the fibula?**

25 cm.

O   **What should be incorporated into the flap to promote viability of the skin paddle?**

A small cuff of soleus and flexor hallicus longus muscle.

O   **Where should the vascular pedicle lie on the new mandible?**

As close as possible to the new mandibular angle.

O   **To which vessels can the peroneal artery be anastomosed?**

Facial or external carotid artery.

O   **What is the purpose of IMF after FFF placement?**

To minimize movement near the vascular pedicle.

O   **If IMF is used, when is it removed?**

2 weeks postoperatively.

O   **What factors are associated with decreased skin paddle survival?**

Short skin island, short bone graft, use of the skin paddle intraorally.

O   **What is the role of angiography prior to FFF?**

Necessary to confirm presence of the peroneal artery and to confirm that it is free of disease and not the dominant source of blood supply to the distal leg.

O   **What are the reconstructive options when the mandibular condyle must be removed during tumor resection?**

Incompletely reconstruct the ramus so it doesn't extend as high as the glenoid fossa.
Attach a prosthetic condyle to the flap.
Shape the end of the flap to simulate the condyle.
Use the resected condyle as a nonvascularized graft mounted onto the end of the flap with a miniplate.

O   **Which method is optimal?**

Autologous condyle transplantation as it preserves occlusion, TMJ function, and vertical facial height without increasing morbidity.

O   **What must be done prior to autologous condyle transplantation?**

Scrapings of the marrow cavity at the cut end should be sent for frozen section to confirm that it is free of tumor.

O   **What problems can occur if a lateral mandibular defect is not reconstructed?**

Contour deformity of the lateral lower 1/3 of the face, displacement of residual mandible toward the side of the defect, malocclusion.

O   **What are THORPs?**

Titanium hollow screw reconstruction plates.

O   **What are AOs?**

Titanium or steel fixation plates that are more malleable than THORPs.

O   **What is the most common complication of segmental mandibulectomy defect reconstruction with plates?**

Plate exposure.

O   **What factors significantly increase the risk of plate exposure?**

Radiation therapy and extensive soft-tissue resection.

O   **What is the primary advantage of using a soft tissue free flap over a pectoralis major flap in conjunction with a mandibular plate?**

Free flap results in a much lower rate of plate exposure.

O   **Which types of osseous free flaps allow enosseous dental implants?**

Iliac crest, scapula, fibula, and radius.

O   **Which of these is most reliable? least reliable?**

Iliac crest, radius, respectively.

O   **What is the optimal flap for reconstruction of pharyngoesophageal defects?**

Tubed RFFF or free jejunal (RFFF is better for base of tongue or oropharynx, free jejunal flap is better for total pharyngoesophagectomies).

O   **Which of theses has a potentially higher fistula rate?**

Tubed RFFF.

O   **What are the major limitations of microsurgical reconstruction in the head and neck?**

Difficult to restore texture/color of facial skin, soft tissue/bony contour of maxilla, functional mobility of tongue/lower lip, and sensation of oral cavity.

O   **What is the most common complication from microsurgical reconstruction?**

36% suffer medical complications (pulmonary problems, prolonged ventilatory support, acute ethanol withdrawal).

O   **When is the risk of thrombosis highest after microsurgical reconstruction?**

15 – 20 minutes after closure.

O   **If a free flap fails, what is the best option for reconstruction?**

If medical condition allows, a second free flap should be performed instead of a locoregional flap.

O   **For reconstruction of oropharyngeal defects, what are the advantages of using a free flap over a pectoralis major flap?**

Lower wound complication rate and shorter hospitalization.

O   **What is the typical order of return of sensation in noninnervated flaps?**

Pinprick, touch, then temperature.

O   **T/F: Significant return of sensation to a free flap occurs even in the absence of neural anastomosis.**

True.

O   **For full thickness defects of the eyelid that cannot be closed primarily, what technique is attempted prior to using any flaps?**

Lateral cantholysis.

O   **What is the primary complication of the temporal advancement flap for reconstruction of the anterior lamella of the eyelid?**

Lateral canthal droop.

O   **What technique is ideal for reconstruction of posterior lamellar defects of the upper lateral eyelid?**

Tarsal rotation flap.

O   **What technique is ideal for reconstruction of large posterior lamella defects of the lower lid?**

Hughes tarsoconjunctival flap.

O   **Where should dissection of the tarsoconjunctival flap begin in relation to the lid margin?**

3 – 4 mm superior to the lid margin.

○ **What is the primary disadvantage of this procedure?**

Requires 6 – 8 weeks of ocular occlusion.

○ **T/F: Auricular cartilage grafts can be used to reconstruct the posterior lamella of the lower lid but should not be used in the upper lid.**

True; placement in the upper lid can cause corneal abrasions.

○ **What 4 composite grafts can provide both rigidity and a mucosal surface for eyelid reconstruction?**

Eyelid margin graft, tarsoconjunctival graft, nasal chondromucosal graft, hard palate mucoperiosteal graft.

○ **What is the primary advantage of the eyelid margin graft?**

Eyelash replacement.

○ **What technique is ideal for repair of large full-thickness defects of the upper lid?**

Cutler Beard or Bridge procedure.

○ **What should be done if the distal portion of the canaliculus is resected?**

The cut end should be marsupialized and stented for at least 3 weeks.

○ **Generally, what size defects of the lower lip can be closed primarily?**

< 1/2 the lip.

○ **Which rotation flap is best suited for lateral defects of the lower lip?**

Estlander flap.

○ **What is the primary advantage of the Karapandzic circumoral rotation flap?**

Orbicularis oris muscle is preserved.

○ **What are the best reconstructive options for total lip defects?**

Radial forearm free flap, groin flap, or scapular flap.

○ **What is the best flap for defects of the oral commissure?**

Estlander flap.

○ **What is the primary complication of this flap?**

Microstomia.

○ **What is the best method of reconstruction for defects between 1/2 to 2/3 of the lower lip, not involving the oral commissure?**

Abbe-Sabattini flap.

O   **How wide should the Abbe-Sabattini flap be?**

1/2 the width of the defect.

O   **What are the disadvantages of the Abbe-Sabattini flap?**

Two-staged procedure, risk of patient injuring the flap by opening the mouth too widely, and risk of microstomia.

O   **What is the best method of reconstruction for defects involving 2/3 or more of the lower lip?**

If centered in the midline, the Webster modification of the Bernard-Burow repair.

O   **How wide are the Burow's triangles designed?**

Bases are equal in width to 1/2 of the lip defect.

O   **What is the best method of reconstruction for defects involving 2/3 or more of the upper lip?**

Burow-Dieffenbach +/- Abbe-Sabattini flap.

O   **What is the primary blood supply of the deltopectoral, temporal, forehead, and nape of neck cutaneous flaps?**

Deltopectoral – internal mammary arteries.
Temporal – superficial temporal artery.
Forehead – supraorbital and supratrochlear arteries.
Nape of neck – random (postauricular, occipital vertebral arteries).

O   **What is the primary blood supply of the pectoralis major (PMM), trapezius, latissimus dorsi, and sternocleidomastoid myocutaneous (SCM) flaps?**

PMM – thoracoacromial, lateral thoracic arteries.
Trapezius – occipital or transverse cervical arteries.
Latissimus dorsi – thoracodorsal artery.
SCM – random (occipital, superior thyroid, transverse cervical arteries).

O   **What is the primary blood supply to the temporalis muscle flap?**

Deep temporal artery.

O   **What vessels is the iliac crest free flap based on?**

Deep circumflex iliac vessels.

O   **What vessels is the rectus abdominus free flap based on?**

Deep inferior epigastric vessels.

O   **What tissues are included in the posterior thigh fasciocutaneous flap?**

The fascia lata, subcutaneous tissue and the descending branch of the inferior gluteal artery.

O   **The greater omentum axial flap is based on what vessels?**

Either the right or the left gastroepiploic artery.

○   **What finding on inspection of a flap signifies venous thrombosis?**

Development of a sharp line of color demarcation.

○   **What is the most potent natural inhibitor of thrombin?**

Hirudin.

○   **Where is this substance found in nature?**

Salivary glands of leeches.

○   **What organism lives in the gut of leeches and is the most common organism associated with wound infections when leeches are applied?**

Aeromonas hydrophila.

○   **What antibiotics is this organism sensitive to?**

3rd-generation cephalosporins, ciprofloxacin, aminoglycosides, sulfa drugs, and tetracycline.

○   **What are the contraindications to leech use?**

Arterial insufficiency, severe immunocompromise, allergic reaction to previous leech application.

ANATOMY FOR COSMETIC SURGEONS

O   **How does the aging process alter facial proportions?**

The area from the subnasale to the menton decreases significantly in size compared to the other areas of the face.

O   **What is the ideal nasofrontal angle?**

125 – 135 degrees.

O   **What is the ideal nasolabial angle?**

90 – 120 degrees.

O   **What is the ideal nasofacial angle?**

36 – 40 degrees.

O   **According to the Goode method for determining the nasofacial angle, a ratio of 0.55 corresponds to what angle?**

36 degrees.

O   **What is the Baum method for determining the nasofacial angle?**

The ratio of a vertical line drawn from the nasofrontal angle to the subnasale to a horizontal line perpendicular to the vertical line that passes through the tip; ideally this ratio is 2:1, which corresponds to a 42 degree angle.

O   **What is Powell's modification of the Baum method?**

The ideal ration is 2.8:1, corresponding to an angle of 36 degrees.

O   **What is the Simons method for determining the nasofacial angle?**

The ratio of the length of the upper lip to the length of the base of the nose is ideally 1:1.

O   **What is the ideal alar to lobular ratio?**

1:1.

O   **How does the ideal supratip break differ between men and women?**

More pronounced in women.

O   **In the female, where should maximum brow elevation occur?**

At a line tangent and vertical to the lateral limbus of the eye.

O   **What is the average upper lip length in males and females?**

24 mm in males, 20 mm in females.

O   **What is the average lower lip length in males and females?**

50 mm in males, 46 mm in females.

O   **What is the ideal ratio of the length of the lower lip to the upper lip?**

2:1.

O   **How does the skin differ between Asians and Caucasians?**

Asians have thicker skin with greater collagen density and are more prone to hypertrophic scarring and prolonged erythema.

O   **How does the skin age differently between Asians and Caucasians?**

Asians develop fewer fine rhytids but more pigmented lesions than Caucasians.

O   **T/F: With aging, Asians will accumulate greater volumes of fat than Caucasians.**

True.

O   **How does the platysma muscle differ between Asians and Caucasians?**

Thicker in Asians, with lower incidence of diastasis.

O   **What are the typical features of the facial structure in Asians?**

Prominent malar imminences with relatively shallow midface, wide prominent mandibular angles, short and posteriorly-inclined chin, broad and flat nasal dorsum with limited tip projection and broad nasal base.

O   **How does the incidence of complications following rhytidectomy differ between Asians and Caucasians?**

Flap necrosis is less common and hypertrophic scarring is more common in Asians.

O   **What does a medial epicanthal fold cover?**

Lacrimal lake.

O   **What is unique about the anatomy of the Asian eyelid?**

Levator muscle lacks attachment to the pretarsal skin, resulting in an absent pretarsal fold.

O   **What is the most common form of acquired eyelid ptosis?**

Levator aponeurosis disinsertion or dehiscence.

O   **What are the physical signs of aponeurosis disinsertion?**

Thin upper lid skin and high lid fold with good levator function (>10 mm).

O **Define mild, moderate, and marked ptosis.**

Mild 1 – 2 mm, moderate 2 – 3 mm, marked >4 mm.

O **How is lower lid laxity defined?**

If >10 mm or >25% of the skin can be gathered without distortion of the rim.

O **What is the significance of a "negative vector" profile?**

Describes patients with protuberant eyes and hypoplastic malar eminence… fat should not be removed from these patients during blepharoplasty.

O **What structure divides the lacrimal gland into 2 lobes?**

Levator aponeurosis.

O **What is Hering's law?**

Unilateral ptosis with contralateral lid retraction… if you cover the ptotic eye with a patch for 30 – 60 min, the retracted eye will settle into the normal position and the ptotic eye will reveal itself.

O **What are the dimensions of the palpebral fissure when the eyes are open?**

30 x 10 mm.

O **What structures make up the middle lamella?**

Orbital septum, capsulopalpebral fascia, posterior surface of orbicularis oculi.

O **What provides static support to the lower lid?**

Tarsal plate and its associated medial and lateral canthal tendons.

O **What provides dynamic support to the lower lid?**

Adhesion of the pretarsal portion of the orbicularis to the tarsal plate.

O **What structure in the lower lid is analogous to the levator aponeurosis of the upper lid?**

Capsulopalpebral fascia.

O **What are the lower eyelid retractors?**

Capsulopalpebral fascia and the inferior tarsal muscle.

O **What lines the posterior surface of the eyelid?**

Palpebral conjunctiva.

O **What creates the gray line in the lid margin?**

The muscle of Riolan.

O   **What does the gray line divide?**

The anterior and posterior lamella.

O   **What structures make up the anterior lamella of the lid?**

Pretarsal orbicularis oculi muscle and the eyelid skin.

O   **What structures make up the posterior lamella of the lid?**

Conjunctiva and the tarsal plate.

O   **What structure forms the medial canthal tendon?**

The superficial head of the pretarsal fibers of the orbicularis oculi muscle.

O   **What is the function of the deep head of the orbicularis oculi?**

Inserts on the posterior lacrimal crest and provides structural support to the lid.

O   **What happens with disruption of the deep head?**

Lateral and anterior displacement of the medial canthal angle.

O   **Where does the lateral canthal tendon insert?**

Orbital tubercle located 5 mm posterior to the lateral orbital rim.

O   **What is the ideal brow position in a woman?**

Medial segment club-shaped and inferior to the lateral segment; peak of arch above the orbital rim at the lateral limbus; lid margin to brow distance >2 cm.

O   **What is the ideal brow position in a man?**

At the level of the supraorbital rim with a less pronounced arch.

O   **Where is the frontal branch of VII most vulnerable during brow lift?**

Just above the lateral brow, 1 – 2 cm from the orbital rim.

O   **Where should subperiosteal undermining begin during brow lift?**

2.5 cm above the lateral orbital rim to avoid injury to the supraorbital nerve.

O   **What muscles draw the eyebrows medially?**

Corrugator supercilii muscles.

O   **What muscle draws the medial edge of the brow inferiorly?**

Procerus.

O   **What muscle creates vertical and oblique rhytids in the medial eyebrow region?**

Corrugator supercilii muscle.

O   **What is the SMAS?**

Tissue plane of the face composed of fibrous and/or muscle tissue that is continuous with the platysma and lacks direct bony insertion.

O   **What is the relationship of the SMAS to the parotid gland?**

Densely adherent to, yet distinct from, the parotid fascia.

O   **Where are the branches of the facial nerve in relation to the SMAS?**

Deep.

O   **When dissecting from the temporal region to the zygomatic arch, where does the deep temporal fascia divide into superficial and deep layers?**

The temporal line of fusion at the level of the superior orbital rim.

O   **What happens to the fascia as dissection continues towards the zygomatic arch?**

The temporoparietal fascia and the superficial layer of the deep temporal fascia fuse 1 cm above the zygomatic arch.

O   **What is the relationship of the SMAS to the zygomatic arch?**

It terminates 1 cm below the zygomatic arch.

O   **What is the relationship of the SMAS to the lower eyelid?**

It merges with the muscle fibers of the periorbital orbicularis oculi.

O   **What is the only location in the face where the SMAS is not covered by the fascial-fatty layer?**

Superior portion of the lower eyelid.

O   **What is the relationship of the frontal branch of VII to the temporoparietal fascia?**

Lies within it.

O   **What plane separates the temporoparietal fascia from the deep temporal fascia?**

Subaponeurotic plane of loose areolar tissue.

O   **What separates the superficial and deep layers of the deep temporal fascia?**

Superficial temporal fat pad.

O   **What fat pad separates the temporalis muscle from the deep temporal fascia and the zygomatic arch?**

The deep temporal fat pad, an extension of the buccal fat pad.

○   **What is the relationship of the frontal branch of VII to the zygomatic arch?**

Travels over it on the surface of the loose areolar layer and superficial layer of the deep temporal fascia.

○   **What are the only mimetic muscles that receive innervation from VII on their superficial surfaces?**

Buccinator, levator anguli oris, and mentalis muscles.

○   **Where are dense fibrous attachments between the superficial and deep facial fascias located?**

Along the zygomatic arch, overlying the parotid gland, along the anterior border of the masseter muscle.

○   **T/F: The buccal fat pad, parotid duct, facial artery and vein, and facial nerve lie in the same anatomic plane in the cheek.**

True.

○   **What are the 2 types of retaining ligaments that support the facial skin?**

Osteocutaneous ligaments and fusion of the superficial and deep fascias.

○   **What ligaments support the malar pad over the zygomatic eminence?**

Zygomatic ligaments.

○   **What ligaments support the soft tissue of the medial cheek?**

Masseteric cutaneous ligaments.

○   **What is the primary cause of midface aging?**

Ptosis of the malar fat pads and diminished tone of the zygomatic musculature.

○   **What is the primary cause of jowls in the elderly patient?**

Attenuation of the masseteric cutaneous ligaments.

○   **What is the significance of the position of the hyoid bone in rhytidectomy?**

Dictates the maximum improvement possible in the cervicomental angle; ideal position is high and posterior.

○   **Ideally, the nasal tip should lead the remainder of the profile by what distance?**

1 – 2 mm.

○   **What is the single most important aesthetic quality of the nasal tip and base?**

Symmetry.

○   **What is the ideal configuration of the alar margin?**

S-shaped, exposing 2 – 3 mm of the caudal columella on lateral view.

○   **What is the anatomic basis of "hanging columella?"**

Excessively high arch of the alae, abnormally extreme curvature of the intermediate and medial crura, or overaggressive surgical removal of the lateral crus and adjacent soft tissue with subsequent cephalic contraction of alar margin.

○   **What are the nasal anatomic subunits?**

Nasal dorsum, nasal sidewalls, nasal tip, alar lobules, depressions of the supra-alar facets.

○   **Which muscles elevate the nose?**

Procerus, levator labii superioris alaeque nasi, anomalous nasi muscles.

○   **Which muscles depress the nose?**

Alar nasalis, depressor septi nasi muscles.

○   **What are the other muscles of the nose (the compressor and dilators)?**

Transverse nasalis, compressor narium minor, dilator naris anterior muscles.

○   **What effect does separation of the upper lateral cartilages from the nasal bones have on the nasal airway?**

Causes the middle of the nasal vault to cave in.

○   **What is the nasal valve?**

The angle between the caudal quadrangular cartilage and the distal upper lateral cartilages.

○   **What structures are found in the nasal valve area?**

Septum, upper lateral cartilages, and anterior head of the inferior turbinates.

○   **What is the normal angle of the nasal valve in Caucasians?**

9 – 15 degrees.

○   **What is the only septal component that is paired?**

The vomer… may be bilaminar owing to its dual embryonic origin.

○   **What is the most important surgical component of the septum?**

Quadrangular cartilage… provides midline support and can significantly influence the external appearance of the nose.

○   **What are the major tip support mechanisms?**

Contour, size, and strength of the lateral crura; attachment of the medial crural footplate to the caudal septum; attachment of the caudal edge of the upper lateral cartilages to the cephalic border of the alar cartilages.

O   **What are the minor tip support mechanisms?**

Nasal tip ligamentous aponeurosis; cartilaginous septum; nasal spine; strength and resilience of the medial crura; thickness of tip skin and subcutaneous tissue; supportive strength of the alar sidewalls.

O   **What are the major anatomic features that determine tip projection?**

Thickness and character of tip skin; shape and strength of alar cartilages; length of infratip lobule and columella; anatomy of the quadrangular cartilage (especially the anterior septal angle); size of the nasal spine and premaxilla.

O   **What are two angles used to determine chin projection?**

Legan angle (normal 12 degrees +/- 4), Merrifield Z angle (normal 80 degrees +/- 5).

O   **Which of these uses the Frankfort horizontal line as a reference?**

Merrifield Z angle.

O   **What is the Gonzales-Ulloa method of determining chin projection?**

Anterior chin should approximate a line perpendicular to the Frankfort horizontal line where it intersects the nasion.

O   **Where should the chin lie in relation to a vertical line dropped from the lips?**

In males, the chin should meet the line; in females, the chin should lie 2-3 mm posterior.

O   **Where is the incision made using the external approach to chin augmentation?**

2 – 3 mm posterior to the submental crease.

O   **What is the difference between microgenia and micrognathia?**

Microgenia is a small mandible with normal occlusion; micrognathia is an underdeveloped mandible with class II occlusion.

O   **What is retrognathia?**

Normal sized mandible with class II occlusion.

O   **What is the normal thickness of the chin pad?**

8 – 11 mm.

O   **What is the normal position of the lower lip in relation to the upper lip and chin?**

The most anterior portion of the white roll should lie slightly posterior to the upper lip and lie in the same plane as the soft tissue chin point.

O   **What are the causes of lower lip eversion?**

Skeletal deep bite, lower tooth procumberance, excess lip weight and bulk.

O   **What measurement can be use to determine deficiency in the malar area?**

The distance from the malar prominence to the nasolabial groove on lateral projection (ideally >5 mm).

O   **What is the normal angle between the ear and the head?**

25 – 30 degrees.

O   **What is the normal incline of the vertical axis of the auricle?**

20 degrees.

O   **What is the normal vertical height of the auricle?**

About 6 cm.

O   **What is the normal width of the auricle?**

About 55% of the length.

O   **What is the normal distance from the helical rim to the skull?**

1 – 2 cm.

O   **What is the normal superior limit of the auricle?**

The level of the brow.

FACIAL DERMATOLOGY

○ **Skin that rarely burns and tans more than average is which Fitzpatrick's class?**

IV.

○ **What are the characteristics of photoaged skin?**

Thicker than normal with wrinkling, roughness, sallowness, telangiectasias, mottled hyperpigmentation, and loss of elasticity.

○ **What are the histologic features of photoaged skin?**

Thickened stratum corneum, thinner atrophic epidermis with atypia, irregular dispersion of melanin, decreased glycosaminoglycans, abnormal elastic fibers in the dermis (solar elastosis).

○ **What is melasma?**

Large, symmetric macules on the cheeks, forehead, upper lip, nose, and chin.

○ **What causes melasma?**

Genetic predisposition, exposure to UV radiation, pregnancy, oral contraceptives, thyroid dysfunction, cosmetics, phototoxic and antiseizure drugs.

○ **T/F: Complete avoidance of sunlight can reverse some of the histologic signs of photoaging.**

True.

○ **What effects do alpha hydroxy acids have on the dermis?**

Increase collagen and glycosaminoglycan production.

○ **What skin preparations have been shown to significantly improve the overall severity of photodamaging but have not been shown to affect wrinkles?**

8 – 10% alpha hydroxy acids.

○ **Which patients are better served by 15 – 20% alpha hydroxy acids?**

Patients with sebaceous, Fitzpatrick type III and IV skin.

○ **What are the clinical effects of tretinoin?**

Decrease in fine wrinkling, roughness, and mottled hyperpigmentation after 6 months of use.

○ **What are the histologic effects of tretinoin?**

Thinner stratum corneum, thickened epidermis, increased collagen, angiogenesis, and more uniform dispersion of melanin granules.

○   **What is the mechanism of action of retinoids?**

Cause a 70% inhibition of AP-1 transcription factor binding to DNA, which decreases the activation of metalloproteases such as collagenase, gelatinase, and stromatolysis.

○   **What is the mechanism of action of hydroquinone?**

Blocks the conversion of dopa to melanin.

○   **What is ochronosis?**

A potential adverse reaction to hydroquinone characterized by a reticulated, sooty pigmentation of the cheeks, forehead, and periorbital regions.

○   **Which bleaching agent is also an effective treatment for acne?**

Azelaic acid.

○   **Which bleaching agent is produced by *Aspergillus* and *Penicillium*?**

Kojic acid.

○   **What are the components of Jessner's solution?**

Resorcinol, salicylic acid, lactic acid, and ethanol.

○   **How deep does Jessner's solution penetrate?**

Remains intraepidermal.

○   **How deep can a 20% TCA solution penetrate?**

Down to the papillary dermis.

○   **What are the 4 levels of TCA peels?**

Level 0 – no frost, skin appears slick and shiny representing removal of the stratum corneum.
Level 1 – irregular light frost with some erythema; 2 – 4 days of light peeling.
Level 2 – pink white frost, full thickness epidermal peel, 5 days of peeling.
Level 3 – solid white frost, papillary dermis.

○   **What are the initial manifestations of systemic phenol toxicity from a chemical facial peel?**

Hyperreflexia and hypertension.

○   **When are cardiac arrhythmias that develop during a phenol peel most likely to occur?**

Within 30 minutes of the start of the procedure.

○   **What is the incidence of positive responses to skin tests for injectable collagen?**

3%.

○   **What are the main indications for collagen injection?**

Glabellar frown lines, nasolabial lines, crow's feet, and saucer-shaped acne scars.

○   **How long does injectable collagen remain in the tissue?**

3 – 6 months.

○   **What is the primary advantage of AlloDerm?**

Semi-permanent (20 – 50% persistence beyond 1 year).

○   **What is isolagen?**

Injectable autologous soft tissue material derived from cultured human fibroblasts.

○   **Which area of the face is CO_2 laser most effective for treating rhytids?**

Periorbital.

○   **What is the major complication of laser resurfacing of darker skinned individuals?**

Dyspigmentation (hyper- or hypo-).

○   **What factors affect the risk of complications after laser skin resurfacing?**

Number of laser passes, energy densities, degree of pulse or scan overlap, preoperative skin condition, anatomic areas.

○   **What are the normal side effects of laser skin resurfacing?**

Erythema, edema, serous discharge, and crusting.

○   **Which laser causes the most intense and prolonged side effects?**

CO_2 laser.

○   **How long do side effects last after CO_2 and Er:YAG laser?**

3 – 6 months after CO_2 laser; 2 – 4 weeks after Er:YAG laser.

○   **What are the mild complications of laser skin resurfacing?**

Prolonged erythema, acne or milia, contact dermatitis, pruritus.

○   **What % of patients develop postinflammatory hyperpigmentation?**

33% (more for darker skin types).

○   **What treatments can be used to help this problem?**

Hydroquinone or retinoic acid plus a topical class I corticosteroid, glycolic acid.

○   **What should be used to prevent this problem?**

Sunscreen (pretreatment regimens have not been proven to help).

○ **What factors increase the risk of prolonged erythema?**

Regular use of tretinoin or glycolic acid, rosacea, multiple passes, inadvertent pulse stacking, aggressive intraoperative rubbing.

○ **What is the purpose of application of topical vitamin C after skin resurfacing?**

To decrease the inflammation associated with prolonged erythema (must wait until reepithelization is complete before applying).

○ **When does hypopigmentation after laser skin resurfacing present?**

6 – 12 months after treatment.

○ **What % of patients develop contact dermatitis after laser resurfacing?**

65%.

○ **How is it treated?**

Bland emollients (avoid topical antibiotics), topical class I corticosteroids, cool and wet compresses.

○ **What % of patients develop HSV despite antiviral prophylaxis?**

2 – 7%.

○ **What is the typical prophylactic antiviral regimen?**

Starting 1 – 2 days preprocedure, 250 mg BID famciclovir for 7 – 10 days (if no history of HSV)... 500 mg BID if history positive for HSV.

○ **How should an outbreak of HSV be treated?**

Switch to a different antiviral and administer the maximum dose.

○ **Which anatomic areas are more prone to scarring after laser treatment?**

Infraorbital area, mandible, and anterior neck.

○ **What other factors increase the risk of scarring?**

Development of wound infection or contact dermatitis, recent use of isotretinoin, history of radiation therapy, history of keloids.

○ **What can be used to treat scarring after laser skin resurfacing?**

Intralesional or topical corticosteroids, 585 nm pulsed-dye laser (2 to 3 treatments at 6 – 8 week intervals).

○ **Patients who have previously undergone blepharoplasty are at increased risk for which complication after laser skin resurfacing?**

Ectropion.

○ **What are the 2 most common complications of dermabrasion?**

Milia and hypopigmentation.

COSMETIC SURGERY

O   **What are the primary theories on the etiology of infraorbital bags?**

1. Congenitally excess fat.
2. Weakening of the orbital septum and attenuation of the orbicularis oculi.
3. Weakening of global support resulting in enophthalmos and lower lid pseudoherniation
4. Weakening and descent of the Lockwood suspensory ligament.

O   **What is the consequence of overly aggressive resection of upper lid skin?**

Loss of crease definition.

O   **Why should extra caution be taken during lateral dissection of the upper lid?**

To avoid prolapsing the lacrimal gland.

O   **What is the most severe, yet rarest complication of blepharoplasty?**

Retrobulbar hemorrhage… incidence 0.04%.

O   **When should lid malposition after blepharoplasty be corrected?**

No sooner than 6 months after the initial surgery.

O   **What happens to the position of the globe when 2.5 cc of fat is removed?**

Globe moves 1 mm inferiorly and 2 mm posteriorly.

O   **How does release of the arcus marginalis affect eye contour?**

Creates a more convex, youthful eye contour.

O   **What are two major limitations of the transconjunctival approach to lower lid blepharoplasty?**

Redundant skin cannot be removed and orbicularis hypertrophy cannot be treated.

O   **Identification of what structure is essential in safely exposing the medial and central fat pads during a transconjunctival lower eyelid blepharoplasty?**

Inferior oblique muscle.

O   **What are the two types of lower lid malposition after blepharoplasty?**

Retraction and ectropion.

O   **Which is more common?**

Retraction.

O   **What is the difference between retraction and ectropion?**

Retraction is vertical lid shortening due to fibrosis in the middle lamellar plane; ectropion is lid eversion caused by shortening of the anterior lamella, skin, and orbicularis oculi.

○   **What is the most common cause of lower lid retraction after blepharoplasty?**

Accumulation of small amounts of blood in the middle lamellar plane.

○   **What are 5 lower lid blepharoplasty techniques that help prevent postoperative retraction?**

1.   Horizontal alignment of lower lid incisions.
2.   Preservation of a strip of orbicularis attached to the tarsal plate.
3.   Draping of the flap medially and superiorly.
4.   Placement of a suspension suture between the deep surface of the orbicularis and the orbital periosteum.
5.   Triamcinolone injection into plane of orbital septum.

○   **What factors predispose to lid malposition after lower lid blepharoplasty?**

Proptosis or unilateral high myopia; preexisting scleral show; malar hypoplasia; lower lid laxity from previous surgery; females >65 years and all males.

○   **What are the relative contraindications to the coronal forehead lift?**

Male-pattern baldness in men and high hairlines in women.

○   **What is the plane of dissection in the coronal forehead lift?**

Subgaleal.

○   **In what region is division of the frontalis muscle prohibited?**

Between the lateral brow and the temporal hair line.

○   **Which patients are good candidates for the pretrichial forehead lift?**

Women with a high hairline and long vertical height to the forehead.

○   **Which patients are good candidates for the midforehead lift?**

Men with deep rhytids in whom a coronal lift is contraindicated.

○   **Which patients are good candidates for direct brow lift?**

Those with brow asymmetries (ie, from facial nerve paralysis) and marked ptosis of the lateral eyebrow.

○   **Which patients are not good candidates for endoscopic brow lift?**

Women with high hairlines, patients with male-pattern baldness or tight, thick skin with extensive bony attachments (more common in Asians and Native Americans).

○   **What is the proper plane of dissection in the temporal region to avoid injury to VII?**

Within the subaponeurotic plane (deep to the temporoparietal fascia).

O   **What is the safest plane of dissection in the temporal region when exposure of the zygomatic arch is necessary?**

Within the superficial temporal fat pad deep to the superficial layer of the deep temporal fascia.

O   **In what region of the face can transection of the SMAS directly injure a branch of VII?**

Temporal region.

O   **What is the safest plane of dissection in the malar region?**

Along the superficial surface of the elevators of the upper lip (zygomaticus major and minor).

O   **How does the facelift incision differ between men and women?**

In women, the incision runs along the posterior margin of the tragus (post-tragal); in men, the incision is placed in the preauricular crease (pre-tragal) so that facial hair does not grow on the tragus postoperatively. Also, a margin of non-hair-bearing skin is preserved around the inferior attachment of the earlobe in men.

O   **What is the difference between SMAS imbrication and SMAS plication?**

Imbrication involves undermining and cutting the SMAS prior to suspension; plication involves folding the SMAS on itself.

O   **What is the difference in outcome between these approaches?**

No significant difference in outcome.

O   **In what direction are the flaps pulled during SMAS suspension?**

Primarily superiorly and partially posterior.

O   **What complication results from pulling too far posteriorly?**

Widening and flattening of the oral commissure.

O   **What effect does SMAS suspension have on the nasolabial folds?**

Deepens them.

O   **Which approach to rhytidectomy improves the nasolabial folds?**

Deep plane rhytidectomy.

O   **In which plane is the neck dissected during deep plane rhytidectomy?**

Pre-platysmal.

O   **In which plane is the lower face dissected during deep plane rhytidectomy?**

Sub-SMAS plane.

O   **In which plane is the midface dissected during deep plane rhytidectomy?**

Subcutaneous for 2 – 3 cm anterior to the tragus, then immediately superficial to the orbicularis and zygomaticus muscles.

○ **Where in the midface is the facial nerve most vulnerable during SMAS undermining?**

Anterior to the parotid gland.

○ **T/F: Closed suction drains are associated with a significantly lower incidence of hematoma after rhytidectomy.**

False.

○ **What is a pixie or satyr earlobe?**

Common complication of rhytidectomy where the earlobe is elongated and directly attached to the facial cheek skin.

○ **What is the most common complication of rhytidectomy?**

Hematoma.

○ **T/F: Hematoma after rhytidectomy is more common in males than females.**

True.

○ **What is the incidence of hematoma after rhytidectomy?**

0.3 – 15%.

○ **When do most major hematomas occur after rhytidectomy?**

First 12 hours postoperatively.

○ **What is the incidence of facial nerve injury during rhytidectomy?**

0.4% – 2.6%.

○ **What is the incidence of temporary facial nerve paralysis after deep plane rhytidectomy?**

3.6%.

○ **What is the most commonly injured nerve during rhytidectomy?**

Greater auricular nerve.

○ **What is the most likely cause of dimpling of the skin following liposuction of the jowls?**

Directing the opening of the extractor towards the skin.

○ **What is the proper plane of dissection during rhinoplasty?**

Deep to the subcutaneous tissue and SMAS layers.

❍   **Reduction of what structure accomplishes the majority of profile changes in patients requesting reduction rhinoplasty?**

Cartilaginous dorsum.

❍   **What are the complications of radical septal resections?**

Columellar retraction, dorsal saddling, airway collapse, increased nasal width, loss of tip support, and septal perforation.

❍   **What effect does excessive surgical reduction of the nasal bridge have on the eyes?**

Pseudohypertelorism.

❍   **What is the most common cause of nasal valve collapse?**

Rhinoplasty.

❍   **Defects of the nasal valve involving what structures can be repaired with a composite graft from the auricle?**

Vestibular skin and alar cartilage.

❍   **How much auricular cartilage can be harvested without affecting the structural integrity of the ear?**

The entire concha can be removed as long as the antihelix is kept intact.

❍   **When should a posterior incision be used to harvest auricular cartilage?**

Small grafts and when epithelial and soft tissues are to be incorporated with the graft.

❍   **What is the advantage of leaving a small amount of soft tissue on the auricular graft?**

More rapid host bed fixation.

❍   **What is one way to improve the stability of a columellar strut?**

Carve the base into a V or fork or rest a large strut on a cartilage platform (plinth).

❍   **What is the most common cause of alar margin elevation?**

Overaggressive resection of the lateral crus.

❍   **What are the different approaches used in septoplasty?**

Complete, partial, hemi- and high transfixion incisions.

❍   **Which major tip support mechanism is violated by the complete transfixion incision?**

Attachment of the medial crura to the caudal septum.

❍   **What effect does the complete transfixion incision have on tip projection and rotation?**

Decreases tip projection and increases tip rotation (resulting in nasal shortening).

○   **What is the difference between the hemitransfixion incision and the Killian incision?**

The hemitransfixion incision is made unilaterally at the junction of the caudal septum and the columella, whereas the Killian incision is made unilaterally 2 – 3 mm cephalic to the mucocutaneous junction.

○   **What is the most crucial factor limiting surgical correction of a congenitally short nose?**

Dorsal skin shortness.

○   **What are the three primary incisions used in tip surgery?**

Intercartilaginous, transcartilaginous, and marginal incisions.

○   **Which major tip support mechanism is violated by the inter- and transcartilaginous incisions?**

Attachment of the caudal edge of the upper lateral cartilages to the cephalic edge of the alar cartilages.

○   **What are the two major approaches to tip surgery?**

Delivery and nondelivery.

○   **What are the two types of nondelivery approaches?**

Transcartilaginous and retrograde.

○   **What are the advantages of using a nondelivery approach?**

Requires minimal dissection ensuring more symmetric and predictable healing; resists cephalic rotation; single incision; preserves existing tip projection; resists tip retrodisplacement and postoperative tip ptosis.

○   **What are the disadvantages of using a nondelivery approach?**

Technically more difficult if inexperienced.

○   **What are the advantages to the open approach?**

Wider exposure, allowing the use of binocular vision, bimanual dissection, and microcautery for hemostasis; enables direct vision of the domes and the nasal profile; can secure tip grafts directly with suture and approach the septum from above-down as well as from below-up.

○   **What are the disadvantages of the open approach?**

Transcolumellar external scar; risk of disturbing normal anatomy in the infratip lobule and caudal aspects of the alar cartilages; prolonged edema in thick-skinned patients; potential for excess trauma to the tip and dorsal skin flap; increased operative time; increased difficulty in judging the exact tip-supratip relationship after skin flap replacement; grafts must be suture-fixated.

○   **When can the transcartilaginous incision not be used?**

In patients with widely divergent intermediate crura where the domes need exposure for narrowing.

○   **Which incisions can be used for exposure and delivery of the alar cartilages?**

Intercartilaginous and marginal incisions.

○   **In the delivery approach, what are the indications for using a complete, rather than hemi-, transfixion incision?**

Severely deviated caudal septum; when access to the nasal spine is necessary; when tip rotation and nasal shortening are desired.

○   **Which technique results in greater cephalic tip rotation: interrupted or complete strip?**

Interrupted strip.

○   **How much cartilage should be preserved during a complete strip procedure?**

At least a 4 – 5 mm strip or 75% of the original cartilage volume.

○   **What techniques can be used to augment the effects of the complete strip, without sacrificing tip projection?**

Medial triangle excision, alternating incomplete incisions, crosshatching, gentle morselization, transdomal suture narrowing.

○   **What are the various interrupted strip techniques?**

Lateral division, medial division, multiple vertical interrupting cuts, both medial and lateral division with a resection of a lateral segment, rotation of a segment of lateral crus into medial crus.

○   **Which of these techniques is best for thick-skinned patients with abundant soft tissue and a wide, under-projected tip?**

Rotation of a segment of lateral crus into the medial crus.

○   **Which technique is ideal for patients with an over-projected tip due to overdeveloped alar cartilages?**

Medial and lateral division with resection of lateral segment.

○   **What are the advantages of lateral interruption techniques?**

Reduced likelihood of uneven tip-defining points becoming evident months after surgery; faster symmetrical healing; less loss of projection; avoidance of notching and pinching.

○   **What are the advantages and disadvantages of medial interruption techniques?**

Useful in more extreme anatomic situations to normalize tip projection but almost always result in a moderate to major loss of tip projection and have the potential for notching and pinching.

○   **What are the major adjunctive procedures for tip rotation?**

Caudal septal shortening, upper lateral cartilage shortening, high septal transfixion with septal shortening, reduction of convex caudal medial crura.

○   **Which of these is preferred when the anatomy of the tip – infratip lobule and related structures is ideal?**

High septal transfixion with septal shortening.

○   **What are the minor adjunctive procedures for tip rotation?**

Complete transfixion incision, wide skin sleeve undermining, excision of excessive vestibular skin, proper tip taping, plumping grafts, columellar strut, division of the septi depressor muscle.

○   **What are the risk factors for developing bossae or horns after rhinoplasty?**

Thin skin, strong cartilages, and bifidity.

○   **What maneuver can be done to help prevent this complication?**

Transdomal suture to narrow the tip.

○   **What can be done for the patient whose lateral crura are concave?**

Dissect lateral crura completely free and reverse them 180 degrees.

○   **What is the Goldman technique for increasing tip projection?**

Interrupted strip; borrowed cartilage from the lateral crus is sutured into the medial crus, resulting in elongation of the medial crura.

○   **What techniques can be used to decrease tip projection?**

Sacrifice of major tip support mechanisms, reduction of a large nasal spine, resection of a small amount of cartilage from the lateral alar crus, softening the domes by serial crosshatching, reduction of overdeveloped cartilaginous dorsum.

○   **What is Binder's syndrome?**

Maxillonasal dysplasia with inadequate projection, absent nasal spine, premaxillary hypoplasia, severe columellar-lobular disproportion.

○   **How do chin implants used in women differ from those used in men?**

More oval in women, squarer and larger in men.

○   **Where should the chin implant lie in relation to the lower incisors?**

The anterior surface should not lie beyond the labial surface of the lower incisors.

○   **What is the significance of the labiomental fold in chin implantation?**

If the fold is high, implantation can enlarge the entire lower face.

○   **Which alloplastic implant material forms a surrounding capsule?**

Solid silicone.

○   **Which alloplastic implant material has been reported to cause the least amount of bony resorption?**

Porous polyethylene.

O   **What is the major problem of using Mersilene mesh for genioplasty?**

High potential for resorption.

O   **What is the average gain in soft-tissue projection after implant placement?**

70% of the size of the implant.

O   **Why is the gain reduced?**

Implant settling, bone resorption, and soft-tissue compression.

O   **What are the advantages and disadvantages of the intraoral approach to chin implantation?**

No visible scars; increased potential for contamination; suture line irritation; requires larger incision than the external approach; unable to stabilize the implant internally.

O   **How is infection managed after chin implantation?**

A 10-day course of antibiotics is given, and if the infection does not resolve, the implant should be removed. If a microporous implant is used, the implant is removed without delay.

O   **What should be done if bony resorption occurs under the implant?**

Nothing.

O   **How much time should be allotted before removing an implant due to improper size?**

At least 3 months.

O   **In which patients is sliding genioplasty indicated?**

In patients with excess or insufficient vertical mandibular height, extreme microgenia, hemifacial atrophy or mandibular asymmetry, and in those who fail alloplastic chin augmentation.

O   **What is the most common complication of submental liposuction?**

Excessive submental wrinkling.

O   **What are the 3 basic categories of auricular defects as defined by Weerda?**

1st, 2nd, and 3rd degree dysplasia.

O   **What is the definition of 1st degree dysplasia?**

Minor deformities that usually do not require additional skin or cartilage for reconstruction.

O   **What is lobule colobomata?**

Bifid lobule.

O   **What is cryptotia?**

Absence of the retroauricular helix.

○   **What is the definition of 2ⁿᵈ degree dysplasia?**

Some structures of a normal auricle are recognizable and partial reconstruction requires the use of additional skin or cartilage.

○   **What is cockleshell ear?**

Type III cup ear where the ear is malformed in all directions.

○   **What is the definition of 3ʳᵈ degree dysplasia?**

None of the structures of a normal auricle are recognizable and total reconstruction requires the use of additional skin and large amounts of cartilage.

○   **What are the 5 stages in the repair of 3ʳᵈ degree microtia?**

I – auricular reconstruction.
II – lobule transposition.
III – atresia repair.
IV – tragal construction.
V – auricular elevation.

○   **What is the ideal age for unilateral microtia correction?**

Age 6.

○   **What does the Converse technique attempt to reconstruct during surgery for the prominent ear?**

Antihelix of the auricle.

○   **What is the basic method of the Converse technique?**

The antihelix is created using an island of cartilage.

○   **What technique involves placing several horizontal mattress sutures along the scapha to create an antihelical sulcus?**

Mustarde technique.

○   **What is the most common complication of otoplasty?**

Inadequate correction.

○   **What is the most feared complication of otoplasty?**

Chondritis.

○   **What complication is caused by too much flexion of the midportion of the antihelix and inadequate flexion at the superior and inferior poles?**

Telephone ear.

❍   **What problem can occur with overzealous tightening of the superior and inferior third of the ear?**

Reverse telephone ear.

❍   **What is the most common cause of hair loss in men and women?**

Androgenetic alopecia or male pattern baldness.

❍   **What is the pathophysiology of androgenetic alopecia?**

Affected scalp follicles inhibit androgen, causing terminal hairs to convert to vellus hairs.

❍   **Which hair follicles are most likely to be involved in androgenetic alopecia?**

Those in the frontotemporal and crown regions of the scalp.

❍   **What is the most commonly used system to classify alopecia?**

Norwood's system.

❍   **What medication used to treat androgenetic alopecia can reduce libido?**

Finasteride.

❍   **What medication used to treat androgenetic alopecia is also used to treat HTN?**

Minoxidil.

❍   **What landmark is used to determine the correct position of the natural hairline?**

The apex of the frontotemporal triangle should fall on a vertical line intersecting the lateral canthus.

❍   **Normally, how many hair follicles are contained within 1 cm^3 of scalp?**

200.

❍   **Approximately what % of hair follicles must be lost before hair loss is noticeable?**

30%.

❍   **How many hairs are contained in a minigraft?**

3 – 8.

❍   **How many hairs are contained in a micrograft?**

1 – 2.

❍   **How long does it take for hair to start growing after transplantation?**

10 – 16 weeks.

❍   **How much time should be allotted between transplantation sessions?**

4 months.

O   **Alopecia in which area of the scalp is not improved by scalp reduction?**

Frontal.

O   **What procedure is normally performed prior to extensive scalp reductions?**

Ligation of the occipital vessels 2 – 6 weeks before the reduction.

O   **Between which layers of the scalp are tissue expanders placed?**

Between the periosteum and the loose areolar tissue.

O   **What transposition flap restores the frontal hairline?**

Juri flap.

O   **What is the blood supply to this flap?**

Superficial temporal artery.

O   **How many stages are required for completion of the Juri flap?**

4.

O   **When should micro and minigrafts be placed in relation to flap or reduction procedures?**

After the flap or reduction procedures have healed.

FACIAL TRAUMA

○ **How much force is required to fracture the frontal sinus?**

800 – 2200 lbs.

○ **What % of the population has a unilateral frontal sinus?**

10%.

○ **Which table of the frontal sinus is thinner?**

Posterior.

○ **What is the significance of the canals of Breschet?**

The mucosa lining these canals can be a potential origin for mucocele formation.

○ **Where is the opening of the nasofrontal duct in the frontal sinus?**

Usually in the posteromedial floor of the sinus.

○ **In what % of the population is the nasofrontal duct a *true* duct?**

15% (in 85% it exists as a foramen draining directly into the nasal cavity).

○ **What is the significance of the presence of a CSF leak when assessing a patient with a frontal sinus fracture?**

Usually associated with a displaced posterior table fracture and a dural tear.

○ **What are the potential complications from untreated nasofrontal duct fractures?**

Meningitis, mucopyocele, intracranial abscess.

○ **What are the absolute indications for surgical repair of frontal sinus fractures?**

Fractures involving the nasofrontal duct and significantly displaced posterior table fractures with or without dural tear and CSF leak.

○ **What is the treatment for a nondisplaced posterior table fracture with a CSF leak?**

Bed rest with head elevation +/- lumbar drain; cranialization considered if not resolved after 5 – 7 days.

○ **What are the indications for frontal sinus obliteration in the presence of a fracture?**

Displaced posterior table fractures with involvement of the nasofrontal duct.

○ **When is cranialization required for treatment of frontal sinus fractures?**

Displaced posterior table fractures with a CSF leak or significantly comminuted posterior table fractures.

O   **What materials can be used to obliterate the frontal sinus?**

Fat, muscle, fascia, or cancellous bone; can also allow spontaneous osteogenesis after burring the inner cortices.

O   **What does survival of a free fat graft in the frontal sinus depend on?**

The number of transferred pre-adipocytes.

O   **What is the indication for surgical treatment of isolated anterior table fractures?**

Cosmetic deformity.

O   **When are bone grafts used in the repair of anterior table fractures?**

When gaps > 4 – 5 mm are present.

O   **Why is the midface inherently prone to deficient projection?**

It lacks good sagittal buttresses.

O   **What are the 3 paired vertical buttresses of the midface?**

Nasomaxillary, zygomaticomaxillary, and pterygomaxillary.

O   **What are the horizontal buttresses of the midface?**

Frontal bar and cranial base, zygomatic arch and temporal process of the zygoma, maxillary palate and alveolus, and the greater wing and pterygoid plates of the sphenoid.

O   **On physical exam, the nose and the maxillary alveolar process are found to be free-floating. What type of fracture has occurred?**

LeFort II.

O   **Which of the LeFort fractures involves the infraorbital rim?**

LeFort II.

O   **What are the sequelae of untreated maxillary fractures?**

Midface retrusion, facial elongation, and anterior open bite deformity.

O   **What are the sequelae of untreated lateral zygomatic arch fractures?**

Increased midfacial width and malar flattening.

O   **What is the best anatomic guide to reconstruction of the length and medial position of the zygomatic arch?**

Lateral orbital alignment.

O   **What do "miniplates" refer to?**

2.0 mm, 1.5 mm, or 1.3 mm screw applications.

○ **What do "microplates" refer to?**

1.0 mm screw applications.

○ **Which tooth has the longest root?**

Canine.

○ **What is the general approach to repair of LeFort III fractures?**

Begin stabilization at the cranium then work caudally.

○ **Your patient has a fracture of the condylar head and mandibular body and a comminuted midface fracture. How do you approach reconstruction?**

First ORIF the midface, then place the patient into MMF, then ORIF the mandibular body fracture.

○ **Your patient has a fracture of the mandibular body and a comminuted midface fracture. How do you approach reconstruction?**

First MMF, then ORIF the mandible, then ORIF the midface.

○ **What is the treatment of choice for an edentulous 40-year-old epileptic man who sustains a LeFort I fracture during a seizure?**

Direct wiring of the zygomaticomaxillary buttresses.

○ **How can one repair a floating palate when the anterior and lateral walls of the maxilla are severely comminuted?**

Replace the comminuted bone with a bone graft fixed to the alveolar ridge and infraorbital rim.

○ **What are the horizontal buttresses of the nasoethmoidal region?**

Superiorly, the frontal bone and bilateral superior orbital rims; inferiorly, the bilateral inferior orbital rims.

○ **What are the vertical buttresses of the nasoethmoidal region?**

The paired "central fragments" arising from the frontal process of the maxilla and internal angular process of the frontal bone.

○ **What are the 3 limbs of the medial canthal tendon?**

Anterior, superior and posterior limbs.

○ **Which of these covers the lacrimal fossa?**

Superior limb.

○ **Which part of the lacrimal system is most vulnerable to injury?**

The inferior canaliculus near the medial canthal tendon.

O   **What makes up the superior portion of the bony nasal septum?**

Perpendicular plate of the ethmoid.

O   **What is the "bowstring sign"?**

An obvious give that occurs with lateral tension on the lower lid, indicating disruption of the medial canthal tendon.

O   **What test is performed to evaluate for entrapment of the extraocular muscles?**

Forced duction test.

O   **What is the normal intercanthal width?**

30 – 35 mm in Caucasians or roughly the width of the alar base.

O   **What is a type I NOE fracture as described by Markovitz et al?**

Single, noncomminuted central segment fracture.

O   **What is a type II NOE fracture as described by Markovitz et al?**

Comminuted, but identifiable, central fragment.

O   **What is a type III NOE fracture as described by Markovitz et al?**

Severely comminuted fracture with disruption of the medial canthal tendon or too small of a central fragment to be repaired directly.

O   **How does Markovitz's classification assist with management?**

Type I fractures usually can be repaired with microplates; type II fractures usually require transnasal wires in addition to plate fixation; type III fractures usually require at least 2 sets of transnasal wires and may require bone grafting.

O   **What is the preferred donor site for bone grafting in the repair of NOE fractures?**

Outer or inner table of the parietal skull.

O   **On physical examination, digital pressure on the nasal tip causes prolapse of the distal nose into the pyriform aperture. Which type of NOE fracture is this according to Gruss' classification of NOE injuries?**

Type II

O   **What is the "workhorse" for exposure of the nasoethmoidal region?**

Coronal approach.

O   **Where should the point of attachment of the medial canthal tendons be directed?**

Posterior and superior to the lacrimal fossa to avoid telecanthus and blunting of the medial canthal area.

O   **In cases of panfacial fractures, when should NOE fractures be repaired?**

Last.

O   **What is the most likely cause of cyclovertical diplopia following repair of a NOE fracture?**

Disruption of the trochlea.

O   **What are the indications for endoscopic optic nerve decompression after facial trauma?**

66% reduction in amplitude of the visual-evoked response, loss of red color vision, bony impingement on the optic canal, afferent papillary defect.

O   **What are the potential complications of endoscopic optic nerve decompression?**

CSF leak, carotid artery injury, transection of the ophthalmic artery, orbital fat herniation.

O   **What post-orbital fracture visual acuity scores are associated with a return to normal acuity after treatment?**

20/400 or better.

O   **What is the most common cause of loss of vision after reduction of facial fractures?**

Increased intraorbital pressure, usually secondary to venous congestion.

O   **What is the most sensitive test to detect optic nerve injury after facial trauma?**

Pupillary reaction to light.

O   **What are the contraindications to orbital exploration after orbital trauma?**

Injury to an only-seeing eye; presence of hyphema, globe injury, or retinal tear; and medical instability.

O   **How far posterior should dissection proceed when placing a Medpor implant for defects of the posterior convex orbital floor?**

4 cm.

O   **Which approach to the inferior orbital rim involves cutting the capsulopalpebral fascia?**

Transconjunctival.

O   **What % of patients with ZMC fractures have other associated facial injuries?**

25%.

O   **What is the most prominent portion of the ZMC?**

Malar eminence.

O   **Where is this located in relation to the lateral canthus?**

2 cm inferior.

○   **What are the 4 bony attachments to the skull radiating from the malar eminence?**

Superior attachment to the frontal bone (frontozygomatic suture); medial attachment to the maxilla (zygomaticomaxillary suture); lateral attachment to the temporal bone (zygomaticotemporal suture); and a deep attachment to the greater wing of the sphenoid (zygomaticosphenoidal suture).

○   **Which of these is strongest?**

Zygomaticofrontal buttress.

○   **What is the weakest part of the entire ZMC complex?**

Orbital floor.

○   **Why are fractures of all 4 segments called "tripod" and not "tetrapod" fractures?**

Some consider the medial attachment to the maxilla and the deep attachment to the sphenoid bone as a single unit.

○   **What is a type A ZMC fracture?**

Isolated to one component of the tetrapod structure (zygomatic arch, lateral orbital wall, or inferior orbital rim).

○   **What is a type B ZMC fracture?**

Injury to each of the 4 supporting structures.

○   **What is a type C ZMC fracture?**

Complex fracture with comminution of the zygomatic bone.

○   **Which of these is least common?**

Type A.

○   **Which radiographic view is best for visualizing the zygomatic arches?**

Submental vertex.

○   **What is the normal inclination of the orbital floor?**

Inclines superiorly at a 30-degree angle from anterior to posterior and at a 45-degree angle from lateral to medial.

○   **What are the indications for surgical exploration after ZMC injury?**

Visual compromise, EOM entrapment, globe displacement, significant orbital floor disruption, displaced or comminuted fractures.

○   **What are the 3 approaches to the frontozygomatic buttress?**

Hemicoronal, lateral brow, and the upper blepharoplasty incisions.

○ **When approaching the frontozygomatic buttress through the hemicoronal incision, how is the temporal branch of the facial nerve avoided?**

Dissection begins just superficial to the superficial layer of the deep temporal fascia; 2 cm above the zygomatic arch, the dissection is carried deep to the superficial layer of the deep temporal fascia.

○ **What is a potential complication of this approach?**

Damage to the temporal fat pad, resulting in temporal wasting.

○ **What are the 3 approaches to the inferior orbital rim/orbital floor?**

Transconjunctival, subciliary, and rim incisions.

○ **What are the 2 transconjunctival approaches?**

Preseptal and retroseptal.

○ **Which of these involves an incision in the fornix directly into the orbital fat?**

Retroseptal.

○ **What are the advantages to the preseptal approach?**

Protection of the inferior oblique muscle and periorbita.

○ **What is the primary disadvantage to the preseptal approach?**

Slightly higher risk of lower-lid entropion.

○ **What are the disadvantages of the retroseptal approach?**

Increased risk of injury to the inferior oblique muscle and prolapse of orbital fat into the surgical field.

○ **What can be done to improve exposure with the transconjunctival approach?**

Lateral canthotomy with cantholysis.

○ **What are the advantages of the subciliary approach?**

More direct, requires less understanding of orbital anatomy, and provides more exposure than the transconjunctival approach.

○ **What are the advantages of using mesh implants for repair of orbital floor fractures?**

No need for a bone or fascial barrier between the orbital contents and the mesh; posterior orbital shape can be simulated more easily than with bone grafts; well tolerated when exposed to open paranasal sinuses; may facilitate survival of bone grafts in the anterior orbit.

○ **What are the advantages of using cranial bone as an autogenous graft compared to other bone grafts for orbital reconstruction?**

Harvested from the same surgical field; little postoperative pain; donor site complications are rare; large amounts can be harvested; less likely to resorb than endochondral grafts.

O   **What are the advantages of using Medpor over other alloplastic materials for orbital reconstruction?**

Semi-rigid; porous allowing fibrous, vascular, and bony ingrowth; minimal inflammatory reaction; infection and extrusion are rare.

O   **What are the 3 approaches to zygomatic arch fractures?**

Direct percutaneous, temporal (Gillies), and hemicoronal approaches.

O   **What are the advantages of the Gillies approach?**

No visible scar, protects the temporal branch of the facial nerve, and allows bimanual reduction.

O   **What is the plane of dissection with the Gillies approach?**

Dissection is carried out between the temporalis muscle and its overlying fascia.

O   **What is the most appropriate approach for exposure of the inferior maxillary buttresses?**

Upper labial buccal sulcus incision.

O   **What are the advantages of using miniplates over wires in reducing fractures of the ZMC?**

Wires only stabilize in the x plane whereas miniplates add stabilization in all 3 spatial planes (x, y, z); wires are difficult to place in free-floating pieces of bone; wires require exposure of the deep surface of the bone.

O   **What determines the projection of the upper face?**

The frontal bar (supraorbital rims and frontal sinuses).

O   **Reduction of which buttresses is essential to restore upper facial width?**

Frontozygomatic buttresses.

O   **Reduction of which buttresses is essential to restore the midfacial length?**

Zygomaticomaxillary and nasomaxillary buttresses.

O   **What is the most serious complication after orbital reconstruction?**

Blindness.

O   **Where are the anterior and posterior ethmoid arteries and optic canal in relation to the anterior lacrimal crest?**

24 – 12 – 6 rule: anterior ethmoid artery is approximately 24 mm posterior to the lacrimal crest; the posterior ethmoid artery is 12 mm posterior to the anterior ethmoid artery; the optic canal is 6 mm posterior to the posterior ethmoid artery.

O   **What is the average depth of the orbit?**

40 – 50 mm.

○ **What is the most common complication after orbital reconstruction?**

Enophthalmos.

○ **What is the incidence of persistent diplopia after orbital reconstruction?**

7%.

○ **When is diplopia likely to persist after orbital reconstruction?**

If diplopia occurs within 30 degrees of the primary position.

○ **What is the incidence of permanent scleral show with the subciliary approach?**

28%.

○ **What is the most effective treatment for entropion that fails to resolve with massage?**

Placement of a spreader graft (ie, palatal mucosal graft) in the posterior lamella.

○ **What is the general approach for repair of panfacial fractures?**

Begin laterally, work medially, and correct NOE and nasal septal fractures last; frontal fractures should be repaired before midface fractures.

○ **T/F: Patients with titanium implants cannot undergo MRI.**

False.

○ **Which plating material has been shown to have significantly less streak artifacts on CT scans?**

Titanium (as compared to stainless steel and vitallium).

○ **What are the weakest areas of the mandible?**

Area around the 3rd molar, socket of the canine tooth, and the condyle.

○ **What is class I occlusion?**

The mesiobuccal cusp of the maxillary 1st molar articulates with the mesiobuccal groove of the mandibular 1st molar.

○ **What is class II occlusion?**

The mesiobuccal cusp of the maxillary 1st molar lies anterior to the mesiobuccal groove of the mandibular 1st molar.

○ **What is class III occlusion?**

The mesiobuccal cusp of the 1st maxillary molar lies posterior to the mesiobuccal groove of the mandibular 1st molar.

○ **What is an anterior crossbite?**

The maxillary incisors are lingual to the mandibular incisors.

○   **What is a posterior crossbite?**

The maxillary or mandibular posterior teeth are either buccal or lingual to normal.

○   **What is an open bite?**

Lack of anterior incisal contact when the posterior teeth are in occlusion.

○   **What is the difference between overbite and overjet?**

Overbite occurs in the vertical plane whereas overjet occurs in the horizontal plane.

○   **In an adult, what # is the left 3rd molar of the mandible?**

17.

○   **In an adult, what # is the right 3rd molar of the mandible?**

32.

○   **How many deciduous teeth are there?**

20.

○   **How are they numbered?**

A to T.

○   **What is a class I mandible fracture?**

Fracture between two teeth.

○   **What is a class II mandible fracture?**

Teeth are present on only one side of the fracture.

○   **What is a class III mandible fracture?**

Fracture in an edentulous area.

○   **Which parts of the mandible are most commonly fractured?**

Condyle (36%), body (21%), and angle (20%).

○   **T/F: The medial pterygoid muscle elevates the jaw.**

True.

○   **What are favorable fractures?**

Fractures where the muscles tend to draw the fragments together.

○ **What is the most likely mechanism of injury for bilateral condylar fractures?**

Anterior blow to the chin.

○ **Anterior open bite suggests which type of fracture?**

Bilateral condylar fractures.

○ **What are the typical physical findings of a unilateral condylar neck fracture?**

Contralateral open bite and ipsilateral chin deviation.

○ **What % of mandible fractures are associated with other injuries?**

40 – 60%.

○ **What % of mandible fractures are associated with cervical spine injury?**

2.6%.

○ **In patients with mandible fractures, what mechanisms of injury are most predictive of an associated cervical spine injury?**

Penetrating high-velocity gunshot injury; high-velocity MVA.

○ **What is the difference in the mechanism of healing between fractures repaired with MMF and fractures repaired with ORIF?**

With MMF, a callus, formed via micromovement of the fractured ends, bridges the fractured ends together; with ORIF, no callus is formed, and the fracture heals via direct bone growth.

○ **Rigid fixation is based on what two means of stabilization?**

Compression and splinting.

○ **The "zone of tension" refers to which area of the mandible?**

Superior border of the mandible.

○ **The "zone of compression" refers to which area of the mandible?**

Inferior border of the mandible.

○ **What does "dynamic compression" refer to?**

Two-plate system (compression and tension plates).

○ **How is stabilization by splinting performed?**

Reconstruction plates with bicortical screws.

○ **When is stabilization by splinting performed?**

When compression is impossible (eg, inadequate fracture surface area, atrophic edentulous fractures, comminuted fractures, and defect fractures).

O   **What are the indications for extraction of teeth in mandibular fracture lines?**

Teeth that are grossly mobile, have fractured roots, have advanced dental caries and periapical pathology, have soft-tissue pathology, or that hinder fracture reduction.

O   **Which mandible fractures require ORIF with bicortical screws?**

Complex open fractures that are displaced, comminuted, or infected.

O   **What factors lead to infection of mandible fractures?**

Moving fragments, foreign bodies, dead bone.

O   **What is the indication for reduction of coronoid process fractures?**

Trismus secondary to impingement of the fractured fragment on the zygoma.

O   **What is normal interincisal opening?**

40 – 50 mm.

O   **What is the optimal treatment for a nondisplaced condylar fracture?**

If occlusion is normal, soft diet and close observation; bilateral fractures or unilateral fractures with malocclusion should be treated with MMF for 3 weeks, then elastics for 2 weeks.

O   **What are the absolute indications for open reduction of a condylar fracture?**

Displacement of the fractured fragments into the middle cranial fossa, inadequate reduction with MMF, lateral extracapsular displacement of the condyle, foreign body (ie, bullet) embedded in the joint.

O   **What are the relative indications for open reduction of a condylar fracture?**

Bilateral condylar fractures in an edentulous patient when MMF is impossible, condylar fractures when MMF is not recommended for medical reasons, bilateral condylar fractures associated with midface fractures.

O   **What are the approaches to ORIF of condylar fractures?**

Submandibular or retromandibular (most common); intraoral; preauricular face lift incision.

O   **How is closed reduction achieved in edentulous patients?**

The patient's dentures are wired to his or her jaws using circummandibular and circumzygomatic wires or screws. Gunning splints are used if dentures are not available.

O   **What sort of plates should be used in the severely atrophic mandible?**

Large reconstruction plates.

O   **What sort of plates should be used with comminuted mandible fractures?**

Large reconstruction plates.

O   **What are the only plates that can bear the stress of mastication during healing?**

Eccentric dynamic compression plates.

O   **Why should compression plates be over-contoured by 3° - 5°?**

Compression at the buccal surface tends to produce spreading on the lingual side; over-contouring will overcome this.

O   **Where are inferiorly positioned plates placed?**

At the inferior border of the mandible to avoid the neurovascular bundle.

O   **What type of screws are used to secure superiorly positioned plates?**

Monocortical to prevent damage to tooth roots.

O   **When should lag screws be used to reduce a fracture?**

For an oblique fracture with an intact inner fragment where the length of the fracture is at least twice the thickness of the bone.

O   **What are miniplates?**

Lightweight, compression-neutral plates designed to be used with self-tapping screws.

O   **What is the incidence of infection after mandible fracture?**

7%.

O   **What are the most common causes of delayed healing and non-union?**

Infection and noncompliance.

O   **What is the most common cause of infection after ORIF?**

Poor plating technique.

O   **What is the treatment for infected extraoral mandibular ORIF?**

Removal of the tooth and the failed plate, debridement of dead bone, placement of a large reconstruction plate, and primary grafting if inadequate bone contact exists.

O   **What material is used for grafting?**

Fresh autogenous particulate marrow.

O   **10 days after ORIF of a mandibular body fracture, your patient presents with an exposed plate and purulent drainage. The reduction is grossly intact. What do you do?**

Open wound, remove involved tooth if applicable; if hardware is loose, replace it with a new plate; if hardware is rigid, continue drainage, wound care.

○   **4 weeks after ORIF of a mandibular body fracture, your patients presents with an exposed plate and purulent drainage. The reduction is grossly intact. What do you do?**

Open wound, remove involved tooth if applicable, remove hardware, and assess union; if nonunion is present, most patients will heal with MMF; other option is plate and bone graft (external approach).

○   **T/F: After mental nerve injury, sensation usually returns even without repair.**

True.

○   **What problem may arise in the edentulous, denture-wearing patient after mandible fracture with mental nerve disruption?**

Patients who wear a complete mandibular denture require gingival sensation; in the presence of bilateral mental nerve paresthesia, it may be impossible for the patient to tolerate a mandibular denture.

○   **What is brisement forcé?**

Forced jaw opening under anesthesia; usually successful for treatment of trismus that does not respond to physiotherapy.

○   **What can be done for trismus that does not respond to brisement forcé?**

Coronoidectomies.

○   **After MMF for a condylar fracture, your patient complains of deviation of his jaw on opening. What should be done?**

The patient should look in the mirror while opening the jaw and practice forcing himself to open without deviation. The deviation can be overcome with these exercises.

○   **A patient presents to you with TMJ ankylosis after repair of a condylar fracture. What should be done?**

Surgical correction (interpositional arthroplasty, costochondral grafting, total joint prosthesis) followed by vigorous physical therapy.

○   **What is the typical long-term interincisal opening after surgical correction of TMJ ankylosis?**

25 – 28 mm.

○   **What would be the optimal treatment for a 25-year-old man with a LeFort I fracture, bilateral dislocated subcondylar fractures, and a comminuted left parasymphyseal fracture?**

ORIF of the parasymphyseal fracture, ORIF of one subcondylar fracture, and MMF for 3 weeks.

○   **When are serial explorations indicated after penetrating injuries to the face?**

For high-energy gunshot or rifle (>1200 ft/s) injuries, shotgun injuries, and high-energy avulsion injuries.

○   **After high-energy avulsion injuries to the face, when is reconstruction of missing bone and soft tissue initiated?**

When no further necrosis is seen at reexploration of the wound.

O   **What are the contraindications to primary closure of bites?**

Any human bite; animal bites seen after 5 hours of injury; all avulsion injuries from any animal bite.

O   **What is the appropriate management for a deep puncture wound from a dog or cat bite?**

Post-exposure rabies prophylaxis should be considered for all bites. If the animal is healthy, it should be quarantined for 10 days to exclude rabies. If the animal is unavailable or suspected rabid, immediate vaccination and immunoglobulin therapy should be administered. In addition, antibiotic coverage to include *Pasteurella multocida*, should be initiated.

O   **What is the proper tetanus prophylaxis for a patient with a tetanus-prone wound, who last received a booster 7 years ago?**

0.5 ml absorbed toxoid.

O   **What is the appropriate tetanus prophylaxis for a patient with a tetanus-prone wound, who has not been previously immunized?**

0.5 ml absorbed toxoid and 250 units of human tetanus immune globulin.

O   **What is the most helpful test for evaluation of aerodigestive injuries caused by transcervical gunshot wounds?**

Esophagram with water-soluble contrast agent followed by barium.

O   **What % of cervical perforations will be missed with water-soluble contrast agents?**

50%.

O   **What % of thoracic perforations will be missed with water-soluble contrast agents?**

25%.

O   **What is the sensitivity of barium in detecting perforations?**

80 – 90%.

O   **What sort of neurologic sequelae usually result from isolated unilateral vertebral artery injury?**

None.

O   **After carotid artery injury, when is it too late to attempt revascularization?**

When coma has occurred beyond 3 hours, if an anemic infarction has occurred, or if no vascular back flow is present.

O   **What is the definition of cerebral perfusion pressure (CPP)?**

CPP = mean arterial pressure (MAP) – intracranial pressure (ICP).

O   **Cerebral perfusion-directed therapy attempts to maintain CPP at or above what?**

70 mm Hg.

O   **Compared to adults, children are at a higher risk for what type of injury after penetrating injuries to the face and neck?**

Neurological injury.

O   **What is the strongest predictor of negative outcome in trauma patients?**

Arterial hypotension <90 mm Hg.

O   **Transcatheter arterial embolization is most useful in the management of what type of neck injury?**

Gunshot wound (GSW) to zone III of the neck.

O   **A supraclavicular stab wound is in which neck zone?**

I.

O   **What is the most common cranial nerve injury after low-velocity GSW to the paranasal sinuses?**

Trigeminal nerve.

O   **What is the major advantage of immediate aggressive reconstruction after a high-energy GSW to the face?**

Less soft tissue scarring and contracture.

O   **What is the craniofacial ratio at birth?**

8:1.

O   **What is the craniofacial ratio in adulthood?**

2:1.

O   **Due to these differences, which facial fractures are more common in children than in adults?**

High facial fractures (orbital roof, temporal bone fractures).

O   **At what ages are deciduous teeth present?**

From 20 months until age 5 – 6.

O   **What are the most common injuries associated with facial trauma in children?**

Dental injuries.

O   **Which part of the mandible is most commonly fractured in children?**

Condyle.

O   **What are the 3 types of condylar fractures?**

Intracapsular crush fractures of the condylar head, high condylar fractures through the neck above the sigmoid notch, and low subcondylar fractures.

O   **Which of these is most common?**

Low subcondylar fracture (often incomplete or "greenstick" injury).

O   **What is the usual treatment of condylar fractures in children?**

Soft diet.

O   **What are the indications for open reduction of condylar fractures in children?**

When the fractured condyle directly interferes with jaw movement; when the fracture reduces the height of the ramus and results in an open-bite deformity; when the condyle is dislocated into the middle cranial fossa.

O   **T/F: A mandible fracture in a child is much more likely to be associated with other injuries than in an adult.**

True.

O   **Among children, which mandible fractures result in the highest incidence of dentofacial abnormalities?**

Intracapsular crush fractures of the condyle.

O   **What is the difference in tooth viability when comparing plates versus wires for fixation of mandible fractures?**

There is a significant increase in the nonviability of teeth in the line and adjacent to fractures of the mandible treated by plates compared to those treated with wires.

O   **What is the best way to treat mandible fractures in infants <2 years of age?**

Acrylic splints x 2 – 3 weeks.

O   **What are the treatment options for children between 2 and 5 years of age?**

Interdental eyelet wiring, arch bars, cap splints, or soft diet.

O   **Which teeth can be used in children between the ages of 5 and 8 for immobilization?**

Deciduous molars.

O   **Which teeth can be used in children between the ages of 7 and 11 for immobilization?**

Primary molars and incisors.

O   **How long should immobilization typically be maintained in children?**

2 – 3 weeks.

O   **In a child, what is the treatment for an incomplete monocortical crack of the mandibular body with normal occlusion and movement?**

Soft diet.

O   **When can bicortical plates be used in children?**

When permanent dentition is present.

HEAD AND NECK ONCOLOGY

○ **What are 5 major approaches of gene transfer, and which is most common?**

Replacement of mutated tumor suppressor genes, introduction of toxic/suicide genes, immunomodulation (most common), delivery of antisense nucleotides, and cytolytic viral therapy.

○ **What are the 2 main categories of gene delivery agents?**

Viral and nonviral/physical.

○ **What are some physical methods of gene transfer?**

Cationic liposomes, plasmid DNA, ballistic particle, calcium-phosphate-induced uptake and electroporation.

○ **What are the problems with physical methods of gene transfer?**

Lack of specificity and extremely low efficiency.

○ **What viruses are employed in head and neck gene therapy?**

Adenovirus, adeno-associated virus, herpes virus, retroviruses, and vaccinia virus.

○ **What are the advantages of using adenovirus?**

Adenovirus is highly infective of both quiescent and actively-dividing cells, has a known tropism for cells of the upper aerodigestive tract, and can carry large genes.

○ **What are the problems with using retroviruses?**

Can only infect actively dividing cells, are permanently integrated into the host cell's genome, and randomly insert into the host genome.

○ **What does the adenovirus vector do once it enters the host cell?**

Forms a nonreplicating, extrachromosomal entity called an episome that persists for 7 – 42 days.

○ **Where does the adeno-associated virus vector insert its DNA in the host cell?**

At the 19q13.4 location.

○ **What problems may result from insertion at this location?**

This location is associated with chronic B-cell leukemias and integration into both copies of chromosome 19 may lead to cell death.

○ **What are the characteristics of an ideal oncolytic virus?**

Selective for infection and lysis of cancer cells; stimulates a potent antitumor response with limited local/systemic toxicity.

O   **What is the most commonly used gene for cytotoxic gene therapy?**

Herpes simplex virus-thymidine kinase gene (HSV-tk).

O   **How does this gene work?**

Expresses a viral thymidine kinase that is foreign to mammalian cells but phosphorylates the drug ganciclovir into a compound that terminates DNA synthesis in tumor cells.

O   **What is a proto-oncogene? oncogene?**

A proto-oncogene participates in normal cellular signaling, transduction, and transcription; an oncogene is a mutant allele of a proto-oncogene.

O   **What are the two most common tumor suppressor genes under investigation for treatment of head and neck cancers?**

p53 and p16.

O   **What is an antisense drug?**

A small single-stranded nucleotide complementary to a target mRNA molecule that binds to mRNA and halts transcription.

O   **What is the function of IL-2?**

Stimulates T and NK cells.

O   **What is immunologic gene therapy?**

Enhancement of an immune response specifically against tumor-associated antigens using viral vectors.

O   **What is adoptive T-cell immunotherapy?**

Ex vivo enhancement of tumor immunogenicity; lymphocytes are removed from the patient then reinfused after in vitro activation against the patient's own tumor cells.

O   **What are some known head and neck tumor antigens?**

MAGE is seen in 71%; others include mutated CASP-8, SCCAg, cytokeratin fragment 19.

O   **What is the role of the MHC (major histocompatability complex) in the development of head and neck cancer?**

Tumor cells can escape early detection by the patient's immune system via decreased expression of class I MHC antigens.

O   **What is an alloantigen?**

A human antigen from a different individual.

O   **What is allovectin-7?**

An alloantigen that encodes for class I MHC HLA-B7. It is plasmid DNA with a liposome vector that is injected directly into the tumor. Partial response without toxicity has been demonstrated in Phase I trials.

O   **What is CD44?**

A cell surface adhesion molecule that plays an important role in the growth and metastasis of several kinds of tumors.

O   **What is the prognostic significance of CD44?**

Down-regulation of CD44v6 in head and neck tumor cells is closely related to metastases and invasion.

O   **What is the most common site of laryngeal cancer?**

Glottis.

O   **T/F: Embryologically, the supraglottis (SG) and glottis are separate entities.**

True.

O   **What is Broyles' tendon?**

Vocalis muscle tendon that inserts into the thyroid cartilage.

O   **What is its significance?**

Serves as a pathway for tumor extension into the thyroid cartilage.

O   **What anatomic structures inhibit malignant invasion by laryngeal cancers?**

Conus elasticus, quadrangular membrane, thyrohyoid membrane, cricothyroid membrane, internal perichondrium of the thyroid lamina.

O   **What are the boundaries of the pre-epiglottic space?**

Epiglottic cartilage posteriorly, thyrohyoid membrane and hyoid bone anteriorly, hyoepiglottic ligament superiorly.

O   **What anatomic feature of the epiglottis facilitates extension of carcinoma into the pre-epiglottic space?**

Fenestrations/dehiscences.

O   **Which portion of the larynx has sparse lymphatic drainage?**

Anterior glottis (epithelium of the TVC).

O   **What are the 7 different types of squamous cell aberrations occurring in the larynx?**

Benign hyperplasia, benign keratosis (no atypia), atypical hyperplasia, keratosis with atypia or dysplasia, intraepithelial carcinoma, microinvasive SCCA, invasive SCCA.

O   **What % of patients with carcinoma in situ of the vocal cord will develop invasive SCCA after a single excisional biopsy?**

1 in 6 (16.7%).

O   **What is "microinvasive" SCCA of the vocal cord?**

Invades through the basement membrane but not into the vocalis muscle.

O   **What is Ackerman's tumor?**

Verrucous carcinoma, thought to be less radiosensitive and less likely to metastasize than SCCA.

O   **What are "carpet carcinomas"?**

Term used by Kleinsasser to describe laryngeal carcinomas with diffuse mucosal spread and limited submucosal infiltration.

O   **What are the two most important factors predicting lymph node metastasis in laryngeal cancer?**

Tumor size and location.

O   **T/F: CT scan of the larynx underestimates the stage of laryngeal cancer.**

True.

O   **T/F: Once invasion of the laryngeal framework occurs, the ossified portions of cartilage have the least resistance to tumor spread.**

True.

O   **What is the significance of vocal cord fixation in laryngeal carcinoma?**

Invasion of the vocalis muscle has occurred, and lymph node metastasis is more likely.

O   **T/F: Any laryngeal tumor with vocal cord fixation is at least stage T3.**

True.

O   **What % of glottic tumors display perineural and vascular invasion?**

25%.

O   **What % of patients with a primary laryngeal cancer will eventually develop a 2nd primary?**

10 – 20%.

O   **What are the boundaries of a glottic carcinoma traversing the anterior commissure associated with normal or limited cord mobility?**

Anterior commissure tendons, vocal ligament, conus elasticus.

O   **What is the 5-year survival of advanced laryngeal cancer without lymph node metastasis?**

50%.

❍   **What is the stage of a transglottic tumor without vocal cord fixation, cartilage invasion, or extension beyond the larynx?**

T2.

❍   **What % of these tumors will metastasize to the cervical lymph nodes?**

25%.

❍   **What is the 5-year survival of advanced laryngeal cancer when lymph node metastasis is present at diagnosis?**

<20%.

❍   **What is the approximate 5-year survival for T2 glottic cancer involving the anterior commissure treated with primary radiotherapy?**

80% (70% for true crossing tumors).

❍   **What is the significance of positive margins after laryngeal surgery?**

Unclear; no correlation exists between recurrence rate and the type of involved margin (gross, close, intraepithelial). Some advocate careful followup instead of further treatment.

❍   **Which type of laryngeal cancer is mostly likely to metastasize distally?**

Supraglottic.

❍   **T/F: Tumor size is related to the likelihood of distant metastasis.**

False.

❍   **What % of patients with distant metastasis and laryngeal carcinoma have cervical metastasis?**

75%.

❍   **T/F: No correlation with distant spread has been found with the age, sex, or general clinical condition of the host.**

True.

❍   **T/F: The degree of differentiation of the primary correlates with distant metastasis.**

False.

❍   **What is the most common site of distant metastasis from laryngeal carcinoma?**

Lungs.

❍   **What are the next 3 most common sites of metastasis?**

In order of frequency, mediastinal lymph nodes, skeletal system, and liver.

❍   **How does metastatic disease to the lungs normally present?**

Multiple small lesions less than 3 mm that are difficult to detect on x-ray.

○   **What are the characteristics of skeletal metastases?**

Osteolytic lesions most frequently found in the lumbosacral spine and ribs.

○   **What are the 2 most common reasons for tumor recurrence after hemilaryngectomy?**

Inability to recognize the inferior tumor margin and spread of tumor through the cricothyroid membrane.

○   **What is the incidence of positive cervical nodes in patients with T3 glottic tumors?**

30 – 40%.

○   **What is the 5-year survival rate for patients with T3 glottic tumors?**

50%.

○   **What is the difference between hemilaryngectomy and vertical partial laryngectomy (VPL)?**

Thyroid perichondrium is preserved in VPL and excised in hemilaryngectomy.

○   **What are the contraindications to VPL and laryngoplasty?**

Fixed vocal cord, involvement of the posterior commissure, invasion of both arytenoids, bulky transglottic lesions, invasion of the thyroid cartilage, subglottic extension >1 cm anteriorly (5 mm posteriorly), transglottic lesions extending to the supraglottis.

○   **What are the contraindications to VPL for treatment of postradiation tumor recurrence?**

Involvement of both vocal cords, involvement of body of arytenoid, subglottic extension >5 mm, fixed vocal cord, cartilage invasion, different tumor type from original primary.

○   **In which circumstance can a hemilaryngectomy be performed in the presence of vocal cord fixation?**

If the tumor does not extend through the cricothyroid membrane or the perichondrium of the thyroid cartilage.

○   **What technique is most effective in preventing postoperative stenosis after VPL?**

Epiglottopexy.

○   **What is an imbrication laryngectomy?**

A through-and-through excision of a horizontal segment of the larynx with anastomosis of the caudal and cephalic laryngeal margins.

○   **What are the treatment options for T$_{is}$, microinvasive, and T1 glottic carcinoma?**

Endoscopic surgical excision, laser excision, thyrotomy and cordectomy, or radiation.

○   **Which parts of the glottis are most difficult to treat with radiation?**

Anterior commissure, posterior 1/3 of the vocal cord.

O **What are the contraindications to laser excision of early glottic carcinoma?**

Involvement of the anterior or posterior commissure, subglottic extension.

O **What is the purpose of vestibulectomy during excision of early glottic cancer?**

Excision of the false vocal cord enhances intraoperative and postoperative visualization of the entire vocal cord.

O **What is CHP? CHEP?**

Cricohyoidopexy and cricohyoidoepiglottopexy.
Conservation laryngeal procedures performed in concordance with a supracricoid partial laryngectomy. Require preservation of at least one functional cricoarytenoid unit (SLN, RLN, arytenoid, cricoid, and cricoarytenoid musculature).

O **What are the indications for a supracricoid partial laryngectomy with CHP or CHEP?**

1. T2 transglottic (TG) or supraglottic (SG) lesions not amenable to SG laryngectomy secondary to ventricular invasion, glottic extension, or impaired TVC motion.
2. T3 TG/SG lesions with TVC fixation or preepiglottic space involvement.
3. T4 TG/SG lesions with limited invasion of thyroid ala without extension through the outer thyroid perichondrium.
4. Selected glottic tumors at the anterior commissure with preepiglottic space or SG involvement.

O **What are the major complications of these procedures?**

Aspiration pneumonia, rupture of the pexis, laryngocele, laryngeal stenosis.

O **What is the incidence of persistent aspiration after hemilaryngectomy?**

6 – 10%.

O **What is the incidence of delayed decannulation after partial laryngectomy?**

3 – 5%.

O **What structures are considered part of the supraglottis?**

Epiglottis, false vocal cords, aryepiglottic folds, and arytenoids.

O **Where does supraglottic carcinoma most often begin?**

Junction of the epiglottis and false cords.

O **What anatomic structure serves as a natural barrier to the inferior extension of supraglottic cancers?**

Ventricle (embryologic development is completely separate from the false cord).

O **Which kind of supraglottic cancers are more likely to extend inferiorly to the anterior commissure or ventricle... ulcerative or exophytic?**

Ulcerative lesions.

O   **What proportion of patients with supraglottic cancer present with advanced disease?**

2/3.

O   **T/F: Stage I lesions of the supraglottis can be controlled equally well with radiotherapy or surgery.**

True.

O   **What is the greatest single cause of failure of supraglottic laryngectomy?**

Lymph node metastasis.

O   **What is the risk of cervical metastases in patients with T1, T2, T3 and T4 tumors of the supraglottis?**

Approximately 20%, 40%, 60%, and 80%, respectively.

O   **What are other significant prognostic factors for supraglottic tumors?**

Positive surgical wound washings, nearness of neoplastic involvement to the margins of surgical resection, stomal recurrence after laryngectomy, regional and distant metastases.

O   **What are the contraindications to supraglottic laryngectomy?**

Vocal cord fixation, extension to apex of pyriform sinus, bilateral arytenoid involvement, extensive involvement of BOT, involvement of the anterior commissure, invasion of the thyroid cartilage, invasion into the interarytenoid space.

O   **T/F: Extension of a tumor in the pyriform sinus below the plane of the laryngeal ventricle is an absolute contraindication to supraglottic laryngectomy.**

True.

O   **What are the advantages of transoral laser resection of early supraglottic cancer?**

Oncologically sound, no tracheostomy or feeding tube is usually necessary, early discharge, rapid resumption of deglutition, more cost effective.

O   **What is the absolute contraindication to endoscopic laser resection of supraglottic SCCA?**

Base of tongue involvement.

O   **Patients with supraglottic cancer who undergo both surgery and radiation therapy (versus surgery alone) are at a significantly higher risk for what?**

Long-term gastrostomy feeding.

O   **What is the most common and serious complication following supraglottic laryngectomy?**

Bronchopneumonia.

O   **What is the supraglottic swallow?**

Patient inhales, takes food into mouth, performs Valsalva to close the glottis, coughs to clear debris from the glottis, swallows, and then exhales.

○   **Why are patients prone to aspiration after supraglottic laryngectomy?**

Secondary to loss of epiglottis and closure of false cords, to decrease in laryngeal elevation and loss of afferent stimulation to the vocal cords with tracheostomy, and to decrease in sensation from loss of superior laryngeal nerves during tumor resection.

○   **What % of patients undergoing supraglottic laryngectomy and unilateral neck dissection will fail in the contralateral neck?**

16%, despite receiving XRT to the area.

○   **What % will fail if bilateral neck dissections are performed?**

9%.

○   **What % of laryngeal tumors are primarily subglottic?**

5%.

○   **What are the differences between primary and secondary subglottic tumors?**

Primary tumors are less common, usually present with stridor or dyspnea and at a more advanced stage, and have a worse survival time than secondary tumors.

○   **What is the primary site of lymphatic drainage from subglottic tumors?**

Paratracheal nodes.

○   **Compared to supraglottic and glottic tumors, subglottic tumors are at a much higher risk for developing what?**

Stomal recurrence.

○   **What is the mortality rate for stomal recurrence?**

Nearly 100%.

○   **What is the treatment of choice for primary subglottic cancer?**

Total laryngectomy, bilateral neck dissection, near total thyroidectomy, paratracheal node dissection and postoperative radiation to the superior mediastinum and stoma; if the anterior cervical esophageal wall is involved, then laryngopharyngectomy with cervical esophagectomy instead of total laryngectomy.

○   **T/F: Chemosensitive tumors are usually radiosensitive.**

True.

○   **Which types of radiation beams are used for superficial tumors and why?**

Electron beams; their finite range spares deeper tissues.

○   **T/F: Proton beams have poorer skin-sparing properties than electron beams.**

False.

O   T/F: It takes the same amount of radiation to reduce a cell population from 100 to 10 cells as it does to reduce it from 10 billion to 1 billion cells.

True.

O   T/F: The dose of radiation necessary to kill hypoxic cells is 2.5 – 3.0 times greater than that required to kill well-oxygenated cells.

True, as free radical formation requires oxygen.

O   T/F: Cells undergoing DNA synthesis in the S phase are much more radiosensitive than cells in other phases of the cell cycle.

False, they are much more radioresistant in the S phase.

O   T/F: The cells responsible for acute radiation injuries are rapidly cycling.

True.

O   Which factors determine the probability of local control with RT?

The number of malignant cells and the proportion of hypoxic cells.

O   Which type of cancer is most sensitive to RT: exophytic, infiltrative, or ulcerated?

Exophytic.

O   Which has a steeper dose-response curve: small well-vascularized tumors or bulky tumors?

Small well-vascularized tumors.

O   When, after RT, is a positive biopsy a reliable indicator for persistent disease?

3 months after treatment.

O   When does mucositis typically appear?

2nd week of RT.

O   When do maximal skin reactions usually appear?

5th week of RT.

O   T/F: Surgery is more effective in salvaging RT failures than RT is in salvaging surgical failures.

True.

O   How do RT failures differ from surgical failures in site of recurrence?

RT failures often occur in the center of areas that were grossly involved with cancer initially; surgical failures often occur at the periphery of the original tumor.

O **What is conventional fractionated radiotherapy?**

1.8 – 2.5 Gy QD, 5 fractions Q week, for 4 – 8 weeks (total dose 60 – 65 Gy for small tumors, 65 – 70 Gy for larger tumors).

O **How is an altered fractionated schedule different?**

Lower dose per fraction, 2 or more fractions QD, decreased overall treatment time, with total dose same or higher.

O **What are the 2 categories of altered fractionation?**

Accelerated and hyperfractionated.

O **What is the difference between these?**

Accelerated: total dose is the same as conventional treatment, but overall treatment time is decreased
Hyperfractionated: overall treatment time is the same as conventional treatment, but total dose is increased, dose per fraction is decreased, and the number of fractions is increased.

O **What impact does hyperfractionated therapy have on locoregional control and survival rates compared to conventional therapy?**

Significantly higher locoregional control and survival rates.

O **What were the results from the EORTC 22851 study comparing accelerated split-course XRT to conventional XRT?**

The accelerated course resulted in significantly higher late side effects without significant locoregional control or survival advantage.

O **What were the results from the RTOG 9003 study evaluating accelerated treatments with concomitant boost?**

This protocol resulted in significantly higher locoregional control and survival rates with somewhat higher rate of late side effects compared to conventional XRT.

O **Radiation is not as effective for tumors with which characteristics?**

High volume, cartilage-destroying, with bulky lymph node disease.

O **What is the maximum dose of radiation to the spinal cord?**

45 Gy (increased risk of radiation myelitis above this level).

O **What are the advantages of planned preoperative RT?**

Unresectable tumors may be made resectable; the extent of surgical resection may be diminished; the treatment portals preoperatively are usually smaller than those used postoperatively; microscopic disease is more radiosensitive preoperatively due to better blood supply; the viability of tumor cells that may be disseminated by surgical manipulation is diminished.

O **What are the disadvantages of planned preoperative RT?**

Wound healing is more difficult, and the dose that can be safely delivered preoperatively is less than that which can be given postoperatively.

O   **What are the advantages of postoperative RT?**

The anatomic extent of the tumor can be determined surgically, making it easier to define the treatment portals required; a greater dose can be given postoperatively than preoperatively; the total dose to be given can be determined on the basis of residual tumor burden after surgery; surgical resection is easier and healing is better in non-irradiated tissue.

O   **How many cells must be present for a positive margin to be detectable?**

10^6.

O   **When should postoperative RT begin?**

3 – 6 weeks postoperatively.

O   **T/F: RT should not be delayed in the presence of a fistula, open wound, or bony exposure.**

True; as long as the carotid artery is not exposed, radiation treatments should never be delayed.

O   **What are the most common late effects of RT to the head and neck?**

Damage to the eyes, hearing loss, endocrine disorders, xerostomia, chondro- and osteoradionecrosis, soft tissue fibrosis and necrosis.

O   **What are the 3 most important factors leading to osteoradionecrosis (ORN)?**

Hypovascularity, hypocellularity, and hypoxia (the "3H's").

O   **What are the three types of ORN?**

Type I occurs soon after radiation therapy; Type II occurs long after radiation therapy and is induced by trauma; Type III occurs long after radiation therapy and occurs spontaneously.

O   **Which bone in the head and neck is most commonly affected by ORN?**

Mandible; it has a relatively tenuous blood supply, and it is stress-bearing.

O   **What is the incidence of ORN after radiation to the head and neck?**

10 – 15%.

O   **What are the risk factors for development of ORN?**

Dose of radiation (>70 Gy), size and extent of primary, post-radiation dental extraction.

O   **How much time must elapse before starting radiation after dental extractions?**

10 days.

O   **T/F: Almost all cases of ORN are secondary to overlying soft tissue necrosis.**

True.

O   **What effects does RT have on the skin?**

Dryness secondary to damaged sebaceous and sweat glands, thinning of the epidermis, telangiectasias.

O   **What is the principle dose-limiting factor of RT?**

Fibrosis of the subcutaneous tissue and muscle.

O   **What are the ocular complications of RT?**

Cataracts, radiation retinopathy, optic nerve injury, lacrimal gland damage, ectropion/entropion.

O   **Cataracts can occur after how much RT?**

6 Gy.

O   **At what doses can radiation retinopathy or optic neuropathy occur?**

50 – 55 Gy.

O   **What effects does RT have on the ears?**

Serous OM; possibly SNHL, although this controversial.

O   **What effects does RT have on the brain or spinal cord?**

Transient radiation myelopathy, transverse myelitis.

O   **What is the principle sign of transient radiation myelopathy?**

Electric shock sensations triggered by flexing the cervical spine (L'Hermitte's sign).

O   **What is the somnolence syndrome?**

Lethargy, nausea, headache, cranial nerve palsies, ataxia presenting 2 – 3 months after RT and lasting 2 – 4 weeks.

O   **What clinical factors increase the risk of radiation injury?**

Male gender, extremes of age, higher doses and fractions, comorbidities.

O   **What is the most common manifestation of acute injury to the peripheral nervous system?**

Paraesthesias.

O   **What % of patients treated with 50 – 60 Gy of RT to the head and neck complain of ageusia?**

Up to 50%.

O   **What is the pathogenesis behind transient radiation myelopathy?**

Demyelination of the posterior columns.

O   **What are the late radiation effects caused by fibroblast injury?**

Atrophy, contraction, and fibrosis of soft tissue.

O   **Which cranial nerve is most commonly damaged by RT to the head and neck?**

XII.

O   **What is most common hormonal deficiency after RT for NPC?**

Growth hormone deficiency.

O   **How is isotretinoin effective in the treatment of SCCA of the head and neck?**

Reduces the incidence of second primary tumors.

O   **What was the first published randomized trial for organ preservation?**

The VA trial for SCCA of the larynx.

O   **What were the treatment arms?**

1. Surgery.
2. 2 cycles of cisplatinum and 5-fluorouracil.
    a. Responders received a 3rd cycle followed by XRT.
    b. Nonresponders had surgery +/- postoperative XRT.

O   **What was the outcome of this study?**

No significant difference in survival among the three arms.

O   **What are the 3 major randomized studies on organ preservation as treatment for laryngeal cancer?**

VA, GETTEC, EORTC.

O   **What conclusions can be made based on meta-analysis of these studies?**

The surgical patients had slightly higher (but not significant) survival advantage (6%). Among patients receiving chemotherapy, 58% were able to keep their larynx. Better outcomes were seen in patients with hypopharyngeal cancer who underwent chemotherapy than in those with laryngeal cancer.

O   **What is the best organ-sparing treatment for a patient with stage III SCCA of the supraglottis?**

Induction chemotherapy followed by radiation therapy.

O   **What is a functional neck dissection?**

Complete cervical lymphadenectomy sparing the sternocleidomastoid muscle, spinal accessory nerve, and internal jugular vein.

O   **What is the primary blood supply to the skin flaps raised in a neck dissection?**

Transverse cervical artery and facial artery.

O   **Which neck dissection incision results in the best cosmetic outcome?**

MacFee incision.

O   **How should this flap be modified if reconstruction with a deltopectoral flap is planned?**

Inferior incision should be as low as possible.

O   **How far apart should the inferior and superior limbs be with the MacFee incision?**

At least 4 fingerbreaths apart.

O   **Why is the superior limb placed 1 cm inferior to the mandible?**

To hide the scar in the shadow of the mandible.

O   **What are the indications for postoperative radiation after neck dissection?**

Multiple nodes or extracapsular spread.

O   **What is the significance of the number of pathologically positive nodes on prognosis?**

Greater than 3 pathologically positive nodes is a negative prognostic indicator.

O   **What are the recommended indications for elective neck dissection by the National Cancer Comprehensive Network?**

When expected incidence of microscopic or subclinical disease surpass 20% (though many use 25% or 30% as the criteria).

O   **What is the gold standard for identification of subclinical disease?**

Histologic examination of the surgical specimen.

O   **What is the incidence of recurrent disease in the treated N_0 neck in the absence of primary site recurrence?**

2 – 4%.

O   **What is the incidence of contralateral neck metastasis after unilateral selective neck dissection (in the N_0 neck)?**

5%.

O   **What can be said of the presence of level V cervical metastases from SCCA of the upper aerodigestive tract?**

Uncommon (7%), and if present, most likely to occur in the presence of level IV metastases.

O   **For SCCA of the tongue, invasion beyond _____ is associated with a significantly higher incidence of lymph node metastasis.**

4 mm (30% versus 7% if 4mm or less invasion).

O   T/F: Disease-free, but not overall, survival is improved in patients with early oral tongue cancer who undergo elective neck dissection.

True.

O   High expression of which growth factor receptor in head and neck SCCA can potentially predict lymph node metastasis?

Epidermoid growth factor receptor (EGFR).

O   When SCCA grossly invades the adventitia of the carotid artery, how will resection of the artery affect survival?

It will not improve long-term survival.

O   T/F: Neck dissections removed in continuity with the tumor specimen are associated with a significantly higher incidence of survival than those removed separate from the tumor.

True.

O   What are the 3 subsites of the hypopharynx?

Pyriform sinus, postcricoid area, and posterior pharyngeal wall.

O   In which of these sites is cancer more common in females?

Postcricoid area.

O   Which structures separate the hypopharynx from the larynx?

Aryepiglottic folds.

O   What structure in the hypopharynx marks the location of the cricoarytenoid joint?

Pyriform apex.

O   What are the boundaries of the pyriform fossa?

Superiorly, the inferior margin of the hyoid; anteriorly, the junction of the anterior and posterior halves of the thyroid cartilage; posteriorly, the posterior edge of the thyroid cartilage; apex, the cricoarytenoid joint.

O   What are the layers of the posterior pharyngeal wall, from superficial to deep?

Mucosa, constrictor muscles, longus colli, retropharyngeal space, prevertebral fascia.

O   T/F: Hypopharyngeal cancer has the worst prognosis of all head and neck cancers

True; 70% of patients present with advanced disease (stage III and IV) and the 5-year disease-specific survival is only 33%.

O   What is Plummer-Vinson syndrome?

Disease of young women characterized by iron-deficiency anemia, glossitis, splenomegaly, esophageal stenosis, achlorhydria, and severe GERD. These patients have a higher incidence of cancer of the postcricoid area.

O   **In what region of the world is Plummer-Vinson syndrome most common?**

United Kingdom and Scandinavia… rare in the US.

O   **What are the most common and least common sites of tumor involvement in the hypopharynx?**

Pyriform sinus is the most common site (75%); postcricoid area is the least common site (3-4%).

O   **How does the behavior of pyriform sinus tumors differ from postcricoid and posterior pharyngeal wall tumors?**

Tumors of the pyriform sinus tend to infiltrate deeply at early stages; those of the postcricoid area and posterior pharyngeal wall tend to remain superficial until achieving an advanced stage.

O   **In which country does postcricoid involvement occur in 50% of hypopharyngeal tumors?**

Egypt.

O   **What are the three most common presenting symptoms of hypopharyngeal cancer?**

Dysphagia, neck mass, and sore throat (in descending order of incidence).

O   **What features of hypopharyngeal tumors distinguish them from other head and neck tumors?**

Propensity for early submucosal spread and skip lesions.

O   **What significance do these features have on treatment?**

Wide surgical margins (4-6 cm inferior to gross, 2-3 cm superior to gross) and wide radiation therapy ports are necessary.

O   **What is the incidence of cervical metastases at the time of presentation of pyriform sinus tumors? What % are bilateral or fixed?**

60%, 25%, respectively.

O   **T/F: The size of the primary lesion is related to the incidence of lymph node metastases in tumors of the hypopharynx.**

False.

O   **Where do posterior pharyngeal wall tumors metastasize?**

Bilaterally to level II cervical nodes, mediastinum, and superiorly to the nodes of Rouviere at the skull base.

O   **Which site of the hypopharynx drains bilaterally into levels IV and VI?**

Postcricoid area.

O   **T/F: The involvement of the medial (as opposed to lateral) wall of the pyriform sinus significantly increases the likelihood of *bilateral* cervical metastasis.**

True.

O   T/F: Due to the high incidence of cervical metastases, treatment of the neck is necessary in all patients with hypopharyngeal cancer.

True.

O   How does one assess for involvement of the prevertebral fascia?

Intraoperative evaluation is most accurate. During endoscopy, one can attempt to mobilize the posterior pharyngeal wall to assess for involvement. Video esophagography and CT scan are also helpful.

O   What is the incidence of a 2nd primary at the time of diagnosis in patients with hypopharyngeal cancer?

5 – 8%.

O   During endoscopic evaluation of a tumor of the hypopharynx, what 4 questions must be answered?

1. Can the larynx be saved?
2. Is a partial or total pharyngectomy necessary?
3. Is a partial or total esophagectomy necessary?
4. Does the tumor extend into the prevertebral fascia?

O   T/F: Superficial lesions of the posterior pharyngeal wall can be resected endoscopically with a laser and left to mucosalize by secondary intention.

True.

O   What is the most direct approach for resection of all other posterior pharyngeal wall tumors?

Suprahyoid.

O   What is the most serious complication of this approach and how can it be avoided?

Damage to the hypoglossal and superior laryngeal nerves; can be avoided if the greater horn of the hyoid is left undissected.

O   What approach is used for resection of posterolateral tumors?

Combined suprahyoid and lateral pharyngotomy.

O   What is the most serious complication of lateral pharyngotomy?

Excessive retraction on the great vessels leading to thrombosis or embolism.

O   Which tumors of the pyriform sinus do not necessarily require total laryngectomy?

2 cm or smaller, located at least 1.5 cm superior to the pyriform fossa apex, with normal vocal cord movement, and no invasion into adjacent sites; patients must also have good pulmonary function.

O   What procedure is performed for resection of these lesions?

Partial laryngopharyngectomy.

O   When is total esophagectomy indicated?

If the inferior margin during resection of a postcricoid tumor extends below the mediastinal inlet or if a second primary is present in the distal esophagus.

○ **What are 2 important techniques to prevent postoperative fistula formation?**

Tension-free closure and perioperative antibiotics.

○ **What are the reconstructive options after partial pharyngectomy?**

Primary closure (if 3 or more cm of tissue is available), skin graft, SCM flap, radial forearm free flap or deltopectoral flap with a de-epithelialized pedicle.

○ **What problem arises when regional or transplanted skin flaps are used for reconstruction of the hypopharynx when the larynx is preserved?**

A large amount of immobile pharyngeal wall interferes with the pharyngeal component of swallowing, making aspiration inevitable.

○ **What are the reconstructive options after total laryngectomy and partial pharyngectomy?**

Primary closure if more than 40% of the pharyngeal circumference is left in situ, regional flap (pectoralis major, deltopectoral), radial forearm free flap, gastric patch, free jejunal patch, tongue base rotation flap.

○ **What are the reconstructive options after total laryngectomy and total pharyngectomy?**

Free jejunal interposition graft, U-shaped pectoralis major + split thickness skin graft, tubed thin flap (radial forearm or de-epithelialized deltopectoral).

○ **During placement of a tubed flap, where should the longitudinal suture line uniting the sides of the flap into a tube be placed?**

Against the prevertebral fascia.

○ **What are the reconstructive options after total laryngopharyngectomy and cervical esophagectomy?**

Gastric pull-up, free jejunal graft.

○ **What is the primary limitation of the gastric pull-up?**

Obtaining enough length to achieve a tension-free closure.

○ **What is the blood supply to the gastric pull-up?**

Right gastroepiploic and right gastric arteries.

○ **What is the blood supply to the jejunum?**

Superior mesenteric arterial arcade.

○ **What electrolyte problem is disproportionately associated with gastric pull-up?**

Hypocalcemia secondary to impaired calcium absorption and inadvertent parathyroid resection during thyroidectomy.

O   **What length of jejunum is normally harvested for reconstruction?**

15 – 20 cm.

O   **What can be done for a large discrepancy between the circumference of the pharyngeal stoma and the jejunal segment?**

The proximal jejunum can be opened longitudinally along its antimesenteric border or a redundant piece of jejunum can be inserted into the proximal segment to widen the lumen.

O   **Where do fistulas most often occur after free jejunal transfer?**

At the superior anastomosis between the jejunum and pharynx.

O   **Where do strictures most often occur after free jejunal transfer?**

At the inferior anastomosis between the jejunum and esophagus.

O   **What can happen if the free jejunal graft is too long?**

Pooling of secretions and dysphagia.

O   **What can be done to prevent functional dysphagia due to neuromuscular incoordination?**

Myotomy of the jejunal musculature.

O   **T/F: TEP is not effective in patients reconstructed with gastric pull-up.**

False, although the voice quality is poor.

O   **What is the fistula rate in patients who have had prior irradiation requiring total laryngectomy and partial pharyngectomy?**

15 – 20%.

O   **What is the fistula rate following free jejunal transfer (non-irradiated patients)?**

10 – 20%.

O   **What is the perioperative mortality rate of gastric pull-up?**

5 – 20%.

O   **What is the rate of major complications after gastric pull-up?**

50%.

O   **What are the most common complications of gastric pull-up?**

Regurgitation, cervical dysphagia, stricture, anastomotic leak.

O   **What % of patients require dilatation after gastric pull-up?**

50%.

O   **What sort of GI complaints do patients have after gastric pull-up?**

Early satiety, emesis, dumping syndrome.

O   **What can be done to treat or prevent dumping syndrome?**

Eating small dry meals, restricting fluid intake during meals, using octreotide (somatostatin analogue).

O   **What is the primary advantage of the midline mandibular osteotomy for resection of oropharyngeal tumors compared to the lateral mandibulotomy?**

Preservation of the inferior alveolar and lingual nerves.

O   **If a marginal mandibulectomy is performed and the bony margin is positive, does one irradiate the remaining bone?**

No, as bone is relatively hypoxic and cannot generate many free radicals with XRT; the patient should be taken back to the OR for mandibulectomy.

O   **T/F: Due to shrinkage, at least 8 – 10 mm of in-situ margin must be taken to achieve a 5 mm pathologically clear margin for tumors of the oral cavity.**

True.

O   **What factors are most strongly related to overall speech function 3 months after surgery for oral or oropharyngeal cancer?**

Closure type, % oral tongue resected, and % soft palate resected.

O   **What is the differential diagnosis for the etiology of stridor in a patient who has undergone total glossectomy and post-op XRT?**

Edema secondary to altered lymphatics; recurrent tumor; GERD; superinfection.

O   **What are the most common presenting symptoms in patients with tumor of the retromolar trigone (RMT)?**

Referred otalgia and trismus.

O   **How many years does it take for a former smoker to have the same probability of developing an oral cavity cancer as a nonsmoker?**

16.

O   **What is the chance that a patient cured of an oral cavity cancer will develop a second primary if they continue to smoke?**

40%.

O   **What is the incidence of cervical metastases from base of tongue (BOT), tonsil, and soft palate SCCA?**

70%, 60%, 40%, respectively.

○   **What is the incidence of malignancy in adults with asymmetric tonsils with normal-appearing mucosa and no cervical lymphadenopathy?**

4.8%.

○   **What % of T3/T4 tumors of the tonsil can be salvaged after failing primary XRT?**

50%.

○   **What is the purpose of using a STSG to cover a small defect after excision of a tonsil cancer?**

If the pterygoid muscles are exposed during resection, placing a STSG will help prevent muscle fibrosis and trismus.

○   **What are the risk factors for developing osteosarcoma in the mandible or maxilla?**

History of ionizing radiation, fibrous dysplasia, retinoblastoma, prior exposure to thorium oxide (radioactive scanning agent).

○   **What chromosomal abnormality do osteosarcoma and retinoblastoma have in common?**

Deletion of the long arm of chromosome 13.

○   **What are the most important prognostic factors in patients with osteosarcoma?**

Tumor size, grade, and surgical margin status.

○   **T/F: There is a much lower risk of distant metastases with osteosarcoma of the head and neck than that of the long bones.**

True.

○   **T/F: A patient with T3N2aM0 SCCA of the BOT has a complete response to external-beam RT both at the primary site and the neck. A planned neck dissection should be done to increase the rate of regional control.**

True.

○   **Which site in the oropharynx is associated with the worst functional outcome after combined surgery and RT regardless of tumor stage?**

BOT.

○   **What are the three most common odontogenic tumors?**

Ameloblastoma, cementoma, odontoma.

○   **What are the three most common odontogenic cysts?**

Radicular cyst (65%), odontogenic keratocyst, dentigerous cyst.

○   **What are odontomas composed of?**

Enamel, dentin, cementin, and pulp.

O   **Where does a radicular or periapical cyst occur?**

Along the root of a non-viable tooth, as the liquefied stage of a dental granuloma.

O   **Where do dentigerous cysts develop?**

Around the crown of an unerupted, impacted tooth.

O   **Multiple odontogenic keratocysts are a manifestation of what syndrome?**

Basal cell nevus syndrome.

O   **What is a Pindborg tumor?**

Calcified epithelial odontogenic tumor that is less aggressive than ameloblastoma and is associated with an impacted tooth.

O   **Which mandibular tumor or cyst produces white, keratin-containing fluid?**

Odontogenic keratocyst.

O   **What is the incidence of recurrence after excision of odontogenic keratocyst?**

62% in the first 5 years.

O   **How does osteosarcoma of the mandible appear radiographically?**

Sunburst appearance, radiating periosteal new bone.

O   **How does chondrosarcoma of the mandible appear radiographically?**

Soft tissue mass with amorphous "popcorn" calcifications.

O   **How does ameloblastoma appear radiographically?**

Displaced surrounding structures, with multiple loculations and a honeycomb appearance.

O   **How does cemento-ossifying fibroma appear radiographically?**

Well-circumscribed lesion with a dense core and lucent rim; the core enlarges and rim diminishes with maturation.

O   **What is the most common cause of death in osteosarcoma of the head and neck?**

Intracranial extension.

O   **What is the optimal treatment for osteosarcoma of the head and neck?**

Surgery and radiation therapy.

O   **What % of parotid gland tumors are benign?**

75 – 80%.

O   **What is the most common site of a salivary gland neoplasm?**

Parotid gland (73%).

O   **What is the least common site of a salivary gland neoplasm?**

Submandibular gland (11%).

O   **What is the most common site of a *malignant* salivary gland neoplasm?**

Minor salivary glands (60%; of these, 40% occur on the palate).

O   **What is the least common site of a malignant salivary gland neoplasm?**

Parotid gland (32%).

O   **Which salivary gland has the best prognosis for malignant tumors?**

Parotid gland.

O   **Which salivary gland has the worst prognosis for malignant tumors?**

Submandibular gland.

O   **What is the most common tumor of the parotid gland?**

Pleomorphic adenoma in adults, hemangioma in children.

O   **How does metastasizing pleomorphic adenoma differ from carcinoma ex-pleomorphic adenoma?**

It is histologically benign, lacking malignant epithelial components.

O   **What is the most common malignant tumor of the parotid gland in adults?**

Mucoepidermoid carcinoma.

O   **What is the histologic appearance of pleomorphic adenoma?**

Morphologically diverse with mucoid, chondroid, osseous, and myxoid elements.

O   **What is the most common complication of parotidectomy?**

Hematoma.

O   **What is the most important prognostic factor for malignant salivary gland neoplasms?**

Stage.

O   **Which salivary gland tumors have the worst prognosis (5)?**

High-grade mucoepidermoid, adenocarcinoma, squamous cell carcinoma, undifferentiated carcinoma, and carcinoma ex-pleomorphic adenoma.

○ **What are the indications for postoperative radiation after parotidectomy?**

High probability of residual microscopic disease; positive margins; advanced stage; high grade; deep lobe tumors; recurrent tumors; presence of regional metastases; angiolymphatic invasion.

○ **What is the rate of lymph node metastasis from SCCA of the parotid gland?**

47%.

○ **What factors are predictors of occult regional disease in parotid cancer?**

Extracapsular extension, preoperative facial paralysis, age >54 years, and perilymphatic invasion.

○ **What are the indications for neck dissection in the treatment of salivary gland malignancies?**

Clinical metastasis, submandibular tumor, SCCA, undifferentiated carcinoma, size >4 cm, and high grade mucoepidermoid carcinoma.

○ **What is the most common site of distant metastasis for adenoid cystic carcinoma?**

Lung.

○ **What is the incidence of subclinical neck disease with adenoid cystic carcinoma of the parotid gland?**

11%.

○ **What is the cell of origin of parotid gland SCCA?**

Excretory duct cell.

○ **Which salivary gland tumor contains both benign and malignant cells?**

Malignant lymphoepithelioma.

○ **Which benign parotid gland tumors are recognized by a high concentration of mitochondria on electron microscopy?**

Warthin's tumor and oncocytoma.

○ **What is the most common salivary gland malignancy following radiation?**

Mucoepidermoid.

○ **What is the most common malignancy of the submandibular and minor salivary glands?**

Adenoid cystic.

○ **What type of tumor comprises 50% of all lacrimal gland neoplasms?**

Adenoid cystic.

O   **What are the 4 types of growth patterns of adenoid cystic carcinoma and which is most common?**

Cribiform (most common... looks like Swiss cheese), tubular/ductular, trabecular, or solid.

O   **Which type of radiation therapy does adenoid cystic carcinoma respond best to?**

Neutron beam.

O   **What is the 5-year survival of patients with malignant parotid gland tumors who present with VIIth nerve paresis?**

18%.

O   **What is the most common salivary gland malignancy to occur bilaterally?**

Acinic cell.

O   **What are the 2 most common malignant tumors of the parotid gland in children younger than 12?**

Mucoepidermoid is the most common, followed by acinic cell.

O   **What cells do mucoepidermoid tumors arise from?**

Epithelial cells of interlobar and intralobar salivary ducts.

O   **What feature distinguishes low-grade from high-grade mucoepidermoid carcinoma?**

The amount of mucin in the tumor.

O   **What is the incidence of cervical metastasis of mucoepidermoid carcinomas?**

30 – 40%.

O   **Your patient has a mucoepidermoid carcinoma of the parotid gland. Histologic evaluation of the biopsy specimen reveals a scant amount of mucin. There is no clinical evidence of regional metastasis. Do you treat the neck?**

Yes.

O   **What is the second most common malignant tumor of the minor salivary glands?**

Adenocarcinoma.

O   **What are the four types of monomorphic adenomas?**

Basal cell, trabecular, canalicular, and tubular.

O   **What is the histologic appearance of Warthin's tumor?**

Abundant lymphoid sheets with distinct germinal centers; bilayer epithelium.

O   **Which salivary gland tumor is more common in Eskimos?**

Malignant oncocytoma.

○ **Which salivary gland tumor is more common in women with a history of breast cancer?**

Mucoepidermoid carcinoma.

○ **What is the treatment of choice for metastatic cutaneous SCCA to the parotid?**

Total parotidectomy with preservation of VII (unless invaded by tumor) and postoperative radiation therapy to the parotid area and ipsilateral neck.

○ **When must the facial nerve be sacrificed during parotidectomy?**

Preoperative facial nerve weakness or paralysis; adenoid cystic carcinoma abutting the nerve; malignant tumor infiltrating the nerve.

○ **What % of malignant tumors of the parotid gland present with facial nerve weakness or paralysis?**

20%.

○ **Which salivary gland tumor has a high propensity for perineural invasion?**

Adenoid cystic carcinoma.

○ **What are the clinical features of salivary duct carcinomas?**

Most commonly involve the parotid gland and present as an asymptomatic mass; higher incidence in males; distant metastases are the most common cause of death.

○ **What is the incidence of false positives for FNA and frozen section of parotid tumors?**

2%.

○ **What does continuous facial nerve monitoring during parotidectomy prevent?**

Short-term paresis.

○ **What factors are associated with the development of temporary facial paresis after parotidectomy?**

Deep lobe tumor; previous parotid surgery; history of sialoadenitis; addition of a neck dissection to the parotid surgery; increased age; diabetes mellitus; increased operative time; history of parotid irradiation; no EMG monitoring.

○ **Which branch of the facial nerve is most commonly paretic after parotidectomy?**

Marginal mandibular.

○ **What is the incidence of immediate onset of facial nerve dysfunction after parotidectomy for benign disease?**

46%.

○ **What are the boundaries of the parapharyngeal space?**

Inferior: hyoid bone.
Superior: petrous bone.
Medial: soft palate, tonsils, superior pharyngeal constrictor.
Lateral: medial pterygoid muscle, ramus of the mandible, posterior belly of the digastric.
Dorsal: vertebral column and paravertebral muscles.
Ventral: pterygomandibular raphe.

○   **What structures are found in the prestyloid compartment of the parapharyngeal space?**

Medial pterygoid muscle, fat, lymphatics, minor nerves and vessels.

○   **What structures are found in the poststyloid compartment of the parapharyngeal space?**

Carotid sheath, IX, X, XII, cervical sympathetic chain.

○   **What space does the parapharyngeal space communicate with dorsally?**

Retropharyngeal space.

○   **Parapharyngeal tumors arising from the deep lobe of the parotid will involve which compartment?**

Prestyloid compartment.

○   **What happens to the carotid sheath with deep lobe parotid tumors extending into the parapharyngeal space?**

It is displaced posteriorly.

○   **How do these tumors appear radiographically?**

As a "dumbbell"; they must traverse through the stylomandibular tunnel to access the parapharyngeal space.

○   **Which compartment are neurogenic tumors most likely to arise in?**

Poststyloid compartment.

○   **What is the most common presentation of a parapharyngeal space tumor?**

Medial displacement of the lateral oropharyngeal wall or as a palpable mass beneath the angle of the mandible.

○   **What is the most common tumor of the parapharyngeal space?**

Pleomorphic adenoma.

○   **What is the best surgical approach for removal of parapharyngeal tumors?**

Transcervical.

○   **What should be done preoperatively for retrostyloid malignancies or tumors suspected to be involving the carotid artery?**

Angiography with balloon occlusion.

○ **What is the incidence of paraganglioma?**

1:30,000.

○ **What % of head and neck paragangliomas are familial?**

7 – 10%.

○ **What are the 2 primary cells of paragangliomas?**

Type I granule-storing chief cells and type II Schwann-like sustentacular cells arranged in a cluster called a Zellballen.

○ **How does one differentiate between a benign and a malignant paraganglioma?**

There are no clear histologic characteristics of malignancy; malignant lesions are defined by the presence of metastases.

○ **What is the most common paraganglioma of the head and neck?**

Carotid body tumor.

○ **What % of carotid body tumors are multicentric?**

10% (30 – 40% in the hereditary form).

○ **What is the inheritance pattern of familial carotid body tumors?**

Autosomal dominant but only the genes passed from the paternal side are expressed.

○ **What is the classic physical finding of carotid body tumors?**

Freely moveable in the lateral direction but fixed in the cephalad-caudal direction.

○ **What is the classic finding on arteriogram of carotid body tumors?**

Splaying of the carotid bifurcation by a well-defined tumor blush ("lyre sign").

○ **What is Shamblin's classification system for carotid body tumors?**

Group I: small and easily excised.
Group II: adherent to the vessels; resectable with careful subadventitial dissection.
Group III: encase the carotid; require partial or complete vessel resection

○ **What is the significance of tumor size on the incidence of complications with resection?**

Tumors larger than 5 cm are associated with a significantly higher rate of complications with removal (67% for tumors >5 cm vs 15% for tumors <5 cm).

○ **What are the advantages of preoperative embolization of paragangliomas?**

Decreased intraoperative blood loss and operative time.

O   **When embolized preoperatively, communication between the external and internal carotid circulation may occur through which vessel?**

Occipital artery.

O   **During resection, which vessel can be sacrificed in most cases?**

External carotid artery.

O   **When is XRT considered in lieu of surgery for treatment of carotid body tumors?**

Very large tumors, recurrent tumors, or poor surgical candidates.

O   **How can one differentiate a vagal paraganglioma from a carotid body tumor?**

Vagal paragangliomas displace the internal carotid anteriorly and medially.

O   **What is the "first bite syndrome"?**

Complication after removal of a carotid body tumor where the patient experiences intense pain with the first bite of food.

O   **What are the two types of temporal bone paragangliomas?**

Glomus jugulare involving the adventitia of the jugular bulb and glomus tympanicum involving Jacobson's nerve (jugulotympanic glomus if unable to discern site of origin).

O   **What are the histologic features of glomus tumors?**

Nests of chief cells with neurosecretory granules, surrounded by fibrovascular stroma and sustentacular cells that are S-100 positive. Chief cells are positive on immunohistochemistry for chromogranin, synaptophysin and neuron-specific enolase neurofilaments.

O   **How do these tumors differ clinically from carotid body tumors?**

More common in females, less likely to secrete catecholamines or metastasize, and are more radiosensitive.

O   **What is the primary advantage of stereotactic radiosurgery for treatment of recurrent glomus jugulare tumors compared to surgery and conventional radiation?**

Lower incidence of cranial nerve injury.

O   **When is stereotactic radiosurgery contraindicated in the treatment of recurrent glomus jugulare tumors?**

For larger tumors (>3.0 – 4.0 cm).

O   **How do most glomus jugulare tumors respond to external beam radiation?**

Less than 50% show tumor regression radiographically; lack of tumor growth is more common.

O   **What is the reported ratio of basal cell to squamous cell cancer in the United States?**

4:1.

○ **After having a basal or squamous cell carcinoma of the skin, what are the chances of developing another one within 5 years?**

50%.

○ **What is basal cell-nevoid syndrome?**

Autosomal dominant disorder characterized by multiple basal cell carcinomas (BCC), odontogenic keratocysts, rib abnormalities, palmar and plantar pits, and calcification of the falx cerebri.

○ **What are some other genetic disorders that are associated with a high risk of cutaneous malignancies?**

Xeroderma pigmentosum, albinism, epidermodysplastic verruciformis, epidermolysis bullosa dystrophica, and dyskeratosis congenital

○ **Which UV light is most responsible for acute actinic damage?**

B.

○ **Other than UV light and genetics, what are some other factors that increase the risk of cutaneous malignancy?**

Long-term immunosuppression after organ transplantation, long-term treatment of psoriasis with photosensitizing chemicals, chronic ulcers, low-dose irradiation.

○ **What is Marjolin's ulcer?**

Burn or ulcer associated with the development of malignancy.

○ **What are the 5 layers of the epidermis from deep to superficial?**

Stratum basale, stratum spinosum, stratum granulosum, stratum lucidum, stratum corneum

○ **What is the most common premalignant skin lesion of the head and neck?**

Actinic keratosis.

○ **What is the name for a skin lesion, most commonly located on the nose, characterized by rapid growth with a central area of ulceration followed by spontaneous involution?**

Keratoacanthoma.

○ **What is Bowen's disease?**

Squamous cell carcinoma-in-situ of the skin.

○ **T/F: Adnexal carcinomas of the skin are very aggressive and have a poor prognosis.**

True.

○ **How do adnexal carcinomas arising from hair follicles classically present?**

A tuft of white hair emerges from the central portion of the tumor.

322   OTOLARYNGOLOGY AND FACIAL PLASTIC SURGERY BOARD REVIEW

○   **Which adnexal skin carcinoma arises from a pluripotential basal cell within or around the hair cells?**

Merkel cell carcinoma.

○   **What is the 5 year survival of patients with Merkel cell carcinoma?**

30%.

○   **Should the N0 neck be treated in patients with Merkel cell carcinoma?**

Yes.

○   **Reconstruction should be delayed after excision of Merkel cell carcinoma until permanent section results are back.**

True.

○   **What is the most common type of skin sarcoma?**

Malignant fibrous histiocytoma.

○   **What are the 5 main types of BCC?**

Nodular, cystic, superficial multicentric, morpheaform, keratotic.

○   **Which of these is most common?**

Nodular.

○   **Which of these is more commonly found on the extremities or trunk?**

Superficial multicentric.

○   **Which of these is a variant of nodular BCC and produces pigment?**

Cystic.

○   **Which of these commonly resembles a scar?**

Morpheaform.

○   **Which of these is the most aggressive?**

Keratotic.

○   **What are the histologic features of BCC?**

Clefting, lack of intracellular bridges, nuclear palisading, and peritumoral lacunae.

○   **What is unique about the path of growth of BCC?**

Follow the path of least resistance, which is typically along embryonic fusion planes.

O   **That being said, which areas of the face are most susceptible to BCC?**

Inner canthus, philtrum, mid-lower chin, nasolabial groove, preauricular area, and retroauricular sulcus.

O   **What are the recommended margins for excision of basal cell skin cancers?**

5 mm.

O   **What percentage of incompletely excised basal cell cancers will recur?**

One-third.

O   **What histologic characteristic of recurrent basal cell cancers has prognostic significance?**

Irregularity in the peripheral palisade.

O   **T/F: Squamous cell carcinoma (SCCA) arising in sun-exposed areas tend to behave less aggressively than those arising *de novo*.**

True.

O   **What % of SCCA arising in areas of actinic change metastasize?**

3 – 5%.

O   **What % of SCCA arising *de novo* metastasize?**

8%.

O   **What % of SCCA arising in areas of scar or chronic inflammation metastasize?**

10 – 30%.

O   **What are the histologic features of SCCA of the skin?**

Keratin pearls in well-differentiated lesions; poorly-differentiated lesions may require identification with a cytokeratin or vimentin.

O   **What are the 5 histopathologic types of SCCA?**

Generic, adenoid, bowenoid, verrucous, and spindle-pleomorphic.

O   **Which of these arises in areas of actinic change?**

Generic.

O   **Which of these is more common in the oral mucosa?**

Verrucous

O   **Which of these is the least common?**

Spindle-pleomorphic.

O   **What factors increase the likelihood of recurrence for SCCA?**

Tumors on the midface, diameter >2 cm or thickness >4 mm, perineural invasion, or regional metastases.

O   **What factors increase the likelihood of regional metastasis of SCCA?**

Tumors arising on the ear, diameter >2 cm or >4 mm thickness, poorly differentiated histology, and recurrent tumors.

O   **What are the indications for MOHS surgery?**

Morpheaform BCC, recurrent BCC, and BCC in cosmetically-sensitive locations.

O   **What are the indications for a prophylactic neck dissection?**

SCCA > 4 cm with deep invasion arising on the cheek, upper neck, or scalp.

O   **What are the indications for postoperative radiation therapy?**

Multiple nodes, extracapsular spread, positive/inadequate margins, or node > 3 cm.

O   **What % of melanomas occur in the head and neck?**

20%.

O   **In what area of the world is the incidence of melanoma the highest?**

Australia.

O   **What % of tumors are not pigmented (amelanotic)?**

5%.

O   **What cells are melanomas comprised of?**

Melanocytes, which are derived from neural crest cells.

O   **Involvement of which areas of the body increases the risk of metastases?**

BANS: back, arms, neck and scalp.

O   **Which classification system is based on histologic layers?**

Clark's.

O   **What are the levels defined in Clark's system?**

Level I: epidermis.
Level II: invasion of basal lamina into the papillary dermis.
Level III: fill the papillary dermis.
Level IV: invasion into the reticular dermis.
Level V: invasion into subcutaneous fat.

O   **Which classification system is based on depth of invasion by millimeters?**

Breslow's.

O **What is the most important prognostic factor of melanomas?**

Depth of invasion.

O **How should a lesion suspicious for melanoma be biopsied?**

A sample should be taken of the tumor and the underlying tissue so that depth can be ascertained; a shave biopsy should never be performed.

O **T/F: Women with melanoma have a better prognosis than men regardless of tumor depth.**

True.

O **What is the incidence of nodal metastases if the depth of the tumor is >4.0 mm?**

>70%.

O **What is the incidence of nodal metastases if the depth of the tumor is <1.50 mm?**

8%.

O **What factor, other than tumor thickness, influences regional metastasis in melanoma?**

Ulceration.

O **What are the risk factors for developing melanoma?**

Family history, multiple atypical or dysplastic nevi, Hutchinson's freckle, presence of large congenital nevi, blond or red hair, marked freckling on upper back, history of 3 or more blistering sunburns prior to age 20, presence of actinic keratoses.

O **What percentage of patients with dysplastic nevus syndrome develop melanoma if a relative has a history of melanoma?**

100%.

O **What is the risk of melanomatous transformation of giant congenital nevi?**

14%.

O **What % of patients with xeroderma pigmentosa develop melanoma?**

3%.

O **What is the chance that a patient with melanoma will develop a second melanoma?**

5%.

O **What are the 4 types of melanoma?**

Superficial spreading, lentigo maligna, acral lentiginous, and nodular sclerosing.

○   **Which is the most common?**

Superficial spreading.

○   **Which has the best prognosis?**

Superficial spreading.

○   **What is the most common form of hereditary cutaneous melanoma?**

Dysplastic nevus syndrome.

○   **Which type of melanoma occurs on palms, soles, nail beds, and mucous membranes?**

Acral lentiginous melanoma.

○   **What is the recommended excisional margin for a 3 cm melanoma?**

2 cm.

○   **What are the indications for parotidectomy in addition to resection of the tumor?**

If the lesion involves the lateral forehead, temporal scalp, preauricular skin, or anterior ear.

○   **When should the submandibular gland be removed with the tumor?**

If the lesion involves the cheek, zygomatic area, nasolabial fold, or upper lip.

○   **Is melanoma radiosensitive?**

It may be sensitive to large dose fractions (600cGy) but not to standard fractionation radiotherapy (180 – 200cGy).

○   **What is the role of large-dose fraction radiotherapy in the management of melanoma?**

Decreases incidence of locoregional recurrence among N0 patients.

○   **What are the boundaries of the cervical esophagus?**

Cricopharyngeus muscle to sternal notch.

○   **What is the arterial supply to the cervical esophagus?**

Thyroid branch of the thyrocervical trunk.

○   **What is the venous drainage of the cervical esophagus?**

Inferior thyroid vein.

○   **What is the risk of developing esophageal cancer in patients who smoke and drink compared to those who don't?**

100 times higher.

O **In which areas of the world is the incidence of esophageal cancer highest?**

Middle East, southern and eastern Africa, and northern China.

O **What are the risk factors for developing esophageal cancer?**

Tobacco, alcohol, achalasia, Plummer-Vinson syndrome, prior head and neck cancer, tylosis, Barrett's disease.

O **What are the clinical features of Plummer-Vinson syndrome?**

Iron deficiency anemia, upper esophageal web, hypothyroidism, glossitis/cheilitis, gastritis, and dysphagia.

O **In patients with Plummer-Vinson syndrome, where is SCCA of the esophagus most likely to occur?**

Post-cricoid area.

O **Metaplasia of the distal esophagus is otherwise known as what?**

Barrett's esophagus.

O **What % of people with GERD have Barrett's esophagus and what % of these people will develop adenocarcinoma?**

5%; 5 – 10% respectively.

O **Cancer of the cervical esophagus is usually what type?**

SCCA.

O **What are the contraindications to surgical resection?**

Presence of distant metastases; involvement of prevertebral fascia, trachea, or carotid arteries.

O **What is the usual cause of death from esophageal cancer?**

Aspiration pneumonia.

O **When do patients with synovial sarcoma usually present?**

Between ages 25 to 36.

O **What is the incidence of regional metastasis in synovial sarcomas of the head and neck?**

12.5%.

O **What is the incidence of local recurrence?**

60 – 90%, usually within 2 years.

O **What are the histopathologic features of synovial sarcoma of the head and neck?**

Poorly differentiated, high grade malignant neoplasms arising from pluripotential mesenchymal cells; biphasic cellular pattern containing spindle cells and epithelioid cells; microcalcifications in 30 – 60%; the existence of monophasic forms, containing either spindle or epithelioid cells, is controversial.

O   **What is the most common cause of death from synovial sarcoma of the head and neck?**

Lung metastases.

O   **Where are most synovial sarcomas of the head and neck located?**

Hypopharynx and parapharyngeal space.

O   **What is the primary mode of treatment?**

Wide surgical excision and postoperative radiation therapy.

O   **What is the 5-year survival rate?**

40 – 50%.

O   **What prognostic significance does the presence of microcalcifications have?**

Better prognosis.

O   **Nasopharyngeal cancer accounts for what % of all cancers diagnosed in the Kwantung province of southern China?**

20%.

O   **What is the incidence of nasopharyngeal cancer among native-born Chinese compared to that among Caucasians?**

118 times higher.

O   **What is the incidence of nasopharyngeal cancer among North American-born Chinese compared to that among Caucasians?**

7 times higher.

O   **What are the classifications of nasopharyngeal cancer designated by the WHO?**

Type I: well-differentiated, keratinizing SCCA.
Type II: poorly differentiated, nonkeratinizing SCCA.
Type III: lymphoepithelioma or undifferentiated.

O   **Which of these is characterized by syncytia (fused multinuclear giant cells)?**

Type III.

O   **Which of these is most common in North America? Least common?**

Most common is type III (70%); least common is type II (10%).

O   **Which of these is not associated with positive EBV titers?**

Type I.

O   **What EBV product is likely to play a role in malignant transformation of nasopharyngeal epithelium?**

Latent membrane protein (LMP-1).

O   **What environmental factor is most strongly linked to NPC?**

Frequent consumption of dried salted fish.

O   **What is the 5-year survival of patients with WHO II or III disease?**

70%.

O   **What is the 5-year survival of patients with WHO I disease?**

30%.

O   **What is the most common site of origin of nasopharyngeal cancer?**

Fossa of Rosenmüller.

O   **Where is the fossa of Rosenmüller?**

Just posterior-superior to the torus tubarius of the eustachian tube orifice.

O   **Which foramina of the skull lie in close proximity to the nasopharynx?**

Foramen lacerum, carotid canal, foramen spinosum, foramen ovale, foramen rotundum, hypoglossal canal, and jugular foramen.

O   **What structure courses through the foramen ovale?**

The mandibular nerve (V3).

O   **What is the relationship of the fossa of Rosenmüller to the parapharyngeal space?**

It lies at the convergence of the fascial planes that separate the parapharyngeal space into its three compartments (prestyloid, retrostyloid, and retropharyngeal).

O   **What kind of epithelium lines the nasopharynx?**

At birth, pseudostratified columnar epithelium; by age 10, the majority is replaced by stratified squamous epithelium. The lateral portion does not change, and the area where these two types meet is lined by transitional epithelium.

O   **After SCCA, what is the 2nd most common malignant tumor of the nasopharynx?**

Lymphoma.

O   **Which nodal groups does nasopharyngeal cancer spread to?**

Retropharyngeal nodes of Rouviere, jugulodigastric nodes, spinal accessory chain.

O   **In the staging system described by Ho, poorer prognosis is associated with cervical metastases to which area of the neck?**

Inferior to a plane spanning from the contralateral sternal head of the clavicle to the ipsilateral superior margin of the trapezius muscle.

O   **T/F: The presence of unilateral compared with bilateral nodal disease in patients with NPC has no prognostic significance.**

True.

O   **What is the incidence of skull base erosion in patients with NPC?**

25%.

O   **What is the most common site of distant metastases?**

Bones.

O   **What % of patients with NPC will have a normal exam by fiberoptic endoscopy at the time of initial evaluation?**

6%.

O   **Smooth, submucosal nasopharyngeal masses located in the midline are most often what?**

Embryologic remnants (Thornwaldt's cysts, pharyngeal bursa remnants).

O   **What is the incidence of cranial nerve palsy at initial presentation in patients with NPC?**

12 – 18%.

O   **What are the most common immunologic findings among patients with NPC?**

Elevated IgA and IgG antibodies against the viral capsid antigen of EBV.

O   **What is the role of ascertaining EBV titers in patients with NPC?**

May be a valuable screening tool in high-risk populations and can help establish the diagnosis of NPC in the patient with an unknown primary. In patients with type I disease, EBV titers are not elevated and have no prognostic significance.

O   **What % of patients with WHO types II and III tumors have abnormally increased titers to EBV VCA and NA?**

80 – 90%.

O   **What test provides prognostic information in patients with NPC?**

Antibody-dependent cellular cytotoxicity (ADCC) assay.

O   **How does this assay predict survival?**

Low levels are associated with worse prognosis.

○   **What factors, described by Ho and Neel, are regarded as important adverse prognostic indicators in patients with NPC?**

Length and symptomatology of disease, extension of tumor outside of the nasopharynx, presence of inferior cervical adenopathy, keratinizing histologic architecture, cranial nerve and skull base extension, presence of distant metastases, and low ADCC titers.

○   **Extension into which space is associated with the worst prognosis in patients with NPC?**

Anterior masticator space.

○   **What is the primary treatment modality for nasopharyngeal cancer?**

Radiation therapy to the nasopharynx (66-70 Gy) and neck (60 Gy).

○   **Why is the clinically negative neck treated?**

Studies have shown improved local control and disease-free survival for prophylactic irradiation of the clinically negative neck in patients with NPC.

○   **What are the complications from radiation overdosage in the treatment of NPC?**

Osteoradionecrosis, brain necrosis, transverse myelitis, hearing loss, hypopituitarism, hypothyroidism, optic neuritis.

○   **What is the role of induction chemotherapy?**

No survival advantage has been proven.

○   **What is the role of concomitant chemotherapy?**

Survival advantage has been found using cisplatinum and 5-flourouracil.

○   **What is the primary problem of using concomitant chemotherapy?**

Poor patient tolerance requiring treatment breaks; split-course radiation therapy has been shown to result in decreased survival compared with continuous course radiotherapy.

○   **How does using cisplatinum avoid this problem?**

Its toxicity (hematologic) does not overlap with that of radiation therapy (mucositis).

○   **How does treatment failure usually manifest in NPC?**

Disease at both the primary site and cervical lymph nodes.

○   **What is the most common site of recurrent/persistent NPC?**

Lateral wall of the nasopharynx.

○   **What are the treatment options for recurrent/persistent NPC at the primary site?**

Reirradiation with larger therapeutic dose than initial treatment; stereotactic radiotherapy; brachytherapy with split palate implantation of radioactive gold grains; surgical resection.

○   **What is the primary contraindication to nasopharyngectomy?**

Tumor involvement of the cavernous sinus or cranial nerves.

○   **What is the anterolateral surgical approach to the nasopharynx?**

The maxillary antrum attached to an anterior cheek flap is developed as an osteocutaneous flap and swung laterally.

○   **What are the most common complications of this approach?**

Trismus and palatal fistula.

○   **What are the advantages of this approach?**

Allows wide exposure of the nasopharynx with low morbidity.

○   **What are other surgical approaches to the nasopharynx?**

Lateral rhinotomy with facial disassembly, transpalatal split, lateral cervical approach with mandibular swing, transparotid temporal bone approach, infratemporal fossa approach.

○   **What is the recommended treatment for neck disease after radiation therapy?**

Radical neck dissection.

○   **What can be done to improve the results of salvage neck dissection?**

Postoperative brachytherapy via hollow tubes placed at the time of surgery.

○   **What is the most common benign sinonasal neoplasm?**

Inverting papilloma.

○   **What is the most common malignant sinonasal neoplasm?**

SCCA, comprising 80% of malignant sinonasal neoplasms.

○   **What is the 2ⁿᵈ most common malignant sinonasal neoplasm?**

Adenocarcinoma.

○   **What are the most common locations of sinonasal SCCA?**

Maxillary sinus, followed by the nasal cavity, then ethmoid sinuses.

○   **Are elective neck dissections warranted in patients with sinonasal SCCA?**

No, as the incidence of occult cervical metastases is 10%.

○   **What percentage of sinonasal tumors can be attributed to occupational exposures?**

Up to 44%.

○   **Where do these tumors most often originate?**

Lateral nasal wall, adjacent to the middle turbinate.

○   **Which substances are thought to predispose to sinonasal neoplasms?**

Nickel, chromium, isopropyl oils, volatile hydrocarbons, organic fibers from wood, shoe, and textile refineries.

○   **Which of these is classically associated with SCCA?**

Nickel.

○   **Which of these are classically associated with adenocarcinoma?**

Hardwood dusts and leather tanning substances.

○   **Which virus is thought to play a role in the etiology of sinonasal tumors?**

HPV, particularly types 6 and 12.

○   **T/F: Smoking by itself is not a significant etiologic factor for sinonasal tumors.**

True.

○   **What is the most common presenting symptom of sinonasal neoplasms?**

Nasal obstruction (50%).

○   **What % of patients with sinonasal tumors are asymptomatic at presentation?**

9 –12%.

○   **What 3 signs are classically present in patients with sinonasal neoplasms?**

Facial asymmetry, tumor bulge in the oral cavity, and nasal mass; the presence of all 3 is seen in about 50% of patients and is significant for advanced disease.

○   **Which nasal masses should not be biopsied in the clinic?**

Masses in children or adolescents and masses suspicious for angiofibroma…some also recommend delaying biopsy of any nasal mass until after imaging has been obtained.

○   **What are the 3 subtypes of Schneiderian papillomas?**

Fungiform, inverting, and cylindrical.

○   **Where do inverting papillomas most commonly arise?**

Lateral nasal wall.

○   **What factor is most related to the chance of recurrence for inverting papilloma?**

Method of removal.

O   **What is the incidence of recurrence after resection of inverting papilloma via lateral rhinotomy/medial maxillectomy?**

13 – 15%.

O   **In patients who undergo resection of inverting papilloma via lateral rhinotomy/medial maxillectomy, what is the most important factor related to risk for recurrence?**

Mitotic index.

O   **What is the differential diagnosis of a small cell sinonasal tumor?**

Esthesioneuroblastoma, plasmacytoma, melanoma, lymphoma, sarcoma, poorly differentiated SCCA, Ewings sarcoma, PNET, and SNUC.

O   **What is a SNUC?**

Sinonasal undifferentiated carcinoma…a very aggressive small cell sinonasal tumor.

O   **What are the poor prognostic factors for SNUC tumors?**

Orbital involvement and neck metastases; tumors in the paranasal sinuses have a worse prognosis than those arising in the nasal cavity.

O   **SNUC tumors have antibodies to what substances?**

Cytokeratin, epithelial membrane antigen, and neuron-specific enolase.

O   **What is the treatment for SNUC?**

Preoperative chemoradiation, followed by surgical resection for those tumors without distant metastases or extensive intracranial involvement.

O   **According to Levine et al, SNUC is most likely a grade 4 variant of what tumor?**

Esthesioneuroblastoma or olfactory neuroblastoma.

O   **In what age group is olfactory neuroblastoma typically seen?**

Bimodal distribution… people in their 20's and 50's.

O   **What histological pattern is characteristic of this tumor?**

Homer-Wright rosettes.

O   **An olfactory neuroblastoma involving the ethmoid sinuses would be classified as what stage by the Kadish system?**

B.

O   **What are the 3 most common malignant bone tumors of the paranasal sinuses?**

Multiple myeloma, osteogenic sarcoma, chondrosarcoma.

○ **What is the pathophysiology of fibrous dysplasia?**

Normal medullary bone is replaced by collagen, fibroblasts, and osteoid.

○ **Where is it most commonly found in the head and neck?**

Maxilla.

○ **How does it appear on MRI?**

On T-1 weighted MRI, mildly hyperintense to hypointense with mild to moderate enhancement; on T-2 weighted MRI, markedly homogenous and hypointense (ground glass appearance).

○ **Where is adenoid cystic carcinoma of the head and neck most commonly found?**

Palate, followed by major salivary glands, then paranasal sinuses.

○ **How are the low-grade and high-grade varieties of adenoid cystic carcinoma defined?**

Low-grade tumors have less than 30% solid anaplastic histology; high-grade tumors have more than 30% solid anaplastic histology.

○ **Where is melanoma most commonly found in the nose and paranasal sinuses?**

Nasal septum.

○ **How does melanoma of the nose differ from cutaneous melanoma?**

More aggressive with a worse prognosis and an unpredictable course… local recurrence is the most common cause of failure.

○ **Where in the head and neck are osteogenic sarcomas most commonly found?**

Mandible.

○ **What is the most common type of lymphoma of the nose and paranasal sinuses?**

Non-Hodgkin's.

○ **How does it appear on MRI?**

Intermediate intensity on T-1 and T-2 weighted images, permeates sinus walls without gross displacement.

○ **What is Ohngren's line and how is it significant?**

Imaginary line from the medial canthus to the angle of the mandible; tumors below the line have a better prognosis than tumors above the line (with the palate as an exception).

○ **What is the most significant prognostic factor in patients with mesenchymal tumors?**

Grade of the tumor.

○ **What factors make a tumor of the nose or paranasal sinuses unresectable?**

Invasion into the frontal lobe, prevertebral fascia, bilateral optic nerves, or cavernous sinus.

O   **Name the tumor--**

Comprises only 3% of Schneiderian papillomas:

Cylindrical papilloma .

Most common type of Schneiderian papilloma, typically seen on the nasal septum:

Fungiform papilloma.

2 – 13% of these benign sinonasal tumors have malignant potential:

Inverting papilloma.

Has a predilection for the mandible and a sunray appearance on X-ray:

Osteogenic sarcoma.

More than 90% will have invaded through at least one wall of the involved sinus at presentation:

SCCA.

Benign tumor, most commonly seen in patients less than 20 years old and has a ground glass appearance on X-ray:

Fibrous dysplasia.

Benign tumor most commonly found in the frontal sinus:

Osteoma.

Encapsulated, benign tumor that arises from the surface of nerve fibers:

Schwannoma.

Unencapsulated tumor that arises from within a nerve; 15% become malignant (when associated with von Recklinghausen's disease):

Neurofibroma.

2nd most common malignant sinonasal tumor; tend to be located superior to Ohngren's line:

Adenocarcinoma.

Arise from pericytes of Zimmerman and considered neither benign nor malignant:

Hemangiopericytoma.

Arise from stem cells of neural crest origin that differentiate into olfactory sensory cells; Homer Wright rosettes are characteristic:

Olfactory neuroblastoma or esthesioneuroblastoma.

First line treatment for this tumor is radiation; 70% present at stage 4:

Lymphoma.

May progress to multiple myeloma:

Extramedullary plasmacytoma.

Most common tumor to metastasize to the sinonasal area:

Renal cell.

Metastasizes to the brain more frequently than any other soft-tissue sarcoma:

Alveolar soft part sarcoma.

O   **Which sinonasal neoplasms remodel rather than erode bone?**

Sarcomas, minor salivary gland carcinomas, hemangiopericytomas, extramedullary plasmacytomas, large cell lymphomas, and olfactory neuroblastomas.

O   **What is the primary modality of treatment for extramedullary plasmacytomas?**

Radiation.

O   **How do you test for multiple myeloma in these patients?**

Measure serum M-protein and urine Bence Jones protein; bone survey; bone marrow biopsy.

O   **What are the four basic surgical procedures used to resect tumors of the midface?**

Medial maxillectomy, suprastructure maxillectomy, infrastructure maxillectomy, and radical maxillectomy.

O   **What are five adjunctive procedures to the above dissections?**

Orbital exenteration, infratemporal fossa dissection, craniotomy, contralateral maxillectomy, rhinectomy.

O   **What are the three basic transfacial approaches to these procedures?**

Lateral rhinotomy, total rhinotomy, midface degloving.

O   **What is the Weber-Fergusson incision?**

Lip-splitting extension of the lateral rhinotomy incision that permits exposure for a radical maxillectomy.

O   **What is the gold standard of treatment for inverting papillomas?**

Medial maxillectomy via lateral rhinotomy.

O   **What area of the sinonasal tract is better visualized with endoscopy as opposed to medial maxillectomy?**

Posterior ethmoid cells, particularly those lateral to the sphenoid sinus and around the optic nerve.

O   **When is a total rhinotomy approach most useful?**

For midline tumors where exposure of the cribriform plate and the bilateral ethmoids is necessary.

○   **What is the primary limitation of the midface degloving approach?**

Limited exposure of the skull base and anterior ethmoid sinuses.

○   **What are the incisions used for the midface degloving approach?**

Sublabial; intercartilaginous; complete transfixion.

○   **What type of resection would be best for a tumor confined to the floor of the maxillary antrum?**

Infrastructure maxillectomy.

○   **What structures are preserved with an infrastructure maxillectomy that would be resected with a total maxillectomy?**

Orbital floor and sometimes the infraorbital nerve.

○   **What are the contraindications to radical maxillectomy?**

Involvement of the sphenoid, nasopharynx, middle cranial fossa, or extensive infratemporal fossa; presence of bilateral cervical metastases or distant metastases.

○   **What are the contraindications to craniofacial resection?**

Poor surgical candidate, presence of multiple distant metastases, invasion of the prevertebral fascia, cavernous sinus (by a high-grade tumor), carotid artery (in a high-risk patient), or bilateral optic nerves/optic chiasm.

○   **According to Larson, what are the indications for orbital exenteration?**

Involvement of the periorbita, posterior ethmoid sinuses or orbital apex.

○   **What is Whitnall's tubercle?**

Insertion site of the lateral canthal tendon.

○   **What happens if the orbital septum is violated during resection of a sinonasal tumor?**

Lid shortening and ectropion.

○   **Why should the inferior turbinate be removed during resection of a sinonasal tumor?**

To prevent interference with a palatal prosthesis.

○   **What should be done during maxillectomy to prevent epiphora postoperatively?**

Dacryocystorhinostomy.

○   **What is the incidence of clinically significant pneumocephalus after anterior craniofacial surgery?**

5 – 12%.

O   **What can cause postoperative pneumocephalus?**

Overly aggressive drainage of CSF via a lumbar drain or ball-valve action of the flaps used to reconstruct the skull base.

O   **What is the treatment of pneumocephalus?**

Emergent drainage with needle aspiration, airway diversion (i.e. tracheostomy), nasal repacking.

O   **According to Levine et al, what treatment protocol has improved both functional and survival outcome for sinonasal malignancies?**

Preoperative radiation (50Gy) +/- chemotherapy (Cytoxan, vincristine) followed by craniofacial resection.

O   **What is the overall 5-year survival for sinonasal SCCA?**

30%.

O   **What is the most common cause of treatment failure?**

Local recurrence.

LARYNGOLOGY AND ENDOSCOPY

○ **What is the most common congenital anomaly of the larynx?**

Laryngomalacia.

○ **Where are vocal nodules most commonly located?**

At the junction of the anterior 1/3 and posterior 2/3 of the vocal fold.

○ **Why are they commonly located there?**

This is the point of maximum velocity of the vocal cords during forceful adduction.

○ **What are the risk factors for developing a vocal fold granuloma?**

Vocal abuse, GERD, prolonged intubation, trauma, surgery.

○ **Where are post-intubation granulomas typically located?**

On the vocal process of the arytenoid.

○ **Compared to men, women have a significantly higher incidence of vocal cord granulomas caused by what?**

Intubation.

○ **Which type of vocal cord granuloma has the worst prognosis?**

Idiopathic.

○ **What is the most useful stroboscopic parameter in differentiating a vocal fold cyst from a polyp?**

Mucosal wave.

○ **What pathologic changes occur in the larynx as a result of GERD?**

Polypoid corditis (Reinke's edema), posterior glottic and arytenoid edema/erythema.

○ **Which of these is most common?**

Posterior glottic edema.

○ **Where is Reinke's edema located?**

Superficial layer of the lamina propria.

○   **What is the most likely cause of prolonged dysphonia and vocal fold stiffness after surgery for Reinke's edema?**

Excessive suctioning of the superficial lamina propria.

○   **Surgical disruption of which layer of the vocal cord is most likely to lead to vocal fold scarring?**

Vocal ligament (highest amount of collagen and fibroblasts).

○   **What are the clinical findings associated with pathologic sulcus vocalis?**

Vocal fold stiffness, fullness, edema, and bowing; capillary ectasia; and vibratory disturbances.

○   **What are the operative and pathologic findings of patients with pathologic sulcus vocalis?**

Loss of superficial lamina propria and fixation of a thinned epithelium to underlying vocal ligament.

○   **What are the physical findings of type 2 sulcus vocalis or "sulcus vergeture"?**

Linear sulcus along the medial edge of the fold separating the superior and inferior lips of the membranous vocal fold by a rigid contracted band.

○   **What are the features of type 3 sulcus vocalis?**

Severe dysphonia, vocal fold stiffness, and a medial pit-shaped sulcus.

○   **What distinguishes type 1 or physiologic sulcus from pathologic sulcus?**

Preservation of vocal cord vibratory activity on videostroboscopy, signifying intact superficial lamina propria (Type I).

○   **What is the best treatment for patients with type 2 sulcus?**

Undermining and segmental slicing (Pontes and Behlau).

○   **What is a laryngocele?**

Abnormal dilatation of the laryngeal saccule.

○   **Where are internal laryngoceles located?**

Beneath the mucosa of the false vocal cord and aryepiglottic folds.

○   **How do laryngoceles become external?**

Penetrate the thyrohyoid membrane at the site of entry of the superior laryngeal artery and nerve.

○   **What are mixed laryngoceles?**

External laryngoceles with a dilated internal component.

○   **What is the normal size (height) of the saccule?**

<8 mm in 75% of normal larynges, 10 – 15 mm in 17%, >15 mm in 8%.

○ **When do most laryngoceles present?**

Can present at any time, but most commonly arise in the sixth decade of life.

○ **Breathiness that progressively worsens as the day wears on is classic for which autoimmune disease?**

Myasthenia gravis.

○ **Which area of the larynx is involved in sarcoidosis?**

Supraglottis.

○ **Which area of the larynx is involved in Wegener's granulomatosis?**

Subglottis.

○ **What condition is characterized by generalized tension in all laryngeal muscles?**

Muscular tension dysphonia.

○ **In which patients is this most commonly seen?**

Untrained occupational and professional voice users.

○ **What are the physical findings in patients with muscular tension dysphonia?**

Vocal cord nodules, posterior glottic chink.

○ **What condition would cause a tense sounding voice, vocal fatigue, and a prolonged closed phase with reduced vibratory and mucosal wave amplitude during videostroboscopy?**

Glottic hyperabduction dysphonia.

○ **What kind of dystonia is spasmodic dysphonia?**

Focal.

○ **What are the characteristics of focal dystonias?**

Inappropriate and excessive efferent activity of motor neurons in small areas.

○ **What are the two types of spasmodic dysphonia (SD)?**

Adductor and abductor.

○ **Which is more common?**

Adductor SD.

○ **Which of these is characterized by a harsh, strained voice with inappropriate pitch breaks, breathiness, and glottal fry?**

Adductor SD.

○   **What are the typical features of abductor SD?**

Breathy, effortful hypnotic voice with abnormal whispered segments of speech.

○   **The inability to sustain vowels during speech is suggestive of what disorder?**

Adductor SD.

○   **Voiceless consonants is suggestive of what disorder?**

Abductor SD.

○   **What % of cases of SD are familial?**

12%.

○   **Which muscles are responsible for adductor SD?**

Thyroarytenoid and lateral cricoarytenoid muscles.

○   **Which muscle is responsible for abductor SD?**

Posterior cricoarytenoid muscle.

○   **What is the preferred method of treatment for SD?**

Chemical denervation with botulinum toxin.

○   **How many serotypes of botulinum toxin exist? Which is the most useful clinically?**

8 serotypes (A through G) with type A being the most useful.

○   **What is the mechanism of action of botulinum toxin?**

Inhibition of acetylcholine release from cholinergic nerve endings.

○   **How is recovery of function accomplished?**

Via sprouting of new nerve terminals and an increase in the number of postjunctional receptors.

○   **What would be the histologic findings on muscle biopsies at the site of botulinum toxin injections?**

Increased unmyelinated axonal sprouts; no change in muscle fibers histologically.

○   **What factors are thought to account for diminished responses to botulinum toxin?**

Formation of antibodies, high cumulative dose, drug interactions.

○   **Which drugs potentiate the effect of botulinum toxin?**

Aminoglycoside antibiotics.

○   **Which drugs limit the effect of botulinum toxin?**

Guanidine and aminopyridines.

○ **What is a MU?**

1 MU is the dose required to kill 50% of a batch of mice.

○ **What is the lethal dose of botulinum toxin for humans?**

2500 to 3000 MU.

○ **What is the starting dose of botulinum toxin for treatment in a patient with harsh, strained voice with intermittent pitch breaks and glottal fry?**

1.0 – 2.5 MU into each thyroarytenoid muscle if administering bilaterally; 5 – 30 MU if administering unilaterally.

○ **What is the starting dose of botulinum toxin for treatment in a patient with a breathy, hypophonic voice with abnormal whispered segments of speech?**

3.75 MU into the most active posterior cricoarytenoid muscle.

○ **What are the onset, peak, and duration of effects of botulinum toxin?**

Onset 24 to 72 hours, peak effect at 10 – 14 days, duration 3 – 6 months.

○ **T/F: Greater duration of symptom control has been demonstrated with unilateral versus bilateral injections.**

True.

○ **What are two ways to deliver botulinum toxin to the posterior cricoarytenoid muscle?**

Transcricoid and retrograde (rotating the larynx away from the side of injection).

○ **How can one confirm placement of the needle in the posterior cricoarytenoid muscle?**

Using EMG guidance, have the patient sniff.

○ **What can be done if symptoms persist after complete paralysis of the posterior cricoarytenoid?**

Inject the contralateral posterior cricoarytenoid muscle with very small increments of toxin or inject the cricothyroid muscle.

○ **How is injection into the cricothyroid muscle accomplished, and how is proper placement confirmed?**

Peroral route; confirm by having the patient sing an ascending scale and observing an increase in EMG activity as the pitch increases.

○ **What are the adverse effects of posterior cricoarytenoid injections?**

Stridor (particularly with exertion), airway compromise, dysphagia and aspiration.

○ **What is adductor laryngeal breathing dystonia?**

Paradoxical adduction of the vocal folds during inspiration, causing inspiratory stridor that worsens with exertion and disappears during sleep.

O   **What effect does adductor laryngeal breathing dystonia have on the voice?**

None.

O   **What syndrome is associated with blepharospasm?**

Meige's syndrome.

O   **Which muscles are involved in blepharospasm?**

Orbicularis oculi, procerus, and corrugator supercilii.

O   **What are the potential adverse effects of botulinum toxin injections into these muscles for treatment of blepharospasm?**

Due to diffusion of the toxin, ptosis, diplopia, epiphora, lagophthalmos.

O   **What muscles are injected when using botulinum toxin to treat hemifacial spasm?**

Zygomaticus major and minor, levator anguli oris, and risorius.

O   **What muscles are injected when using botulinum toxin to treat oromandibular dystonia?**

Masseter, temporalis, medial and lateral pterygoid muscles.

O   **What % of laryngectomy patients who fail voice restoration following tracheoesophageal puncture (TEP) suffer from cricopharyngeal spasm?**

12%.

O   **What is the best test to differentiate between cricopharyngeal spasm and stricture in patients who fail voice restoration following TEP?**

Contrast videofluoroscopy.

O   **How is the cricopharyngeus muscle identified with EMG?**

Electrical activity occurs at rest and diminishes or stops with swallowing.

O   **What are the 2 most common causes of vocal cord paralysis in adults?**

Surgical trauma (#1), and lung cancer (#2).

O   **In patients with unilateral vocal cord paralysis, which side is most commonly involved?**

Left.

O   **What position will the vocal cord be in if the nerve is damaged at or above the nodose ganglion?**

Lateral.

○ **What position will the vocal cord be in if the nerve is damaged below the nodose ganglion?**

Paramedian, due to innervation from the superior laryngeal nerve.

○ **What accounts for vocal fold bowing observed with vocal fold paralysis?**

Denervation atrophy of the thyroarytenoid muscle.

○ **What problems are seen in patients with vocal cord paralysis due to a brainstem disorder?**

Breathiness; pitch changes; chronic aspiration; VPI.

○ **What effect does damage to the superior laryngeal nerve have on voice?**

Decreased range of pitch.

○ **If the vocal cord is in the paramedian position, why is aspiration less likely?**

Indicates that the superior laryngeal nerve is intact, and hence, laryngeal sensation is intact.

○ **What test should be done if the history and physical exam do not explain the etiology of vocal cord paralysis?**

CT scan from skull base to A-P window.

○ **What are the indications for panendoscopy in patients with vocal cord paralysis?**

If history, physical exam, CT scan, electrolytes, RPR, TFT's do not reveal etiology.

○ **What % of patients with unilateral vocal cord paralysis require surgical treatment?**

40%.

○ **What is the primary purpose of laryngeal EMG in patients with vocal cord paralysis?**

To distinguish paralysis from mechanical fixation.

○ **Which laryngeal muscles are typically analyzed with EMG?**

Thyroarytenoid and cricothyroid muscles.

○ **How does the pattern of the EMG wave appear in the presence of a neuropathy?**

Decreased frequency with normal amplitude.

○ **How does the pattern of the EMG wave appear in the presence of a myopathy?**

Decreased amplitude, normal frequency.

○ **What is the significance of a "picket fence" pattern on EMG?**

Indicates partial reinnervation (polyphasic action potentials).

○ **What are the features of a denervation pattern on EMG?**

Sharp waves or fibrillation potentials, complex repetitive discharges, and little or no electrical activity during attempts at voluntary contraction.

○   **What is the significance of a denervation pattern 1 year after injury?**

Spontaneous recovery is very unlikely.

○   **What disease does a fatiguing pattern on EMG suggest?**

Myasthenia gravis.

○   **What is the difference in impedance values and stimulus response thresholds between intramuscular needle electrodes and endotracheal tube-mounted surface wire electrodes for recording laryngeal muscle activity?**

No significant difference.

○   **Your patient has a unilateral vocal cord paralysis after thyroidectomy for goiter. What are the indications for surgical intervention?**

If the paralysis is well tolerated (e.g. no aspiration and voice quality acceptable to the patient), 12 months is allowed for spontaneous recovery before proceeding with surgery. If the symptoms are severe, early surgery, typically a reversible procedure, is indicated.

○   **What is the best way to successfully restore the airway in a one-stage procedure in patients with bilateral vocal fold paralysis (other than tracheostomy)?**

Bilateral laser cordotomy.

○   **What are some of the surgical options for treatment of bilateral vocal cord paralysis?**

Tracheostomy, horizontal cordotomy, arytenoidectomy, lateral cordotomy.

○   **Approximately what % of patients with bilateral vocal cord paralysis never require tracheostomy?**

50%.

○   **In what % of patients with bilateral vocal cord paralysis is decannulation possible after one of these procedures?**

70%.

○   **What are the 4 main categories of procedures for unilateral vocal cord paralysis?**

Medialization thyroplasty, arytenoid adduction, intracordal injection, and laryngeal reinnervation.

○   **What substances can be used for temporary vocal cord medialization?**

Autologous fat, Gelfoam, collagen, micronized alloderm.

○   **When is Teflon paste used?**

Only in patients who are terminally ill with a permanent vocal cord paralysis.

○   **T/F: Previous Teflon injection is a contraindication to medialization thyroplasty.**

False

○   **T/F: When injecting Teflon in the vocal fold, it should be placed as far medial as possible.**

False; it should be placed as far lateral as possible.

○   **T/F: During medialization thyroplasty, the resected fragment of thyroid cartilage should be replaced in its original position after graft insertion.**

False.

○   **When is medialization thyroplasty appropriate for the treatment of vocal cord paralysis?**

Any stable, definitive paralysis in a patient without surgical contraindications.

○   **What symptom, other than hoarseness, is most likely to be improved by medialization thyroplasty and arytenoid adduction?**

Dysphagia.

○   **Into which plane is the implant placed during medialization thyroplasty?**

Subperichondrial.

○   **What are the advantages of performing this procedure under local?**

Desired voice quality can be precisely obtained and airway can be continually evaluated.

○   **What is the aim of arytenoid adduction?**

To pull the muscular process of the arytenoid laterally, resulting in adduction and lowering of the vocal process.

○   **What % of patients develop a granuloma after Teflon injection?**

About 35%.

○   **What is the aim of laryngeal reinnervation?**

To prevent atrophy of the thyroarytenoid muscle.

○   **What are the 2 primary techniques of laryngeal reinnervation?**

End-to-end anastomosis of the recurrent laryngeal nerve to the ansa hypoglossi or nerve-muscle pedicle flap to the thyroarytenoid muscle (using the ansa and a small piece of strap muscle).

○   **What % of patients experience improvement in voice after nerve-muscle implantation?**

76%.

○   **What would be the best treatment for a 60-year-old woman who experiences severe dysphagia and aspiration after removal of a high right vagal schwannoma?**

Right medialization thyroplasty, arytenoid adduction.

○   What is the optimal treatment for presbylaryngeus?

Speech therapy for 1 year; if that fails, then bilateral medialization thyroplasty.

○   T/F: Arytenoid adduction is contraindicated for the treatment of presbylaryngeus.

True; arytenoid adduction is contraindicated in any patient with mobile vocal folds.

○   In which situations is medialization laryngoplasty most efficacious in the treatment of vocal fold scarring?

When arytenoids are mobile, glottic gap is >1.5 mm, and soft tissue deficiency is confined to the anterior 1/3 of the vocal fold.

○   What is the most common complication after insertion of a Blom-Singer indwelling voice prosthesis?

Granulation tissue.

○   What is the disadvantage of the indwelling voice prosthesis compared to the non-indwelling prosthesis?

Higher rate of fungal colonization.

○   What are the contraindications to percutaneous endoscopic gastrostomy?

Inability to perform upper endoscopy safely; inability to transilluminate the abdominal wall; presence of ascites, coagulopathy, or intra-abdominal infection.

○   When should PEG be performed when done as part of an oncologic resection?

After the primary resection to avoid inadvertent spread of tumor cells to the gastrostomy site.

○   What is the incidence of complications after PEG?

9 – 15%.

○   In which part of the world is Zenker's diverticulum most common?

Northern Europe.

○   What is the test of choice for diagnosis of Zenker's diverticulum?

Barium swallow.

○   What factor is most important regarding the risk of surgical complications in patients undergoing Zenker's diverticulectomy?

Size of the diverticulum.

○   What are the primary advantages of endoscopic versus open resection for Zenker's diverticulum?

Shorter operative time with no significant difference in complication rate; absence of skin incision; minimal postoperative pain; quicker resumption of oral feeding; shorter hospital stay.

○   **T/F: Cricopharyngeal myotomy as an adjunctive procedure to diverticulectomy has been shown to significantly decrease the incidence of recurrence.**

False.

○   **What are the primary limitations to endoscopic diverticulectomy?**

Size of the sac; difficult to perform in very small or large sacs (<2 cm or >10 cm); limitations in access due to anatomic factors (ie, inability to extend the neck or limited jaw excursion).

○   **What is the incidence of mediastinitis after diverticulectomy?**

<5%.

○   **Which complication is most likely to be avoided with endoscopic diverticulectomy versus open diverticulectomy?**

Damage to the recurrent laryngeal nerve.

○   **What is the greatest advantage of bronchoscopic visualization during percutaneous dilational tracheostomy?**

Fewer major complications occur.

○   **What are the contraindications to percutaneous dilatational tracheostomy?**

Large thyroid goiter or other neck mass, marked obesity, coagulopathy, previous neck surgery, neck trauma including burns, and inadequate access to the trachea.

○   **What are the clinical criteria for pediatric decannulation?**

Recovery from the original indication for tracheotomy, cessation of mechanical ventilation for at least 3 months, minimal present oxygen requirement, and an absence of frequent pulmonary infections or severe swallowing dysfunction.

○   **When is polysomnography indicated to determine readiness for decannulation in children?**

When the tracheotomy was performed due to a dynamic airway disorder (OSA, craniofacial anomalies, pharyngeal hypotonia).

○   **What is the incidence of tracheoinnominate fistula after tracheostomy?**

2%.

○   **What % of all instances of tracheal bleeding developing 48 hours or longer after surgery are caused by tracheoinnominate fistulae?**

50%.

○   **What % of patients with tracheoinnominate fistulae survive?**

25%.

O   **What are the risk factors for innominate artery rupture after tracheostomy?**

Placement of trach below the 3rd ring; aberrant course of the innominate artery; use of a long, curved tube; overhyperextension of the neck during the procedure; prolonged pressure by inflated cuff; and tracheal infection.

O   **Which patients are at a higher risk of pneumothorax after tracheostomy?**

Children.

O   **What is the most common cause of mortality in pediatric patients who undergo tracheostomy?**

Plugging or accidental decannulation in children <1 year of age.

O   **What should be done if the posterior tracheal wall is disrupted during tracheostomy?**

Tracheostomy tube should be replaced with an endotracheal tube.

O   **Subcutaneous emphysema may prelude what condition after tracheostomy?**

Tension pneumomediastinum.

O   **What % of patients with long-term tracheostomies are colonized with *Pseudomonas*?**

>60%.

O   **What effect does tracheostomy have on the incidence of pneumonia?**

Patients on a ventilator are at a higher risk of pneumonia after tracheostomy and also tend to develop more serious pneumonias (*Pseudomonas*) secondary to antibiotic resistance.

O   **What is the tracheal wall mucosal capillary pressure?**

20 – 30 mm Hg.

O   **How soon will deep mucosal ulcerations and exposure of tracheal cartilage occur when cuff-to-tracheal wall tension exceeds mucosal capillary tension?**

Within 1 week.

O   **What precaution should be taken for a patient with a tracheostomy undergoing general anesthesia?**

Nitrous oxide should be avoided as it diffuses into the cuff and can increase the pressure by up to 40mm Hg. If it used during induction, the cuff should be deflated temporarily.

O   **What are the signs of a tracheoesophageal fistula after tracheostomy?**

Copious secretions, food aspiration, and air leak around the cuff with abdominal distension.

O   **What is Schaefer's classification system of laryngeal injuries?**

Group I: minor hematomas or lacerations, no fractures, and minimal airway compromise.
Group II: moderate edema, lacerations, mucosal disruption without exposed cartilage, nondisplaced fractures, and varying degrees of airway compromise.

Group III: massive edema, mucosal disruption, displaced fractures, cord immobility, and varying degrees of airway compromise.

Group IV: same as III but with 2 or more fracture lines and/or skeletal instability or significant anterior commissure trauma.

○   **What structure is most likely to be fractured after blunt trauma to the anterior neck?**

Thyroid cartilage.

○   **When is CT scan indicated in the evaluation of these patients?**

Only for group I and II patients where there is questionable fracture.

○   **Which types of laryngeal injuries are best managed medically?**

Edema; small hematoma with intact mucosa; small glottic or supraglottic lacerations not involving the free margin of the vocal cords or the anterior commissure and without cartilage exposure; single nondisplaced thyroid cartilage fractures.

○   **What does medical management of laryngeal injuries consist of?**

24 hours or more of airway observation, voice rest, elevation of the head, humidified air, H2 blockers, steroids; antibiotics if lacerations are present.

○   **Which types of laryngeal injuries require open exploration and repair?**

Lacerations involving the free margin of the vocal cord or anterior commissure; large mucosal lacerations with exposed cartilage; multiple displaced cartilage fractures; avulsed or dislocated arytenoids; vocal cord immobility.

○   **When should open exploration be performed after injury?**

Within 24 hours.

○   **What are the indications for endolaryngeal stenting after open repair of laryngeal injuries?**

Disruption of the anterior commissure, multiple displaced cartilage fractures, and multiple, severe lacerations.

○   **What injuries are more commonly associated with laryngotracheal separation than with other laryngeal injuries?**

Subglottic stenosis and bilateral recurrent laryngeal nerve injury.

○   **Which types of laryngeal injuries are more common in children than adults?**

Soft tissue injury with edema, arytenoid dislocation, and recurrent laryngeal nerve injury; telescoping injuries where the cricoid becomes displaced under the thyroid.

○   **What is the most common immediate complication after repair of laryngeal injuries?**

Granulation tissue.

○   **In what age groups is caustic ingestion most common?**

18 – 24 months, 20 – 30 years.

O   **What are the 3 stages of injury after caustic ingestion?**

1.   Necrosis, bacterial invasion, sloughing of the mucosa.
2.   Granulation tissue and reepithelialization (day 5 – several weeks).
3.   Scar formation and contraction.

O   **How does the injury differ after ingestion of acidic substances versus ingestion of basic substances?**

Acidic substances cause coagulation necrosis; the eschar limits the depth of injury. Basic substances cause liquefaction necrosis and are likely to cause deeper injury.

O   **Where is the most likely site of injury after ingestion of an acidic caustic agent?**

Stomach.

O   **After caustic ingestion, what sign is most likely to signal the development of a complication?**

Drooling.

O   **What is the most likely consequence of ingesting hair relaxer?**

No long-term sequelae.

O   **What % of patients without oropharyngeal burn will have evidence of esophageal injury?**

8 – 20%.

O   **What is the test of choice in the evaluation of caustic ingestion?**

Endoscopy.

O   **When is the ideal time to perform endoscopy after ingestion?**

24 – 48 hours post-ingestion.

O   **Once the ABC's have been stabilized, what is the acute management of caustic ingestion injury?**

Prevent ongoing injury with irrigation of eyes, skin, and mouth, +/- flushing of the esophagus and stomach with water or milk <15 mL/kg (NGT placement is controversial).   Surgical exploration is indicated for perforation, mediastinitis, or peritonitis.

O   **What should be done for the patient who has ingested a battery?**

If the battery is still in the esophagus (confirmed by radiographs), immediate esophagoscopy is indicated. If it has passed into the stomach, it can be allowed to pass.

O   **T/F: Inducing emesis and activated charcoal are contraindicated in the management of caustic ingestion.**

True.

O   **What is the management of patients with evidence of grade 1 injury (superficial) on endoscopic exam?**

No intervention; schedule for esophagogram in 3 weeks.

O   **What is the management of patients with evidence of grade 2 or 3 injury (transmucosal or transmural) on endoscopic exam?**

Esophageal rest (NPO), reflux precautions, +/- steroids, +/- antibiotics, +/- lathyrogens, +/- subcutaneous heparin, +/- NGT, +/- prophylactic bougienage.

O   **What are the contraindications to steroid use?**

Grade 3 burns, esophageal or gastric perforation.

O   **What are lathyrogens?**

Substances that interfere with the cross-linking of collagen.

O   **What are some examples of lathyrogens?**

Penicillamine, beta aminopropionitrile, N-acetylceptine.

O   **What % of children with esophageal burns will develop esophageal stricture?**

7 – 15%.

O   **Why should all patients with history of caustic ingestion be followed for life with repeated esophagograms and endoscopy?**

Risk of SCCA of the esophagus is 1000 times that of the general population.

O   **What % of patients with esophageal stricture will develop esophageal cancer?**

1 – 4%.

O   **What are the typical features of esophageal cancer occurring after esophageal stricture from burn injury?**

Usually SCCA, with onset 25 – 70 years post-injury, occurring within the scar tissue, with a lower incidence of distant metastases and higher chance of cure with surgical resection.

O   **What is felt to be the safest way to address severe esophageal strictures with dilatation?**

Retrograde technique using Tucker dilators over a guide string.

O   **What factors are associated with the highest success with esophageal dilatation for treatment of strictures secondary to caustic ingestion?**

Age <8, injuries caused by agents other than lye, injuries limited to the upper 1/3 of the esophagus and <5 cm long.

O   **What is the premise behind pursuing long-term dilatation therapy?**

"The native esophagus is the best esophagus."

O   **What are the indications for esophageal bypass?**

Complete esophageal stenosis and failure to establish a lumen with dilatation.
Irregularity and diverticuli of the esophagus.
Mediastinitis secondary to dilatation.
Fistula formation.
Inability to maintain a lumen of 40 Fr or greater with dilatation.
Patient intolerance of frequent procedures.

O   **What is the most common esophageal bypass procedure?**

Colon interposition.

O   **What is the difference in using the right versus left colon?**

The right colon is interposed in an isoperistaltic fashion whereas the left colon is interposed in an antiperistaltic fashion.

O   **What is the mortality from colon interposition?**

4 – 15%.

O   **What is the most significant early complication of this procedure?**

Cervical anastomotic leak (50%).

O   **What is the most significant late complication of this procedure?**

Cervical anastomotic stricture (44%).

O   **What % of patients are eventually able to swallow well after this procedure?**

92%.

O   **After 3 months of voice therapy, what % of benign vocal cord lesions will reduce in size or resolve?**

46% will reduce in size and 11% will completely resolve.

O   **What % of patients with glottic insufficiency will attain complete closure after voice therapy?**

20%.

O   **What are the available treatments for cricopharyngeal dysphagia?**

Mechanical dilation, pharyngeal plexus neurectomy, cricopharyngeal myotomy, or botulinum toxin.

O   **What are the 4 etiologies of vocal cord immobility?**

Paralysis, synkinesis, cricoarytenoid joint fixation, and interarytenoid scar.

O   **What are the most common manifestations of laryngopharyngeal reflux (LPR)?**

Dysphonia (71%), chronic cough (51%), globus (47%), chronic throat clearing (42%), dysphagia (35%).

THYROID AND PARATHYROID DISORDERS

○ **What is the embryologic origin of the thyroid gland?**

The median downgrowth of the first and second pharyngeal pouches in the area of the foramen cecum.

○ **What is the most common thyroid abnormality in hospitalized patients with non-thyroidal illness?**

Low T3 concentration.

○ **What is the major cause of a decreased T3 concentration in patients with a critical illness?**

Impaired peripheral conversion of T4 to T3 secondary to inhibition of the deiodination process.

○ **What clinical sign is the hallmark of thyroid storm?**

Fever.

○ **What are the hemodynamics of thyroid storm?**

Tachycardia, increased cardiac output and decreased systemic vascular resistance (SVR).

○ **What is the initial treatment of thyroid storm?**

Intravenous fluids, hypothermia, acetaminophen, propranolol, propylthiouracil (PTU) and iodine.

○ **What are the CNS manifestations of myxedema?**

Depression, memory loss, ataxia, frank psychosis, myxedema and coma.

○ **What are the most common causes of hypothyroidism?**

Hashimoto's thyroiditis, pituitary tumor, thyroidectomy, and radioactive I^{131} treatment for thyrotoxicosis.

○ **What test is used to distinguish a hypothalamic defect from a pituitary defect in a patient with hypothyroidism?**

The TRH stimulation test.

○ **What are the most common causes of hyperthyroidism?**

Graves' disease, toxic multinodular goiter, relapsing thyroiditis, amiodarone-induced thyrotoxicosis, autonomous toxic nodule, subacute thyroiditis, pituitary tumor.

○ **A 45-year-old female presents with a 2 year history of diffuse, tender thyroid enlargement, lethargy and a 20-pound weight gain. What is the most likely diagnosis?**

Hashimoto's thyroiditis.

O   **What is the appropriate treatment for the above patient?**

Thyroid hormone replacement therapy.

O   **What is the most common inflammatory disease of the thyroid?**

Hashimoto's thyroiditis.

O   **What antibodies are specific for Hashimoto's thyroiditis?**

Antimicrosomal and antithyroglobulin.

O   **How do patients with Hashimoto's thyroiditis present?**

Firm, diffusely enlarged goiter and hypothyroidism.

O   **What infectious diseases can cause chronic thyroiditis?**

Actinomycosis, TB, and syphilis.

O   **What thyroid disorder is characterized by replacement of the thyroid gland with fibrous tissue?**

Reidel's struma (invasive fibrous thyroiditis, woody thyroiditis).

O   **What is the preferred treatment for patients with toxic multinodular goiter?**

Thyroid resection (lobectomy to total thyroidectomy) because I^{131} treatment often requires repeated doses, does not reduce goiter size and may even cause acute enlargement.

O   **What are the indications for surgical treatment of Graves' disease?**

Extremely large glands, presence of a dominant nodule, failure of I^{131}, massive enlargement with compressive symptoms, pregnant women intolerant to antithyroid drugs, women of childbearing age and patients who are opposed to radioiodine.

O   **What is the treatment of choice for patients over 40 with Graves' disease?**

Radioactive I^{131}.

O   **What medications are used for the routine treatment of hyperthyroidism?**

Propylthiouracil (PTU) and methimazole.

O   **What medication is most commonly used to treat hyperthyroidism during pregnancy?**

PTU.

O   **What is the best agent for rapid surgical preparation of thyrotoxic patients?**

Long acting beta-blocker.

O   **What % of thyroid cancers are well-differentiated?**

>90%.

○   **What % of thyroid nodules are malignant?**

<5%.

○   **What % of thyroid nodules are malignant in patients with a history of radiation exposure?**

30 – 50%.

○   **What is the average lag time between radiation exposure and development of thyroid cancer?**

15 – 25 years.

○   **What is the most common thyroid nodule?**

Follicular adenoma.

○   **What is the significance of age with thyroid nodules?**

More likely to be malignant in women over 50 and men over 40 and in both men and women under 20.

○   **What % of solitary thyroid nodules in children are malignant?**

50%.

○   **What is the significance of size with thyroid nodules?**

More likely to be malignant if >4 cm in diameter.

○   **What is the difference in incidence of malignancy between solitary and multiple nodules?**

Incidence of malignancy in solitary nodules is 5 – 12%; incidence is 3% in multiple nodules.

○   **What % of the normal population will have a positive Chvostek's sign?**

10%.

○   **T/F: The incidence of parathyroid adenoma is higher in the presence of a thyroid nodule.**

True.

○   **What is the purpose of obtaining a preoperative thyroglobulin level?**

Thyroglobulin has been shown to correlate well with histologic tumor type and is useful as a marker for tumor recurrence.

○   **T/F: Thyroglobulin levels should be obtained prior to performing FNA.**

True; FNA will falsely elevate thyroglobulin levels.

○   **What lab test should be obtained in patients with a family history of medullary thyroid cancer?**

Calcitonin.

○   **What is the most sensitive method for detecting thyroid nodules?**

Ultrasound.

○   **What are the advantages of ultrasound in the evaluation of thyroid nodules?**

Can detect nodules as small as 2 –3 mm, can differentiate between solid, cystic, or mixed nodules with >90% accuracy, can detect presence of lymph node enlargement.

○   **What are the disadvantages of ultrasound in the evaluation of thyroid nodules?**

Cannot accurately distinguish benign from malignant nodules.

○   **What % of cold, warm/cool, and hot nodules are malignant?**

17%, 13%, and 4%, respectively.

○   **What is the most useful application of thyroid scanning in patients with thyroid cancer?**

To detect residual thyroid tissue or occult distant metastases after thyroidectomy.

○   **Which cardiovascular medication will interfere with radioiodine scanning?**

Amiodarone.

○   **What % of FNAs of thyroid nodules are either nondiagnostic or suspicious?**

27%.

○   **What % of nodules with an indeterminate FNA are malignant?**

16.7%.

○   **What is the incidence of false positives with FNA of thyroid nodules?**

<5%.

○   **What factors significantly increase the risk of sampling error from FNA?**

Very small (<1 cm) or very large (>4 cm) nodules, hemorrhagic nodules, or multinodular glands.

○   **Most false positives of FNA are due to what disease?**

Hashimoto's thyroiditis.

○   **Which thyroid tumors cannot be diagnosed as malignant with FNA?**

Follicular and Hurthle cell.

○   **What % of nodules diagnosed as having follicular or Hurtle cells, are malignant?**

10 – 20%.

○   **What test should be ordered in a patient with an elevated TSH?**

Antimicrosomal antibody (antithyroperoxidase level) to rule out Hashimoto's thyroiditis.

O **What % of malignant nodules are suppressible by exogenous TSH?**

16%.

O **What % of benign nodules are suppressible by exogenous TSH?**

21%.

O **What level of TSH is optimal during suppression therapy?**

0.1 – 0.5 mIU/L.

O **When is exogenous T4 used in patients with thyroid carcinoma?**

Postoperatively in patients with TSH-dependent carcinomas (follicular, papillary, and Hurtle cell).

O **What are the 3 types of well-differentiated thyroid malignancies?**

Follicular, papillary, and Hurthle cell.

O **Which of these is associated with iodine-deficiency?**

Follicular.

O **Which of these is more likely to be seen in a 30-year-old?**

Papillary.

O **Which of these is more likely to be seen in a pregnant woman?**

Follicular.

O **Which of these is the most common type of thyroid cancer?**

Papillary.

O **Which of these has the best prognosis?**

Papillary.

O **Which of these is relatively unresponsive to ablation with radioactive iodine?**

Hurthle cell.

O **A 65-year-old female presents with a cervical lymph node that is found to have well-differentiated thyroid tissue but the thyroid has no palpable abnormality. What is the next step in management?**

Total thyroidectomy and modified radical neck dissection.

O **What factor best correlates with the presence of lymph node metastases in papillary carcinoma?**

Age.

O   **T/F: Microscopic lymph node involvement does not change the long-term survival in patients with papillary thyroid cancer.**

True.

O   **What are the histologic features of papillary thyroid cancer?**

Calcified laminated bodies called psammoma bodies, elongated, pale nuclei with a ground glass appearance (Orphan Annie-eyes).

O   **What percentage of patients with papillary carcinoma (greater than 1 cm) are found to have multicentric disease on pathologic examination of the entire thyroid?**

70 to 80%.

O   **A 36-year-old female presents with a 3 cm papillary carcinoma and no clinical evidence of lymph node involvement. She was treated with a total thyroidectomy. What adjuvant therapy is indicated?**

TSH suppression with thyroid hormone, radioiodine ablation with I^{131}, follow-up scan 6 months after ablation with thyroglobulin levels and physical examination.

O   **What is the most common site of metastasis from follicular thyroid cancer?**

Bone.

O   **What are the histologic features of follicular thyroid cancer?**

Cuboidal epithelial cells with large nuclei in a well-structured follicular pattern.

O   **How is the definitive diagnosis of follicular thyroid cancer made?**

By demonstration of capsular invasion at the interface of the tumor and the thyroid gland.

O   **What is the most important prognostic indicator of follicular thyroid cancer?**

Degree of angioinvasion.

O   **What are the histologic features of Hurthle cell thyroid cancer?**

Large polygonal thyroid follicular cells with abundant granular cytoplasm and numerous mitochondria.

O   **T/F: Follicular cell carcinoma is more aggressive than Hurthle cell.**

False.

O   **What % of patients with Hurtle cell carcinoma present with distant metastases?**

15%.

O   **What are the 3 most well-known prognostic systems for well-differentiated thyroid cancer?**

GAMES, AMES, and AGES .

O   **What are the indications for adjuvant thyroid hormone in patients with well-differentiated thyroid carcinoma?**

All patients with well-differentiated carcinoma should be treated with thyroid hormone to suppress TSH for life, regardless of the extent of their surgery.

O   **Which cells in the thyroid gland secrete calcitonin?**

Parafollicular or C-cells.

O   **What are the histological features of medullary thyroid carcinoma (MTC)?**

Nests of small, round cells; amyloid; dense, irregular areas of calcification.

O   **In what 4 settings does MTC arise?**

Sporadic, familial, and in association with multiple endocrine neoplasia IIa or IIb.

O   **Which of these has the best prognosis?**

Familial.

O   **Which of these has the worst prognosis?**

Sporadic.

O   **Which of these tends to occur unilaterally?**

Sporadic.

O   **Which of these presents earliest?**

MEN IIb (mean age 19).

O   **What % of MTC occurs sporadically?**

70 – 80%.

O   **What are the characteristics of familial MTC?**

Autosomal dominant inheritance pattern; not associated with any other endocrinopathies.

O   **What other disorders are present in patients with MEN IIa?**

Pheochromocytoma, parathyroid hyperplasia.

O   **What is the mean age of presentation of MTC in patients with MEN IIa?**

27.

O   **T/F: All patients with MEN IIa will have MTC.**

True.

O   **What other disorders are present in patients with MEN IIb?**

Pheochromocytoma, multiple mucosal neuromas, marfanoid body habitus.

O   **What laboratory workup is necessary in patients with MTC?**

Basal and pentagastrin stimulated calcitonin levels, serum calcium, 24-hour urine catecholamines, VMA, and metanephrine, +/- CEA.

O   **What are the histochemical characteristics of MTC?**

Congo red dye positive, apple-green birefringence consistent with amyloid; immunohistochemistry positive for cytokeratins, CEA and calcitonin.

O   **What % of MTCs secrete CEA?**

50%.

O   **What genetic mutation is associated with medullary thyroid cancer?**

Mutation of the RET proto-oncogene.

O   **What is the false-negative rate of the RET analysis?**

5%.

O   **When is prophylactic thyroidectomy recommended in patients with the RET mutation?**

By age 5 or 6.

O   **What is the surgical treatment for medullary thyroid carcinoma (MTC)?**

Total thyroidectomy with central node dissection, lateral cervical lymph node sampling of palpable nodes and a modified radical neck dissection, if positive.

O   **What % of patients have had well-differentiated cancer before developing anaplastic thyroid cancer?**

47%.

O   **What % of patients have had benign thyroid disease before developing anaplastic cancer?**

53%.

O   **What are the 2 types of anaplastic thyroid cancer?**

Large cell and small cell.

O   **Which is more common?**

Large cell.

○   **Which of these is usually responsive to radiation therapy?**

Small cell.

○   **What is the appropriate management for a patient with an anaplastic thyroid carcinoma?**

Debulking and tracheostomy may be performed for palliation of airway obstruction.

○   **What is the best treatment for primary non-Hodgkin's lymphoma of the thyroid gland?**

Chemoradiation.

○   **A 44-year-old male presents with a 5 cm thyroid nodule. FNA returns fluid, the nodule disappears and the cytology is benign. What is the next step in management?**

Total thyroid lobectomy with isthmusectomy should be considered because there is an increased chance of malignancy in large cysts.

○   **A 56-year-old male with no risk factors presents with a thyroid nodule. The FNA is non-diagnostic. What is the treatment of choice?**

Total thyroid lobectomy with isthmusectomy.

○   **When performing a thyroid resection, where should the inferior thyroid artery be ligated?**

It should not be ligated. Branches should be ligated individually at the capsule.

○   **What is the incidence of permanent recurrent laryngeal nerve injury after total thyroidectomy?**

1 – 4%.

○   **What is the incidence of permanent hypoparathyroidism after total thyroidectomy?**

1 – 5%.

○   **T/F: The overall rate of survival is the same after subtotal or total thyroidectomy.**

True.

○   **The local recurrence rate is higher after subtotal than after total thyroidectomy.**

True.

○   **What are the indications for postoperative radioiodine ablation therapy?**

Significant uptake after a total or near-total thyroidectomy, extrathyroidal uptake, metastatic disease.

○   **What medication can be substituted for levothyroxine prior to radioiodine therapy?**

Liothyronine (Cytomel/T3).

○   **What is the optimal TSH value prior to radioiodine therapy?**

30 mU/L.

○ **After ablation therapy, how often are repeat scans performed?**

6 – 12 months after ablation, then every 2 years.

○ **How often are serum thyroglobulin levels measured?**

Every 6 months for the first 3 years, then annually.

○ **T/F: The sensitivity of thyroglobulin testing and radioiodine scans is higher when a patient is off TSH suppression.**

True.

○ **How are patients with MTC managed postoperatively?**

Receive L-thyroxine and 2 weeks of calcium and vitamin D supplementation; serial measurements of calcitonin and CEA.

○ **What is the single most effective chemotherapeutic agent for anaplastic thyroid cancer?**

Doxorubicin.

○ **What are the functions of PTH?**

Stimulates osteolysis and release of calcium and phosphorus from the bone; increases reabsorption of calcium and magnesium and the excretion of phosphorus and bicarbonate in the kidney; enhances intestinal absorption of calcium by stimulating the activation of vitamin D in the kidney.

○ **What % of the population has more than 4 parathyroid glands?**

10%.

○ **What % of the population has only 3 parathyroid glands?**

3%.

○ **What % of parathyroid glands are located in the mediastinum?**

2%.

○ **T/F: The inferior glands vary in location more than the superior glands.**

True.

○ **Where are the inferior parathyroids typically located?**

Inferior and anterior to the inferior thyroid artery.

○ **Where are the superior parathyroids typically located?**

Superior and posterior to the inferior thyroid artery and more likely to extend posteriorly and inferiorly or be found retroesophageally.

○   **From which pharyngeal pouches are the inferior parathyroid glands derived?**

3rd.

○   **What is the primary blood supply of the parathyroid glands?**

The superior and inferior parathyroid arteries, which are usually branches of the inferior thyroid artery.

○   **What are the 3 types of cells comprising the parathyroid glands?**

Chief cells, clear cells, and oxyphil cells.

○   **Which cells produce PTH?**

Chief cells.

○   **What % of a parathyroid gland is composed of fat?**

20 – 30%.

○   **A 48-year-old male has a serum calcium of 13 mg/dl and a serum PTH of 400 mEq/ml. What is the most likely diagnosis?**

Primary hyperparathyroidism secondary to a parathyroid adenoma.

○   **A 35-year-old female has a serum calcium of 8.5 mg/dl, a serum PTH of 400 mEq/ml and a serum creatinine of 5.6 mg/dl. What is the most likely diagnosis?**

Secondary hyperparathyroidism.

○   **What is the most common cause of hypercalcemia?**

Primary hyperparathyroidism.

○   **What is the most common cause of primary hyperparathyroidism?**

Parathyroid adenoma.

○   **What % of cases of primary hyperparathyroidism are due to diffuse hyperplasia?**

14 – 16%.

○   **Which cell is most commonly proliferated in diffuse parathyroid hyperplasia?**

Chief cell.

○   **What % of cases of primary hyperparathyroidism are due to carcinoma?**

3%.

○   **What is the most common cause of secondary hyperparathyroidism?**

Chronic renal failure.

○   **What is the pathophysiology behind secondary hyperparathyroidism from chronic renal failure?**

Chronic hypocalcemia results from decreased production of $1,25(OH)_2$ vitamin D_3, bone resistance to PTH, and decreased clearance of PTH and phosphate, resulting in parathyroid hyperplasia and increased levels of PTH.

○   **What enzyme activates vitamin D in the kidney?**

Renal alpha 1 – hydroxylase.

○   **What % of patients with secondary hyperparathyroidism require parathyroidectomy?**

<5%.

○   **What is tertiary hyperparathyroidism?**

Parathyroid hyperplasia results in autonomous hypersecretion such that hyperparathyroidism continues despite correction of the underlying renal disease.

○   **Which type of multiple endocrine neoplasia is not associated with hyperparathyroidism?**

MEN IIb.

○   **What is the significance of elevated preoperative levels of alkaline phosphatase in patients with chronic renal failure undergoing parathyroidectomy?**

Correlates with a good chance of amelioration of bone pain after parathyroidectomy.

○   **Which terminal of parathyroid hormone (PTH) is active?**

N-terminal.

○   **What is the most accurate test for diagnosis of primary hyperparathyroidism?**

Measurement of intact PTH.

○   **Why is measurement of the C-terminal of PTH not accurate for diagnosis of secondary hyperparathyroidism?**

C-terminal fragments are cleared by the kidney; elevation may indicate either renal insufficiency or hyperparathyroidism.

○   **What is the classic bony change associated with hypercalcemia?**

Osteitis fibrosa cystica; manifested as subperiosteal bone resorption in the phalanges, pelvis, distal clavicles, ribs, femur, mandible, or skull.

○   **What is the earliest radiographic lesion seen in osteitis fibrosa cystica?**

Irregularity of the radial aspect of the second digit middle phalanx

○   **What is another cause of bone disease in patients with renal failure that should be ruled out prior to parathyroidectomy?**

Aluminum bone disease.

○   **What is calciphylaxis?**

Severe soft tissue calcification that can result in deep nonhealing ulcers and gangrene.

○   **What is the medical management of secondary hyperparathyroidism?**

Dietary phosphate restriction, phosphate binders, calcium and vitamin D supplementation (calcitriol), sodium bicarbonate (for metabolic acidosis), charcoal hemoperfusion (for pruritus), bisphosphonates.

○   **What are the indications for parathyroid exploration in patients with asymptomatic or minimally symptomatic hyperparathyroidism?**

Age less than 50.
Serum calcium 1 mg/ml above the upper limits of normal for the lab.
Creatinine clearance reduced by 30% or more compared with age-matched normal persons.
24-hour urinary calcium excretion >400mg.
T-score at lumbar spine, hip, or distal radius <-2.5.
Poor follow-up expected.
Coexistent illness complicating conservative management.

○   **What disease should be ruled out on all patients with hypercalcemia?**

Familial benign hypocalciuric hypercalcemia (FHH).

○   **What is the difference in the Ca/Cr clearance ratio in someone with FHH and someone with primary hyperparathyroidism?**

Ca/Cr clearance <0.01 in FHH; >0.02 in primary hyperparathyroidism.

○   **What are the indications for parathyroidectomy in patients with secondary hyperparathyroidism?**

Bone pain (most common indication), intractable pruritus, calcium-phosphate product over 70 despite medical treatment, calciphylaxis, and osteitis fibrosa cystica.

○   **What is the most common cause of persistent hyperparathyroidism after parathyroidectomy?**

Undiscovered or supernumerary parathyroid gland.

○   **During exploration for primary hyperparathyroidism, 3 normal parathyroid glands are found but the fourth cannot be identified. What is the next step in management?**

Extend the exploration through the existing incision, to include the central neck compartment between the carotids, posteriorly to the vertebral body, superiorly to the level of the pharynx and carotid bulb and inferiorly into the mediastinum.

○   **What intraoperative modality may assist in locating an intrathyroidal parathyroid gland?**

Ultrasound.

○   **What is the most reliable method of differentiating a parathyroid adenoma from parathyroid hyperplasia?**

Visual inspection of all 4 parathyroid glands.

O   **What intraoperative modality confirms adequate removal of parathyroid tissue in patients with hyperparathyroidism?**

Rapid intraoperative PTH assay (expect a decrease of at least 50%).

O   **What is the treatment of choice for patients with hyperparathyroidism associated with MEN-I or MEN-IIa?**

Subtotal (3 1/2 gland) parathyroidectomy or total parathyroidectomy with autotransplantation.

O   **What is the treatment of choice for patients with parathyroid carcinoma?**

Radical resection of the involved gland, the ipsilateral thyroid lobe and the regional lymph nodes.

O   **What study should be performed prior to re-operation for persistent or recurrent hyperparathyroidism?**

^{99}Tc sestamibi is 85% sensitive in experienced centers; more accurate is patient is placed on cytomel to suppress the thyroid.

O   **A 25-year-old pregnant female, in her 2nd trimester, presents with hyperparathyroidism and a serum calcium of 12 mg/dl. What is the treatment of choice?**

Prompt parathyroid exploration.

O   **What is the surgical treatment of choice for patients with secondary hyperparathyroidism?**

Subtotal (3 1/2) parathyroidectomy or total parathyroidectomy with autotransplantation.

O   **What is the first line therapy for patients with marked hypercalcemia and/or severe symptoms?**

Intravenous hydration followed by furosemide.

O   **What are the indications for calcium supplementation after thyroid or parathyroid surgery?**

Circumoral paresthesias, anxiety, positive Chvostek's or Trousseau's sign, tetany, ECG changes or serum calcium less than 7.1 ml/dl.

O   **What is the immediate treatment for patients with acute symptomatic hypocalcemia?**

Intravenous calcium gluconate.

O   **What is the most common presentation of severe hypercalcemia?**

Extreme lethargy.

O   **In a non-acute setting, what is the maximum useful amount of calcium supplementation?**

2 grams of calcium/day.

O   **What is the appropriate calcium supplementation if the maximum amount of calcium has already been given and the patient is still hypocalcemic?**

Calcitriol or other vitamin D preparations should be added.

○   **What genetic defect results in either Jansen's chondrodystrophy or Blomstrand's chondrodystrophy?**

Mutation of the type 1 parathyroid hormone receptor.

○   **Which of these is lethal prenatally?**

Blomstrand's chondrodystrophy.

COMPLICATIONS

○ **What are the consequences of air embolism?**

>50 cc of air causes intensive pulmonary artery vasoconstriction, pulmonary edema, and cor pulmonale. >200 cc of air is fatal.

○ **What are the signs of air embolism?**

Audible sucking sound in the wound, machine-like cardiac murmur, dysrhythmias, sudden systemic hypotension, decreased end expiratory CO_2, increased CVP.

○ **What is the treatment for air embolism?**

Pack wound, compress jugular veins, aspirate air if right atrial catheter is in place, insert needle into right ventricle from under the xiphoid, switch to 100% O_2 and stop nitrous, place patient in left lateral Trendelenburg position.

○ **What is the only preoperative factor to significantly increase the risk of postoperative pulmonary complications?**

Recent smoking history.

○ **What is the most common organism identified in patients with pneumonia after major surgical resection of the upper aerodigestive tract?**

Staphylococcus aureus.

○ **What factor best predicts the risk of a major complication following head and neck oncologic surgery?**

10% loss of baseline body weight.

○ **What are the most commonly isolated bacteria from wound infections following major contaminated head and neck surgery?**

Staph aureus and beta-hemolytic streptococci.

○ **What are the 2nd most commonly isolated bacteria?**

Gram-negative aerobic bacteria.

○ **What is the rate of wound infection following contaminated head and neck surgery with use of perioperative antibiotics consisting of ampicillin/sulbactam or clindamycin?**

15%.

○ **What is the most effective duration for perioperative antibiotic administration?**

24 hours.

O   **What is the initial treatment for a chyle leak diagnosed 3 days after neck dissection?**

Maintain drains and begin medium-chain triglyceride tube feedings.

O   **If the leak does not resolve, what is the next step in management?**

TPN.

O   **Two weeks after undergoing salvage surgery on the neck, a patient loses 800 cc of blood from the operative site. If a bleeding source is not found on carotid arteriogram, what is the next step in management?**

Venous angiography with endovascular occlusion.

O   **What is the incidence of CVA and mortality from carotid blowout?**

10% CVA and 1% mortality if volume is repleted prior to going to the OR. 50% CVA and 25% mortality if volume is not repleted prior to going to the OR.

O   **What is meant by "carotid blowout precautions"?**

Establish IV access with 2 large bore IVs, type and cross 2 units PRBCs, have an intubation tray at the bedside, and educate nursing staff.

O   **What structure is most at risk during removal of a 1st branchial arch sinus?**

Facial nerve.

O   **What is the most serious complication of lateral pharyngotomy?**

Excessive retraction on the great vessels leading to thrombosis or embolism.

O   **What are 2 important techniques to prevent postoperative fistula formation?**

Tension-free closure and perioperative antibiotics.

O   **What electrolyte problem is disproportionately associated with gastric pull-up?**

Hypocalcemia secondary to impaired calcium absorption and inadvertent parathyroid resection during thyroidectomy.

O   **Where do fistulas most often occur after free jejunal transfer?**

At the superior anastomosis between the jejunum and pharynx.

O   **Where do strictures most often occur after free jejunal transfer?**

At the inferior anastomosis between the jejunum and esophagus.

O   **What is the fistula rate in patients who have had prior irradiation requiring total laryngectomy and partial pharyngectomy?**

15 – 20%.

O   **What is the fistula rate following free jejunal transfer (non-irradiated patients)?**

10 – 20%.

O   **What is the perioperative mortality rate of gastric pull-up?**

5 – 20%.

O   **What is the rate of major complications after gastric pull-up?**

50%.

O   **What are the most common complications of gastric pull-up?**

Regurgitation, cervical dysphagia, stricture, anastomotic leak.

O   **What is the most common complication of parotidectomy?**

Hematoma.

O   **What are the complications from radiation overdosage in the treatment of NPC?**

Osteoradionecrosis, brain necrosis, transverse myelitis, hearing loss, hypopituitarism, hypothyroidism, optic neuritis.

O   **What is the incidence of SNHL after radiation therapy for nasopharyngeal cancer?**

14%.

O   **What is the incidence of clinically significant pneumocephalus after anterior craniofacial surgery?**

5 – 12%.

O   **What can cause postoperative pneumocephalus?**

Overly aggressive drainage of CSF via a lumbar drain or ball-valve action of the flaps used to reconstruct the skull base.

O   **What is the treatment of pneumocephalus?**

Emergent drainage with needle aspiration, airway diversion (i.e. tracheostomy), nasal repacking.

O   **What are the most common complications of acoustic neuroma resection?**

SNHL, paralysis of VII, CSF leak (10-35%), meningitis (1-10%), intracranial hemorrhage (0.5-2%).

O   **What % of laryngectomy patients who fail voice restoration following tracheoesophageal puncture (TEP) suffer from cricopharyngeal spasm?**

12%.

O   **What is the best test to differentiate between cricopharyngeal spasm and stricture in patients who fail voice restoration following TEP?**

Contrast videofluoroscopy.

O   **What is the incidence of complications after PEG?**

9 – 15%.

O   **Which complication is most likely to be avoided with endoscopic diverticulectomy versus open diverticulectomy?**

Damage to the recurrent laryngeal nerve.

O   **What is the incidence of tracheoinnominate fistula after tracheostomy?**

2%.

O   **What % of all instances of tracheal bleeding developing 48 hours or longer after surgery are caused by tracheoinnominate fistulae?**

50%.

O   **What % of patients with tracheoinnominate fistulae survive?**

25%.

O   **What are the risk factors for innominate artery rupture after tracheostomy?**

Placement of trach below the 3rd ring; aberrant course of the innominate artery; use of a long, curved tube; overhyperextension of the neck during the procedure; prolonged pressure by inflated cuff; and tracheal infection.

O   **Which patients are at a higher risk of pneumothorax after tracheostomy?**

Children.

O   **What is the most common cause of mortality in pediatric patients who undergo tracheostomy?**

Plugging or accidental decannulation in children <1 year of age.

O   **What is the most common complication after orbital reconstruction?**

Enophthalmos.

O   **What is incidence of persistent diplopia after orbital reconstruction?**

7%.

O   **What is the most common cause of infection after ORIF?**

Poor plating technique.

O   **What is the treatment for infected extraoral mandibular ORIF?**

Removal of the tooth and the failed plate, debridement of dead bone, placement of a large reconstruction plate, and primary grafting if inadequate bone contact exists.

O   **10 days after ORIF of a mandibular body fracture, your patient presents with an exposed plate and purulent drainage. The reduction is grossly intact. What do you do?**

Open wound, remove involved tooth if applicable; if hardware is loose, replace it with a new plate; if hardware is rigid, continue drainage, wound care.

O   **4 weeks after ORIF of a mandibular body fracture, your patients presents with an exposed plate and purulent drainage. The reduction is grossly intact. What do you do?**

Open wound, remove involved tooth if applicable, remove hardware, and assess union; if nonunion is present, most patients will heal with MMF; other option is plate and bone graft (external approach).

O   **What are the most common complications of lateral tympanoplasty?**

Anterior blunting, lateralization, epithelial pearls, canal stenosis.

O   **What is the most common postoperative complication of pressure equalizing tube insertion?**

Persistent otorrhea.

O   **What is the management of injury to the sigmoid sinus during mastoidectomy?**

Apply gentle pressure, place a Surgicel or Gelfoam patch, and continue with surgery.

O   **What is the management of injury to the dura with CSF leak during mastoidectomy?**

Repair with temporalis fascia held in place with sutures or packing and continue with surgery; small tears can be managed with a Surgicel or Gelfoam patch.

O   **Unbeknownst to the surgeon, the dura is torn during mastoidectomy, and postoperatively, the patient develops a severe headache, followed by hemiplegia and coma. What has likely happened?**

Pneumocephalus; torn dura can create a ball valve-like effect and trap air from the middle ear. Influx of air may occur during Valsalva or as a result of high intracranial negative pressure due to the rapid escape of CSF through the tear.

O   **What is the most common location for iatrogenic labyrinthine fistula formation during mastoidectomy?**

Lateral semicircular canal.

O   **What is the management of intraoperative violation of the labyrinth?**

Immediate application of a Gelfoam patch or other tissue seal (other than fat).

O   **Where is the facial nerve most commonly injured during mastoid surgery?**

Near the 2nd genu as it enters the mastoid cavity.

O   **During stapedectomy, the entire stapes footplate falls into the vestibule. What should be done?**

It should be left in the vestibule, as attempts to retrieve it are more likely to cause damage than leaving the footplate where it is.

O   **What is a "perilymph gusher"?**

Rapid release of perilymph after stapes footplate fenestration due to pressure and fluid from the CSF compartment venting through the inner ear.

O   **Which patients are at greater risk for a "perilymph gusher"?**

Patients with congenital stapes fixation and a patent cochlear aqueduct or a large vestibular aqueduct.

O   **What is the management of a "perilymph gusher"?**

Reduction of CSF pressure with mannitol and/or a lumbar drain, application of a tissue seal over the oval window fistula using fascia, perichondrium, or fat and secured with a stapes prosthesis, and postoperative hospitalization with continued reduction in CSF pressure.

O   **Ten days after stapedectomy, your patient complains of progressive hearing loss and vertigo that does not respond to steroids. What do you do?**

Take the patient back to the OR to explore for a granuloma. If one is found, remove the granuloma and place a new prosthesis with a tissue seal over the oval window.

O   **What are the symptoms and signs of a poststapedectomy perilymph fistula?**

Episodic vertigo, especially with exertion, sensorineural hearing loss, loss of speech discrimination, and nystagmus with changes of air pressure on the TM.

O   **What is the most common complication of stapedotomy?**

Prosthesis displacement.

O   **What is the incidence of significant SNHL after revision stapedotomy?**

3 – 30% (up to 14% profound).

O   **What surgical procedure is the most common cause of iatrogenic vocal cord paralysis in children?**

Tracheo-esophageal fistula repair.

O   **What is the incidence of clinically significant VPI after adenoidectomy?**

1:1500 – 3000.

O   **What is the treatment for post-adenoidectomy VPI?**

If it persists beyond 2 months, speech therapy; beyond 6 – 12 months, palatal pushback, pharyngeal flap surgery, or sphincter pharyngoplasty.

O   **What are the most common complications of pharyngeal flap surgery?**

Bleeding, airway obstruction, obstructive sleep apnea.

O   **What is the recurrence rate following excision of a TGDC without removal of the midportion of the hyoid and the ductal remnant?**

38%.

○ **What is the most common complication of segmental mandibulectomy defect reconstruction with plates?**

Plate exposure.

○ **What is the most common complication from microsurgical reconstruction?**

36% suffer medical complications (pulmonary problems, prolonged ventilatory support, acute ethanol withdrawal).

○ **What is the incidence of permanent recurrent laryngeal nerve injury after total thyroidectomy?**

1 – 4%.

○ **What is the incidence of permanent hypoparathyroidism after total thyroidectomy?**

1 – 5%.

○ **A patient develops a CSF leak after resection of an acoustic neuroma. A pressure dressing and lumbar drain are placed with no improvement. Wound exploration and reclosure are performed, and the leak recurs. What is the next step?**

It the tympanic membrane is intact and hearing is present, plug the eustachian tube via a middle fossa approach. If the tympanic membrane is not intact and hearing is not present, perform a blind sac closure of the external auditory canal and obliterate the middle ear and eustachian tube.

BIBLIOGRAPHY

BOOKS/ARTICLES

Adler SC, Rousso D. Evaluation of past and present hair replacement techniques. *Arch Facial Plast Surg.* 1999;1: 266-271.

Albert B. Management of the complications of mandibular fracture treatment. *Operative Techniques in PRS.* 1998;5: 325-333.

Ali MK, Streitmann MJ. Excision of rhinophyma with the carbon dioxide laser: A ten-year experience. *Ann Otol Rhinol Laryngol.* 1997; 106: 952-955.

Anderson JE, *Grant's Atlas of Anatomy*, Eighth Edition, Williams & Wilkins: 1983

Anson BJ et al. Surgical anatomy of the facial nerve. *Arch of Otolaryngol.*1972; 97: 201-213.

Antonelli PJ et al. Diagnostic yield of high-resolution computed tomography for pediatric sensorineural hearing loss. *Laryngoscope.* 1999; 109: 1642- 1647.

Asakage T et al. Tumor thickness predicts cervical metastasis in patients with Stage I/II carcinoma of the tongue. *Cancer.* 1998;82: 1443-1448.

Apuzzo, *Brain Surgery*, Vol 1-2, Chirchill Livingston

Bailey, Byron J., ed. Head and Neck Surgery-Otolaryngology. Philadelphia, PA: J.B. Lippincott Co., 1993.

Backous DD et al. Trauma to the external auditory canal and temporal bone. *Otolaryngol Clin of N Amer.* 1996; 29: 853-866.

Barash, PG, *Clinical Anesthesia*, Third Edition, JB Lippincott: Philadelphia, 1997

Bartlett JG. Antibiotic-associated diarrhea. *NEJM.* 2002;346:334-339.

Bauer CA, Coker NJ. Update on facial nerve disorders. *Otolaryngol Clin of N Amer.* 1996; 29: 445-454.

Bayles SW et al. Mandibular fracture and associated cervical spine fracture, a rare and predictable injury. *Arch Otolaryngol HNS.* 1997; 123: 1304-1307.

Beekhuis GJ. Blepharoplasty. *Otolaryngol Clin of N Amer.* 1982; 15: 179-193.

Benninger MS et. Adult chronic rhinosinusitis: definitions, diagnosis, epidemiology, and pathophysiology. *Otolaryngol-HNS.* 2003;129:S1-S32.

Beppu M et al. The osteocutaneous fibula flap: An anatomic study. *J of Reconstructive Microsurg.* 1992; 8: 215-223.

Bernstein L, Nelson RH. Surgical anatomy of the extraparotid distribution of the facial nerve. *Arch Otolaryngol.* 1984;110: 177-182.

Bhupendra CK et al. Management of complex orbital fractures. *Facial Plastic Surg.* 1998; 14: 83-103.

Biavati MJ et al. Predictive factors for respiratory complications after tonsillectomy and adenoidectomy in children. *Arch Otolaryngol HNS.* 1997;123: 517-521.

Blackwell KE et al. Lateral mandibular reconstruction using soft-tissue free flaps and plates. *Arch Otolaryngol-HNS.* 1996;122: 672-678.

Boyd JB. Use of reconstruction plates in conjunction with soft-tissue free flaps for oromandibular reconstruction. *Clin in Plastic Surg.* 1994;21: 77.

Brackmann PE, ed. *Otologic Surgery,* W.B.Saunders, Philadelphia, 1994.

Breckler, GL, Maull, KI, ed. *General Surgery, Pearls of Wisdom,* Boston Medical Publishing, Lincoln, NE, 1998.

Buckingham ED et al. Connective tissue disease. *Dr. Quinn's Online Textbook of Otolaryngology;* Feb 16, 2000.

Buckingham ED et al. Mohs surgery and reconstruction after Mohs surgery. *Dr. Quinn's Online Textbook of Otolaryngology;* Nov 10, 1999.

Burt JD, Byrd HS. Cleft lip: Unilataral primary deformities. *PRS.* 2000; 105: 1043-1055.

Byers RM et al. Can we detect or predict the presence of occult nodal metastases in patients with squamous carcinoma of the oral tongue? *Head & Neck.* 1998; 20: 139-144.

Byers RM et al. Frequency and therapeutic implications of 'skip metastases' in the neck from squamous carcinoma of the oral tongue. *Head & Neck.* 1997;19: 14-19.

Cady B, Rossi R. An expanded view of risk-group definition in differentiated thyroid carcinoma. *Surgery.* 1988; 104: 947-953.

Chang CY, Cass SP. Management of facial nerve injury due to temporal bone trauma. *Am J Otol.* 1999; 20: 96-113.

Chow JM et al. Radiotherapy or surgery for subclinical cervical node metastases. *Arch Otolaryngol HNS.* 1989; 115: 981-984.

Civetta JM, *Critical Care,* Third Edition, New York, Lippencott-Raven Publishers, 1997

Clark CP. Office-based skin care and superficial peels: The scientific rationale. *PRS.* 1999; 104: 854-864.

Clark N et al. High-energy ballistic and avulsive facial injuries: Classification, patterns, and an algorithm for primary reconstruction. *J of Plastic & Reconstructive Surg.* 1996; 98: 583-601.

Cohn KH et al. Biologic considerations and operative strategy in papillary thyroid carcinoma: Arguments against the routine performance of total thyroidectomy. *Surgery.* 1984; 96: 957-971.

Cordes S et al. Surgery for exophthalmos. *Dr. Quinn's Online Textbook of Otolaryngology;* April 26, 2000.

Cordes S et al. Refinement of the nasal tip. *Dr. Quinn's Online Textbook of Otolaryngology;* Feb 16, 2000.

Cordes S, Quinn FB. Epistaxis. *Dr. Quinn's Online Textbook of Otolaryngology;* October 16, 1996.

Cordes S et al. Congential aural atresia. *Dr. Quinn's Online Textbook of Otolaryngology;* Nov 17, 1999.

Cordes S et al. Genetic hearing loss. *Dr. Quinn's Online Textbook of Otolaryngology*; April 5, 2000.

Cotton RT. Pediatric laryngotracheal reconstruction. *Operative Tech in Otolaryngol HNS*. 1992; 3: 165-172.

Cotton RT et al. Pediatric laryngotracheal reconstruction with cartilage grafts and endotracheal tube stenting: The single stage approach. *Laryngoscope*. 1995; 105: 818-821.

Cotton RT et al. Four-quadrant cricoid cartilage division in laryngotracheal reconstruction. *Arch Otolaryngol HNS*. 1992; 118: 1023-1027.

Decherd ME, Bailey BJ, Quinn FB. Sleep disorders for the Otolaryngologist. *Dr. Quinn's Online Textbook of Otolaryngology;* May 23, 2001.

Decherd ME, Newlands SD. Maxillary and periorbital fractures. *Dr. Quinn's Online Textbook of Otolaryngology*; Jan 26, 2000.

Debry C et al. Drainage after thyroid surgery: A prospective randomized study. *J of Laryngol Otol*. 1999; 113: 49-51.

Derkay CS et al. Management of children with von Willebrand disease undergoing adenotonsillectomy. *Am J Otolaryngol*. 1996;17: 172-177.

Dettelbach MA et al. Effect of the Passy-Muir valve on aspiration in patients with tracheostomy. *Head & Neck*. 1995;17: 297-300.

Dorn MT et al. Pathologic quiz case 1. *Arch Otolaryngol HNS*. 1999; 125: 694-697.

Dorn MT et al. Stridor, aspiration, and cough. *Dr. Quinn's Online Textbook of Otolaryngology*. Jan 19, 2000.

Dorn MT et al. Tonsillitis, tonsillectomy, and adenoidectomy. *Dr. Quinn's Online Textbook of Otolaryngology*; Dec 1, 1999.

Doyle PW and Woodham JD. Evaluation of the microbiology of chronic ethmoid sinusitis. *J Clin Microbio*. 1991;29:2396-2400.

Dyer RK, McElveen JT. The patulous eustachian tube: Management options. *Otolaryngol-HNS*. 1991;105: 832-835.

Eckel HE. Endoscopic laser resection of supraglottic carcinoma. *Otolaryngol HNS*. 1997;117: 681-687.

Eden BV et al. Esthesioneuroblastoma. *Cancer*. 1994; 73: 2556-2562.

Eliashar R et al. Can topical mitomycin prevent laryngotracheal stenosis? *Laryngoscope*. 1999; 109: 1594-1600.

Faust, RJ, *Anesthesiology Review*, Second Edition, Churchill Livingstone: New York, 1994

Ferguson BJ. Definitions of fungal rhinosinusitis. *Otolaryngol Clin of N America*. 2000; 33: 227-235.

Fedok FG. Comprehensive management of nasoethmoid-orbital injuries. *J of Cranio-Maxillofacial Trauma*. 1995;1: 36-48.

Franceschi D et al. Improved survival in the treatment of squamous carcinoma of the oral tongue. *Am J of Surg*. 1993; 166: 360-365.

Gacek RR et al. Adult spontaneous cerebrospinal fluid otorrhea: Diagnosis and management. *Am J Otol.* 1999; 20: 770-776.

Gantz BJ et al. Surgical management of Bell's palsy. *Laryngoscope.* 1999; 109: 1177-1188.

Gates, GA. *Current Therapy in Otolaryngology – Head and Neck Surgery*, 6th ed. St. Louis: Mosby – Year Book; 1998.

Geiger DG, Thompson NW. Thyroid tumors in children. *Otolaryngology Clin, North Am.* 1996: 29:711-720

Gerber ME et al. Selected risk factors in pediatric adenotonsillectomy. *Arch Otolaryngol HNS.* 1996;122: 811-814.

Goodman, AG, Rall, TW, Nies, AS, Taylor, P., *Goodman and Gilman's the Pharmacological Basis of Therapeutics*, Eighth Edition, Pergamon Press: New York, 1990

Gormley PK et al. Congenital vascular anomalies and persistent respiratory symptoms in children. *Internatl J of Ped Otolaryngol.* 1999; 51: 23-31.

Gosain AK et al. Surgical anatomy of the SMAS: A reinvestigation. *PRS.* 1993;92: 1254-1263.

Grant CS et al. Local recurrence in papillary thyroid carcinoma: Is extent of surgical resection important? *Surgery.* 1988; 104: 954-962.

Green SM. *Pocket Pharmacopoeia.* Tarascon, 2004.

Greenfield, Lazar J., *Scientific Principles and Practice*, Second Edition, Lippincott-Raven, 1997.

Grillo HC et al. Laryngotracheal resection and reconstruction for subglottic stenosis. *Ann Thor Surg.* 1992;53:54-63.

Haberkamp TJ, Tanyeri HM. Management of idiopathic sudden sensorineural hearing loss. *Am J Otol.* 1999; 20: 587-595.

Haddadin KJ et al. Improved survival for patients with clinically T1/T2, N0 tongue tumors undergoing a prophylactic neck dissection. *Head & Neck.* 1999;21: 517-525.

Har-El G et al. Resection of tracheal stenosis with end-to-end anastomosis. *Ann Otol Rhinol Laryngol.* 1992; 102: 670-674.

Harrison LB et al. Long term results of primary radiotherapy with/without neck dissection for squamous cell cancer of the base of tongue. *Head & Neck.* 1998;20: 669-673.

Harrison TR, *Principles of Internal Medicine*, Eleventh Edition, New York: McGraw-Hill Book Company, 1987

Hay ID et al. Ipsilateral lobectomy versus bilateral lobar resection in papillary thyroid carcinoma: A retrospective analysis of surgical outcome using a novel prognostic scoring system. *Surgery.* 1987; 102: 1088-1094.

Hidalgo DA. Condyle transplantation in free flap mandible reconstruction. *PRS.* 1994; 93: 770-781.

Hidalgo DA. Fibula free flap: A new method of mandible reconstruction. *PRS.* 1989; 84: 71-79.

Hoffman JF. Naso-orbital-ethmoid complex fracture management. *Facial Plastic Surg;* 14; 67-76.

Hoie J, Stenwig AE. Long-term survival in patients with follicular thyroid carcinoma. *J Surg Oncol.* 1992; 49: 226-230.

Holinger, PH. Clinical Aspects of Congenital Anomalies of the Larynx, Trachea, Bronchi and Esophagus. *J. Laryngol Oto.,* 1961;75:1-44

Houck JR, Medina JE. Management of cervical lymph nodes in squamous carcinomas of the head and neck. *Sem in Surg Oncol.* 1995; 11: 228-239.

Hsu J et al. Antimicrobial resistance in bacterial chronic sinusitis. *Am J Rhin.* 1998;12:243-248.

James DG. Differential diagnosis of facial nerve palsy. *Sarcoidosis Vasculitis and Diffuse Lung Diseases.* 1997; 14: 115-120.

Johnson TM et al. The Rieger flap for nasal reconstruction. *Arch Otolaryngol-HNS.* 1995; 121: 634-637.

Kashima ML et al. Latex allergy : an update for the Otolaryngologist. *Arch Otolaryngol-HNS.* 2001 ;127 :442-446.

Katzenmeyer K et al. Neoplasms of the nose and paranasal sinuses. *Dr. Quinn's Online Textbook of Otolaryngology*; June 7, 2000.

Katzenmeyer K et al. Medical management of vestibular disorders and vestibular rehabilitation. *Dr. Quinn's Online Textbook of Otolaryngology*; April 12, 2000.

Kroll SS et al. Costs and complications in mandibular reconstruction. *Ann Plast Surg.* 1992; 29: 341-347.

Kryger MH, Roth T, Dement WC. *Principles and Practice of Sleep Medicine,* 3rd ed. Philadelphia: WB Saunders; 2000.

Kuhn FA, Javer AR. Allergic fungal rhinosinusitis: perioperative management, prevention of recurrence, and role of steroids and antifungal agents. *Otolaryngol Clin of N America.* 2000; 33: 419-431.

Kushner GM, Alpert B. Open reduction and internal fixation of acute mandibular fractures in adults. *Facial Plastic Surg.* 1998;14: 11-21.

Larson DL, Sanger JR. Management of the mandible in oral cancer. *Sem in Surg Oncol.* 1995;11: 190-199.

LeBoeuf HJ, Quinn FB. Granulomatous diseases of the head & neck: evolution and current concepts. *Dr. Quinn's Online Textbook of Otolaryngology*; Nov 24, 1999.

LeBoeuf HJ et al. Evaluation of the hoarse patient. *Dr. Quinn's Online Textbook of Otolaryngology*; May 17, 2000.

Lee, K.J. *Essential Otolaryngology,* 6th ed. Stamford: Appleton & Lange; 1995.

Leipzig B, Hokanson JA. Treatment of cervical lymph nodes in carcinoma of the tongue. *Head & Neck.* 1982; 5: 3-9.

Li KK et al. The importance of mandibular position in microvascular mandibular reconstruction. *Laryngoscope.* 1996; 106: 903-907.

Liening DA et al. Hypothyroidism following radiotherapy for head and neck cancer. *Otolaryngol HNS.* 1990; 103: 10-13.

Lindberg R. Distribution of cervical lymph node metastases from squamous cell carcinoma of the upper respiratory and digestive tracts. *Cancer.* 1972; 29: 1146-1149.

Lindner HH. The anatomy of the fasciae of the face and neck with particular reference to the spread and treatment of intraoral infections (Ludwig's) that have progressed into adjacent fascial spaces. *Ann Surg.* 1986; 204: 714.

Lippy WH et al. Far-advanced otosclerosis. *Am J Otol.* 1994;15: 225-228.

Lutz CK et al. Supraglottic carcinoma: Patterns of recurrence. *Ann Otol Rhinol Laryngol.* 1990; 99: 12-17.

Manson PN et al. Subunit principles in midface fractures: the importance of sagittal buttresses, soft-tissue reductions, and sequencing treatment of segmental fractures. *PRS.* 1999; 103: 1287- 1306.

Maran AGD et al. The parapharyngeal space. *J of Laryngol Otol.* 1984;98: 371-380.

Marx SJ. Hyperparathyroid and hypoparathyroid disorders. *New Eng J of Med.* 2000;343: 1863-1875.

McGraw-Wall B. Frontal sinus fractures. *Facial Plastic Surg.* 1998; 14: 59-66.

McGraw B, Cole R. Pediatric maxillofacial trauma: age-related variations in injury. *Arch Otolaryngol Head Neck Sur.* 1990;116:41.

McGregor AD, MacDonald G. Routes of entry of squamous cell carcinoma to the mandible. *Head & Neck.* 1998; 10: 294-301.

McHenry C et al. Selective postoperative radioactive iodine treatment of thyroid carcinoma. *Surgery.* 1989; 106: 956-959.

Minor LB. Intratympanic gentamicin for control of vertigo in Meniere's disease: Vestibular signs that specify completion of therapy. *Am J of Otology.* 1999; 20: 209-219.

Monhian N et al. The role of soft-tissue implants in scar revision. *Facial Plast Surg Clin of N Amer.* 1998; 6: 183-190.

Montgomery WW. Suprahyoid release for tracheal anastomosis. *Arch Otolaryngol HNS.* 1974; 99: 255-260.

Moscoso JF et al. Vascularized bone flaps in oromandibular reconstruction. *Arch Otolaryngol-HNS.* 1994; 120:36-43.

Mueller RF et al. Congential non-syndromal sensorineural hearing impairment due to connexin 26 gene mutations - molecular and audiologic findings. *Internatl J Ped Otolarygnol.* 1999; 50: 3-13.

Muller C et al. Thyroid cancer. *Dr. Quinn's Online Textbook of Otolaryngology;* Oct 6, 1998.

Myers JN et al. Squamous cell carcinoma of the tongue in young adults: increasing incidence and factors that predict treatment outcomes. *Otolaryngol HNS.* 2000; 122: 44-51.

Nelson RA. *Temporal Bone Surgical Dissection Manual,* 2nd ed. House Ear Institute, 1991.

Nosan DK et al. Current perspective on temporal bone trauma. *Otolaryngol-HNS.*1997; 117: 67-71.

Onerci M et al. Atlantoaxial subluxation after tonsillectomy and adenoidectomy. *Otolaryngol HNS.* 1997; 116: 271-273.

Pachigolla R et al. Assessment of peripheral and central auditory function. *Dr. Quinn's Online Textbook of Otolaryngology*; March 15, 2000.

Pachigolla R et al. Geriatric otolaryngology. *Dr. Quinn's Online Textbook of Otolaryngology;* November 3, 1999.

Pachigolla R et al. Chin and malar augmentation. *Dr. Quinn's Online Textbook of Otolaryngology*; April 17, 2000.

Packman KS, Demeure MJ. Indications for parathyroidectomy and extent of treatment for patients with secondary hyperparathyroidism. *Surg Clin N Amer*. 1995;75: 465-483.

Paradise JL et al. Efficacy of tonsillectomy for recurrent throat infection in severely affected children. *New Engl J Med*. 1984; 310: 674-682.

Pauw BKH et al. Utricle, saccule, and cochlear duct in relation to stapedotomy. *Ann Otol Rhinol Laryngol*. 1991;100: 966-970.

Persky MS, Lagmay VM. Treatment of the clinically negative neck in oral squamous cell carcinoma. *Laryngoscope*. 1999; 109: 1160-1164.

Piepergerdes JC et al. Keratosis obturans and external auditory canal cholesteatoma. *Laryngoscope*. 1980; 90: 383-391.

Pollock WF. Surgical anatomy of the thyroid and parathyroid glands. *Surg Clin of N Amer*. 1964; 44: 1161-1173.

Pou AM et al. Laryngeal framework surgery for the management of aspiration in high vagal lesions. *Am J of Otolaryngol*. 1998; 19: 1-7.

Pransky SM et al. Intralesional cidofovir for recurrent respiratory papillomatosis in children. *Arch Otolaryngol HNS*. 1999; 125: 1143-1148.

Prater ME et al. Preoperative evaluation of the aesthetic patient. *Dr. Quinn's Online Textbook of Otolaryngology*; May 10, 2000.

Prater ME et al. Clefts of the lip, alveolus, and palate. *Dr. Quinn's Online Textbook of Otolaryngology*; March 3, 2001.

Riechelmann J et al. Total, subtotal, and partial surgical removal of cervicofacial lymphangiomas. *Arch Otolaryngol HNS*. 1999; 125: 643-648.

Rohrich RJ, Zbar RIS. The evolution of the Hughes tarsoconjunctival flap for lower eyelid reconstruction. *PRS*. 1999; 104: 518-522.

Rombeau, John L., Caldwell, Michael, *Clinical Nutrition*, Enteral and Tube Feeding, Second Edition, W.B. Saunders, 1990

Rosen EJ, Quinn FB. Microbiology, infections, and antibiotic therapy. *Dr. Quinn's Online Textbook of Otolaryngology*; March 22, 2000.

Rosen EJ et al. Infections of the labyrinth. *Dr. Quinn's Online Textbook of Otolaryngology*; May 24, 2000.

Sataloff RT. Office evaluation of dysphonia. *Otolaryngol Clin of N America*. 1992; 25: 843-855.

Schaefer SD, Close LG. Acute management of laryngeal trauma. *Ann Otol Rhion Laryngol*. 1998:98;104.

Schuknecht HF et al. Pathology of secondary malignant tumors of the temporal bone. *Ann Otol, Rhino, Laryngology*. 1968; 77: 5-22.

Schusterman MA et al. Use of the AO plate for immediate mandibular reconstruction in cancer patients. *PRS*. 1991;88: 588-593.

Schusterman MA et al. The osteocutaneous free fibula flap: Is the skin paddle reliable? *PRS*. 1992; 90: 787-793.

Schwartz, Seymour I., *Principles of Surgery*, Sixth Edition, McGraw-Hill, 1994

Schweinfurth JM, Koltai PJ. Pediatric mandibular fractures. *Facial Plastic Surg*. 1998; 14: 43.

Secor CP et al. Auricular endochondral pseudocysts: Diagnosis and management. *PRS*. 1999; 103: 1451-1457.

Shah JP et al. The patterns of cervical lymph node metastases from squamous carcinoma of the oral cavity. *Cancer*. 1990; 66: 109-113.

Shaha AR. Preoperative evaluation of the mandible in patients with carcinoma of the floor of mouth. *Head & Neck*. 1991; 13: 398-402.

Sheehy JL. Diffuse exostoses and osteomata of the external auditory canal: A report of 100 operations. *Otolaryngol-HNS*. 1982;90: 337-342.

Sheehy JL, Brackmann DE. Surgery of Chronic Otitis Media. Otolaryngology, Vol 1., Chapter 20. J.B. Lippincott Co, Philadelphia, 1994.

Shorr N, Enzer Y. Considerations in aesthetic eyelid surgery. *J Dermatol Surg Oncol*. 1992; 18: 1081-1095.

Shumrick KA, Smith TL. The anatomic basis for the design of forehead flaps in nasal reconstruction. *Arch Otolaryngol-HNS*. 1992; 118: 373-379.

Spira M. Otoplasty: What I do now – a 30-year perspective. *PRS*. 1999; 104: 834-840.

Stammberger HR, Kennedy DW. Paranasal sinuses: Anatomic terminology and nomenclature. *Ann Otol Rhinol Laryngol-Suppl*. 1995;167: 7-16.

Stierman K, Quinn FB. Laryngeal trauma. *Dr. Quinn's Online Textbook of Otolaryngology*; Oct 6, 1999.

Stoeckli SJ et al. Role of routine panendoscopy in cancer of the upper aerodigestive tract. *Otolaryngol-HNS*. 2001; 124: 208-212.

Strong EB, Sykes JM. Zygoma complex fractures. *Facial Plastic Surg*. 1998; 14: 105-115.

Stroud RH et al. Cutaneous malignancy. *Dr. Quinn's Online Textbook of Otolaryngology*; Feb 9, 2000.

Stucker FJ et al. Management of animal and human bites in the head and neck. *Arch Otolaryngol HNS*. 1990; 116: 789-793.

Stuzin JM et al. Anatomy of the frontal branch of the facial nerve: The significance of the temporal fat pad. *PRS*. 1989; 83: 265-271.

Stuzin JM et al. The relationship of the superficial and deep facial fascias: Relevance to rhytidectomy and aging. *PRS*. 1992; 89: 441-449

Tardy ME. *Rhinoplasty: the art and the science*. Philadelphia: Saunders; 1997.

Tatum SA, Kellman RM. Cranial bone grafting in maxillofacial trauma and reconstruction. *Facial Plastic Surg*. 1998; 14:117-129.

Tharp ME, Shidnia H. Radiotherapy in the treatment of verrucous carcinoma of the head and neck. *Laryngoscope*. 1995; 105: 391-396.

Ulualp SO et al. Possible relationship of gastroesophagopharyngeal acid reflux with pathogenesis of chronic sinusitis. *Am J of Rhinolog*. 1999;13: 197-202.

Urban KG, Terris DJ. Percutaneous endoscopic gastrostomy (PEG): indications and technique. *Operative Techniques in Otolaryngol – HNS*. 1997;8:77-84.

Urken ML et al. Functional evaluation following microvascular oromandibular reconstruction of the oral cancer patient: A comparative study of reconstructed and nonreconstructed patients. *Laryngoscope*. 1991; 101: 935-950.

Utley DS et al. The failing flap in facial plastic and reconstructive surgery: role of the medicinal leech. *Laryngoscope*. 1998; 108: 1129-1136.

Vincent R et al. Malleus ankylosis: A clinical, audiometric, histologic, and surgical study of 123 cases. *Am J Otol*. 1999;20: 717-725.

Wagner HE, Seiler C. Recurrent laryngeal nerve palsy after thyroid gland surgery. *Br J Surg*. 1994 ;81: 226-228.

Weiser, Martin R., Hill, James, Lindsey, Thomas, Hechtman, Herbert B., *Eicosanoids in Surgery*, Scientific American – Surgery Series, 1995

Wiessler MC, Pillsbury HC. *Complications of Head and Neck Surgery*. New York: Thieme Medical Publishers; 1995.

Williams and Rengachary, *Neurosurgery*, Vol 1-3, Second Edition, McGraw Hill

Wilson DP et al. Eyelid reconstruction. *Dr. Quinn's Online Textbook of Otolaryngology*; Oct 28, 1998.

Wolfensberger M, Dort JC. Endoscopic laser surgery for early glottic carcinoma: A clinical and experimental study. *Laryngoscope*. 1990; 100: 1100-1105.

Yoo J et al. Parathyroid disease. *Dr. Quinn's Online Textbook of Otolaryngology*; Feb 12, 1997.

Youmans, *Neurological Surgery*, Vol 1-5, Fourth Edition, Saunders

Yousif NJ et al. The nasolabial fold: an anatomic and histologic reappraisal. *PRS*. 1994; 93: 60-65.

COURSES/CONFERENCES

Annual Symposium in Otolaryngology, Stanford, CA; June 20-21, 2003.

Contemporary Surgical Concepts and Technologies in Snoring and Sleep-Disordered Breathing. Burlingame, CA; April 11-12, 2003.

Annual Symposium in Otolaryngology, Stanford, CA; June 21-22, 2002.

The Art of Rhinoplasty. San Francisco, CA; Nov 2-5, 2001.

Contemporary Surgical Concepts and Technologies in Snoring and Sleep-Disordered Breathing. Burlingame, CA; April 27-28, 2001.

The Home Study Course in Otolaryngology – Head and Neck Surgery. American Academy of Otolaryngology – Head and Neck Surgery 1998/99; 1999/2000; 2000/01

International Conference on Head and Neck Cancer. San Francisco, CA; July 29-August 2, 2000.

San Francisco Otology & Neurotology Update 2000. San Francisco, CA; October 26-28, 2000.

Update of Office Procedures in Otolaryngology 2000. Galveston, TX; June 9-10, 2000.

NOTES

NOTES

NOTES

NOTES

NOTES

NOTES

NOTES

NOTES

NOTES

NOTES

www.ingramcontent.com/pod-product-compliance
Lightning Source LLC
Chambersburg PA
CBHW080702220326
41598CB00033B/5277